Integrative Cardiology

Weil Integrative Medicine Library

Published Volumes

SERIES EDITOR

ANDREW T. WEIL, MD

Donald I. Abrams and Andrew T. Weil: *Integrative Oncology*
Timothy P. Culbert and Karen Olness: *Integrative Pediatrics*
Victoria Maizes and Tieraona Low Dog: *Integrative Women's Health*
Randy Horwitz and Daniel Muller: *Integrative Rheumatology*
Daniel A. Monti and Bernard Beitman: *Integrative Psychiatry*

Integrative Cardiology

EDITED BY

Stephen Devries, MD, FACC, FAHA

Associate Professor of Medicine,
Division of Cardiology
Feinberg School of Medicine
Northwestern University

James E. Dalen, MD, MPH, FACC

Executive Director, The Weil Foundation
Dean Emeritus and Professor Emeritus of Medicine and Public Health
University of Arizona College of Medicine

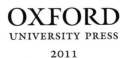

OXFORD
UNIVERSITY PRESS
2011

OXFORD
UNIVERSITY PRESS

Oxford University Press, Inc., publishes works that further
Oxford University's objective of excellence
in research, scholarship, and education.

Oxford   New York
Auckland   Cape Town   Dar es Salaam   Hong Kong   Karachi
Kuala Lumpur   Madrid   Melbourne   Mexico City   Nairobi
New Delhi   Shanghai   Taipei   Toronto

With offices in
Argentina   Austria   Brazil   Chile   Czech Republic   France   Greece
Guatemala   Hungary   Italy   Japan   Poland   Portugal   Singapore
South Korea   Switzerland   Thailand   Turkey   Ukraine   Vietnam

Published by Oxford University Press, Inc.
198 Madison Avenue, New York, New York 10016
www.oup.com

Library of Congress Cataloging-in-Publication Data
Integrative cardiology / edited by Stephen Devries and James Dalen.
p.; cm. – (Weil integrative medicine library)
Includes bibliographical references.
ISBN 978-0-19-538346-1
1. Cardiovascular system—Diseases—Alternative treatment. 2. Integrative medicine.
I. Devries, Stephen R. II. Dalen, James E., 1932- III. Series: Weil integrative medicine library.
[DNLM: 1. Cardiovascular Diseases—therapy. 2. Complementary Therapies–methods.
3. Integrative Medicine—methods. WG 166 I607 2010]
RC684.A48I58 2010
616.1–dc22   2010014554

ISBN 978-0-19-538346-1

1 3 5 7 9 8 6 4 2
Printed in the United States of America
on acid-free paper

To my father, Robert Devries, of blessed memory—who taught by example to care deeply about others and to go beyond.

Stephen Devries

CONTENTS

FOREWORD

Cardiovascular disease is the leading cause of death worldwide. It is multifactorial in origin, with a complex interplay of genetic and lifestyle influences. A strong relationship exists between diet and heart health. Stress and other mental/emotional factors play roles as well. Given this complexity, integrative medicine is ideally suited to both prevent and treat diseases of the heart and blood vessels.

When I was a medical student in the late 1960s, I was taught that atherosclerosis was irreversible. We now know that is reversible, by lifestyle change or drug therapy or a combination of the two. Practitioners of integrative medicine understand the innate healing capacity of the organism and are not surprised that many cardiovascular conditions can be stabilized or reversed through creative application of conventional and unconventional therapies. Because they are trained in lifestyle medicine and whole person medicine, they are able to design broader, more effective, and more cost-effective treatment plans than those relying solely on drugs or the techniques of invasive cardiology.

I am especially pleased to introduce this volume in the Oxford University Press *Integrative Medicine Library* series because the editors are longtime friends and colleagues. Dr. James E. Dalen, an eminent cardiologist and leader in American academic medicine, was Dean of the University of Arizona's College of Medicine in the early 1990s, when I first proposed creating a fellowship program in integrative medicine. As the first medical school dean to encourage such a program, he took a risk and withstood much criticism. Today, the Arizona Center for Integrative Medicine is a Center of Excellence of the College of Medicine and the world leader in training physicians and allied health professionals in medicine of the future. Jim Dalen continues to be a staunch proponent of integrative medicine and its application to his own specialty. His co-editor, Dr. Stephen Devries, was one of the first cardiologists to graduate from the Arizona Center's fellowship training and is now a leading practitioner of integrative cardiology.

Together Drs. Devries and Dalen have assembled an outstanding team of contributing authors and a wealth of useful information for clinicians interested in using the philosophy and practices of integrative medicine to maintain optimum heart health and to manage cardiovascular disease most effectively. I am certain you will find this book as useful as I do.

Andrew T. Weil, MD
Series Editor
Tucson, Arizona
May, 2010

CONTRIBUTORS

James E. Dalen, MD, MPH, FACC
Executive Director, The Weil
    Foundation
Dean Emeritus and Professor Emeritus
    of Medicine and Public Health
University of Arizona College of
    Medicine

Stephen Devries, MD, FACC, FAHA
Preventive Cardiologist
Associate Professor of Medicine
Division of Cardiology
Feinberg School of Medicine
Northwestern University

Tieraona Low Dog, MD
Director of the Fellowship
Arizona Center for Integrative Medicine
Clinical Associate Professor
Department of Medicine
University of Arizona

Thomas B. Graboys, MD, FACC
Clinical Professor of Medicine
Brigham and Women's Hospital and
    Harvard Medical School
President Emeritus
Lown Cardiovascular Research
    Foundation

Mimi Guarneri, MD, FACC
Medical Director
Scripps Center for Integrative Medicine
Division of Integrative Medicine and
    Cardiovascular Diseases
Scripps Clinic

Mark C. Houston, MD, MS, FACP, FAHA
Associate Clinical Professor of
    Medicine
Vanderbilt University School of
    Medicine
Director, Hypertension Institute and
    Vascular Biology
Saint Thomas Hospital

Elizabeth Kaback, MD
Cardiologist
Scripps Center for Integrative Medicine
Division of Integrative Medicine and
    Cardiovascular Diseases
Scripps Clinic

Rauni Prittinen King, RN, BSN, MIH,
HN-BC, CHTP/I
Director of Programs and Planning
Scripps Center for Integrative
    Medicine
Scripps Clinic

Mary Jo Kreitzer, PhD, RN
Director
Center for Spirituality & Healing
University of Minnesota

Kim R. Lebowitz, PhD
Assistant Professor of Psychiatry and
    Surgery
Feinberg School of Medicine
Director of Cardiac Behavioral Medicine
Bluhm Cardiovascular Institute
Northwestern University

Lee Lipsenthal, MD
Internist
Omega Institute for Holistic Studies

John Longhurst, MD, PhD
Professor of Medicine, Physiology and
    Biophysics, Pharmacology and
    Biomedical Engineering
Lawrence K Dodge Chair in
    Integrative Biology
Susan Samueli Dodge Chair in
    Integrative Medicine
Director, Susan Samueli Center for
    Integrative Medicine
University of California, Irvine

Kenneth M. Riff, MD
Vice President
Data Strategy and Clinical Research
Center for Spirituality & Healing,
    University of Minnesota

Gulshan K. Sethi, MD, FACC
Professor of Surgery and Medicine
Medical Director
Circulatory Sciences Program
Director of Clinical Services
Arizona Center of Integrative
    Medicine
University of Arizona

**Stephen T. Sinatra, MD, FACC,
FACN, CNS**
Cardiologist
Assistant Clinical Professor of
    Medicine
University of Connecticut School of
    Medicine

Craig S. Smith, MD
Director
Coronary Care Unit
University of Massachusetts Memorial
    Medical Center
Assistant Professor of Medicine
University of Massachusetts Medical
    School

Christopher Suhar, MD
Cardiologist
Scripps Center for Integrative
    Medicine
Division of Integrative Medicine and
    Cardiovascular Diseases
Scripps Clinic

Andrew T. Weil, MD
Lovell-Jones Professor of Integrative
    Rheumatology
Clinical Professor of Medicine,
    Professor of Public Health, and
    Director of the Arizona Center for
    Integrative Medicine
University of Arizona

PREFACE

Cardiovascular disease is the most prevalent chronic condition and most common cause of death in the United States. Treatment of cardiovascular disorders now consumes more than 10 percent of our health care expenditures (Lloyd-Jones et al., 2009). How did we get to where we are now—and where are we going?

Before World War II, nearly all patients with heart disease were diagnosed as "cardiacs" and treatment was essentially the same for all: a low salt diet, digitalis, and restricted activity. Over the ensuing decades, the marriage of medicine and technology has allowed the cardiologist to accurately diagnose and treat almost every possible type of heart disease.

As a result of these advances, heart disease mortality decreased by an incredible 64 percent from 1950 to 2005 (National Center for Health Statistics, 2008). From 1994 until 2004, deaths due to stroke and heart disease decreased by 25 percent. By comparison, cancer deaths decreased by only 5 percent during the same time period (Rosamond et al., 2007).

This incredible progress, resulting from the infusion of advanced technology into cardiac care, has come at a price. The first is the impact on health care costs. The high-tech treatment of heart disease is very expensive, and is one of the major causes of the escalation of health care costs, stranding millions of Americans with inadequate or no health insurance (Dalen and Alpert, 2008). Lack of adequate health insurance is a significant barrier to preventive health care in the U.S., and is one of the main reasons that the American health outcomes trail other Western nations (OECD).The World Health Association ranked U.S. health care 39th among 191 countries in 2000 (Blendon et al., 2001)

The second significant side effect of high-tech cardiac care is that it has become very impersonal. Most initial visits to a cardiologist are made by patients who already have symptoms of heart disease. In fact, many patients first meet a cardiologist when they are admitted on an emergency basis for an acute coronary syndrome or for congestive heart failure. The cardiologist is seen as the person who orders (and performs) a variety of invasive procedures. The patient may be rushed to a catheterization laboratory for a percutaneous coronary intervention procedure. By necessity, there is usually minimal time to explain the reason for the procedures or to discuss alternative therapies.

At discharge, patients frequently leave with prescriptions for multiple expensive medications. Many fail to take all the prescribed medications because of the expense, or because they do not fully understand the reasons why they are necessary. To compound the problem, patients may experience side effects from medication and are often reluctant to continue them. Consequently, they may be regarded as "noncompliant."

Despite the many successes, conventional cardiac care often leaves patients feeling overwhelmed and confused. Patients may be led to believe that their fate rests with an endless series of complex diagnostic tests and expensive medications—leaving them little control of their own health destiny.

And there is evidence that we are losing ground in the fight against cardiac disease. A recent study compared the prevalence of risk factors in American adults aged forty to seventy-four in 1988 and in 2006 (King et al., 2009). Obesity increased from 28 percent to 36 percent. Those eating a healthy diet decreased 16 percent. Regular exercise decreased 10 percent. Especially sadly, the percentage of smokers did not decline, remaining at 26 percent in 2006. Clearly we must do much better.

What Is Integrative Medicine?

Integrative medicine is the intelligent combination of conventional medicine and other healing modalities not commonly taught in Western medical schools, with an emphasis on maximizing opportunities to promote health and healing. In addition to incorporating all of the incredible advances of medication and technology, integrative medicine emphasizes nutrition, lifestyle, and attention to mind–body influences. And most importantly, the focus of integrative approaches is directed at prevention. The style of integrative medicine is heavily accented on collaboration—that is, seeking to obtain the best possible outcome taking into account the intangible, but vital, nuances of each patient's culture, beliefs, and preferences.

Cardiology is ideally suited for an integrative approach. Heart disease is largely preventable. The influence of nutrition, physical activity, metabolic factors, and emotional state on heart health is unmistakable. The wide-angle lens of integrative medicine is a perfect model to address these multifaceted needs. One of the major benefits of an integrative approach to cardiovascular care is that patients take an active role in their treatment.

The meteoric rise of integrative medicine is a clear message that patients are not satisfied with the status quo (Eisenberg et al., 1998, Nahin et al., 2009). In growing numbers, patients are pursuing scientifically valid options that include, but go beyond the usual of prescriptions and procedures. They want to know about a broader range of options for treatment—but even more, they are pursuing preventive measures with an intensity that is not matched by offerings of conventional medicine.

This book provides the interested health care practitioner with the tools needed to begin the journey toward an integrative approach to cardiology. It is not intended as a comprehensive cardiology text, but more as a starting point from which to develop integrative strategies focused on maintaining heart health.

Authors were selected because they are leaders in their respective areas and share the common background of academic medicine. Yet all are clinicians who have been asked to share their best practices. The charge to each of the authors was to focus on the approaches they have found most effective in their own practice, and to support their contributions with the best scientific evidence available.

The first section of the book describes the core elements of integrative cardiology, beginning front and center with a discussion of nutrition. Foundational chapters that follow discuss exercise, botanicals, aspirin, metabolic cardiology, acupuncture, spirituality, mind–body approaches, and energy medicine.

Andrew T. Weil, in his chapter on nutrition, focuses on the primacy of food as medicine for maintaining heart health. Current nutritional trends are placed in geographic and chronological perspective. Dr. Weil emphasizes the value of a Mediterranean style antiinflammatory diet for heart health and distills complex nutrition science into very practical strategies.

In the chapter on exercise, Craig S. Smith reviews the latest in maintaining heart health, and reviews tips on how to incorporate exercise into a successful heart health program.

The role of botanicals in the prevention and treatment of cardiovascular disease is discussed by Tieraona Low Dog in Chapter 3. Dr. Low Dog reviews the science showing that botanicals can lower blood pressure, improve lipid profiles, and reduce symptoms of congestive failure. The potential for both synergy and adverse reactions involving botanicals and prescription therapy is emphasized.

Although the value of nonprescription therapy is challenged by some, over-the-counter aspirin is, without a doubt, one of the most potent therapies available in all of medicine. James E. Dalen describes how to use this time honored therapy most effectively in Chapter 4.

Metabolic cardiology, as discussed by Stephen T. Sinatra in Chapter 5, describes how biochemical interventions with nutritional supplements can promote energy production in the heart. The role of coenzyme Q_{10}, l-carnitine, d-ribose, and magnesium for support of cardiac systolic and diastolic function is highlighted.

John Longhurst, in Chapter 6, reviews the scientific underpinnings of the 2000-year-old therapy of acupuncture. He describes how acupuncture may be a useful adjunct in the treatment of hypertension, and outlines the promise of its expanded future role in cardiology.

In Chapter 7, Mary Jo Kreitzer and Ken Riff discuss how spiritual practices such as prayer, meditation, journaling, and interacting with nature can have important health benefits for patients with cardiovascular disease. We are reminded that the potential to incorporate spiritual belief for healing is immense, yet largely untapped.

Kim R. Lebowitz, in Chapter 8, emphasizes the mind–body connection, and reviews the evidence that depression, anxiety, and stress are not only risk factors for the development of cardiovascular disease, but lead to adverse outcomes, including cardiac death. She describes techniques to deal with depression, anxiety, and stress using stress management programs, relaxation therapy, and physical activity—therapies that can be as effective as drugs in some patients.

The role of energy medicine in the care plan of patients with cardiovascular disease is reviewed by Rauni Prittinen King in Chapter 9. The historical origins of "hands-on healing" techniques such as therapeutic touch and Qigong date back to Hippocrates. These approaches can be highly successful in addressing an aspect of healing that is often neglected, yet powerful and without side effects.

The second section of this book illustrates how the core elements of integrative cardiology described in the first half can be best utilized for prevention and treatment. This section leads with an overview of integrative approaches to prevention, and continues with chapters on hypertension, coronary artery disease, congestive heart failure, arrhythmias, and cardiac surgery. Emphasis has been placed on practical, clinically useful approaches backed by the best available literature.

Prevention is the cornerstone of integrative medicine. In Chapter 10, Stephen Devries highlights powerful opportunities afforded by nutritional approaches, lifestyle changes, and supplements—combined with conservative use of medication. The importance of evaluation for inherited risk factors that go beyond traditional cholesterol tests is reviewed.

In Chapter 11, Stephen T. Sinatra and Mark C. Houston discuss the role of integrative approaches for the patients with hypertension, especially in patients with borderline hypertension, and in those who do not tolerate prescription medication. Drawing on their extensive experience, they offer a focused view of the simplest and most successful strategies.

Conventional treatment of coronary artery disease is typically confined to pills and procedures. An expanded, integrative approach is provided by Mimi Guarneri, and Christopher Suhar in Chapter 12, with special attention paid to lifestyle changes and awareness of mind–body interactions.

No patients in cardiology are more complex than those with congestive heart failure. In Chapter 13, Elizabeth Kaback, Lee Lipsenthal, and Mimi Guarneri illustrate how the diverse needs of these patients can be optimally addressed by combining conventional care with nutritional supplements and a mindful, openhearted approach that acknowledges and strengthens their physical as well as their spiritual heart.

Arrhythmias are a nuisance for some and life-threatening for others. Thomas B. Graboys puts the current emphasis on high-technology treatment for arrhythmias in a broader perspective in Chapter 14. He advocates for an integrative approach that is simple in delivery, yet steeped in the wisdom of a seasoned clinician.

Patients who undergo cardiac surgery are often overwhelmed by the procedure, especially when it is required on an emergent basis. In Chapter 15, Gulshan K. Sethi, a senior cardiovascular surgeon, describes how integrative techniques can be implemented in the care of patients facing major surgery. The results of this integration are an improvement in the overall patient experience, as well as the surgical outcome.

We hope that you find this book a useful guide for your jouney into the rapidly expanding, and enormously satisfying, field of integrative cardiology.

REFERENCES

Blendon, R. J., Kim, M., Benson, J. M. 2001. The public versus the World Health Organization on health system performance. *Health Aff (Millwood)*, 20, 10–20.

Dalen, J. E., Alpert, J. S. 2008. National Health Insurance: could it work in the US? *Am J Med*, 121, 553–4.

Eisenberg, D. M., Davis, R. B., Ettner, S. L., Appel, S., Wilkey, S., Van Rompay, M., Kessler, R. C. 1998. Trends in alternative medicine use in the United States, 1990-1997: results of a follow-up national survey. *JAMA*, 280, 1569–75.

King, D. E., Mainous, A. G., 3rd, Carnemolla, M., Everett, C. J. 2009. Adherence to healthy lifestyle habits in US adults, 1988-2006. *Am J Med*, 122, 528–34.

Lloyd-Jones, D., Adams, R., Carnethon, M., DE Simone, G., Ferguson, T. B., Flegal,K., Ford, E., Furie, K., Go, A., Greenlund, K., Haase, N., Hailpern, S., Ho, M., Howard, V., Kissela, B., Kittner, S., Lackland, D., Lisabeth, L., Marelli, A., McDermott, M., Meigs, J., Mozaffarian, D., Nichol, G., O'Donnell, C., Roger, V., Rosamond, W., Sacco, R., Sorlie, P., Stafford, R., Steinberger, J., Thom, T., Wasserthiel-Smoller, S., Wong, N., Wylie-Rosett, J., Hong, Y. 2009. Heart disease and stroke statistics–2009 update: a report from the American Heart Association Statistics Committee and Stroke Statistics Subcommittee. *Circulation*, 119, e21–181.

Nahin, R. L., Barnes, P. M., Stussman, B. J., Bloom, B. 2009. Costs of complementary and alternative medicine (CAM) and frequency of visits to CAM practitioners: United States, 2007. *Natl Health Stat Report*, 1–14.

OECD Health at a Glance 2009, OECD Publishing.

Pleis JR, Lucas JW, Ward BW. Summary health statistics for U.S. adults: National Health Interview Survey, 2008. National Center for Health Statistics. *Vital Health Stat* 10(242). 2009.

Rosamond, W., Flegal, K., Friday, G., Furie, K., Go, A., Greenlund, K., Haase, N., Ho, M., Howard, V., Kissela, B., Kittner, S., Lloyd-Jones, D., McDermott, M., Meigs, J., Moy, C., Nichol, G., O'Donnell, C. J., Roger, V., Rumsfeld, J., Sorlie, P., Steinberger, J., Thom, T., Wasserthiel-Smoller, S., Hong, Y., Committee, F. T. A. H. A. S., Stroke Statistics Subcommittee 2007. Heart Disease and Stroke Statistics–2007 Update: A Report From the American Heart Association Statistics Committee and Stroke Statistics Subcommittee. *Circulation*, 115, e69–171.

Integrative Cardiology

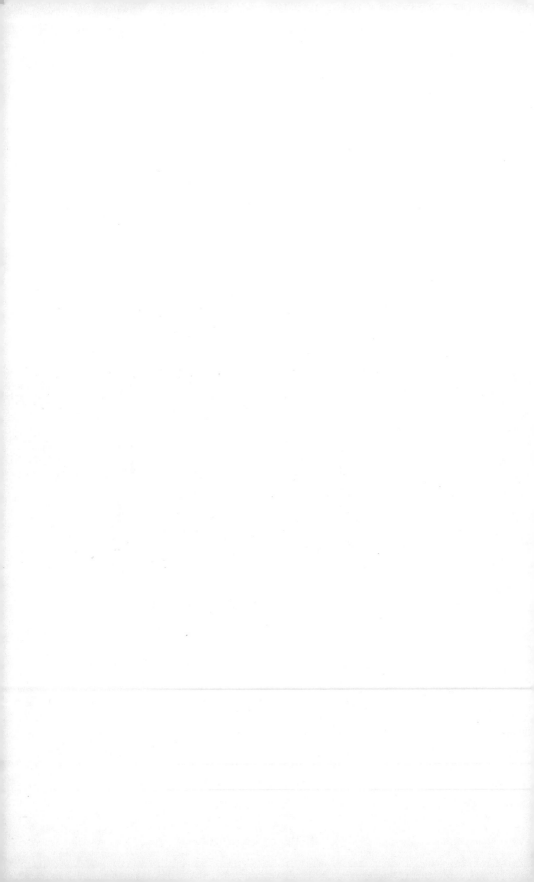

I

The Foundations of Integrative Cardiology

1

Nutrition and Cardiovascular Health

ANDREW T. WEIL

KEY CONCEPTS

- The mainstream North American diet promotes the development of obesity, insulin resistance, metabolic syndrome, and cardiovascular disease.
- Refined, processed, and manufactured foods are the chief culprits; they are full of unhealthy fats and high-glycemic-load carbohydrate.
- An antiinflammatory diet, based on the Mediterranean diet, offers the best protection against cardiovascular disease and also promotes optimum health, without sacrificing the pleasures of good food.
- It is more important to eat the right kinds of fat and right kinds of carbohydrate than to limit intake of either fat or carbohydrate to low percentages of total caloric intake.

■

Understanding of the relationship between dietary habits and cardiovascular health has developed slowly and changed greatly in recent years. Epidemiological data first brought to light significant correlations between diet and incidence of atherosclerosis, coronary heart disease, and myocardial infarction (MI), all rare conditions in many parts of the world that became epidemic in Western, industrialized societies in the twentieth century.

The atherogenic effect of high intake of saturated fat was suggested by a dramatic decrease in heart attacks in Holland, Belgium, Denmark, and other European countries suffering the deprivations of the Second World War, followed by a dramatic increase in heart attacks with the return of peace and prosperity, along with meat, butter, and other animal-derived foods (Malmros 1980). The incidence of myocardial infarction, especially in middle-aged men, was at an all-time high in the U.S. in the middle of the last century, and treatment for it was often ineffective. More alarming was the finding that early atherosclerotic changes could be found at autopsy in healthy American men under twenty who had been killed in accidents or war, changes that were absent in most men of all ages in Asia, Africa, and many other parts of the world (Beaglehole and Magnus 2002).

As the evidence for saturated fat as a cause of elevated serum cholesterol and arterial disease grew, physicians urged patients to substitute margarine for butter, cook with safflower and other polyunsaturated vegetable oils, and decrease consumption of whole-milk products and eggs.

Medical focus on elevated serum cholesterol as the main risk factor for MI and on dietary saturated fat as the main driver of elevated serum cholesterol led, by the 1970s, to condemnation of dietary fat in general as the most harmful element in the Western diet, the one responsible for epidemic atherosclerosis in our population. It followed that a healthy, heart-protective diet was primarily a low-fat diet. A few prominent physicians advocated ultra-low-fat diets, even advising patients to avoid olive oil and oily fish because of presumed adverse effects on serum cholesterol. Ornish (1990) demonstrated reversal of coronary atherosclerosis in patients who followed a strict program of group support, moderate exercise, stress management, and an ultra-low-fat, vegetarian diet. The dietary component of his program has never been evaluated apart from the other interventions.

More recent data on the rising incidence in China and Japan of "Western" diseases, including type 2 diabetes and cardiovascular disease, as people in those countries have moved away from traditional diets in favor of Western ones, strongly suggests the importance of nutritional influences relative to other risk factors. When I lived in Japan as an exchange student in 1959, most Japanese ate traditional breakfasts of miso soup, steamed rice, a small portion of broiled salmon or other fish, seaweed, steamed and pickled vegetables, and green tea. When I returned in the mid-1970s, I found it hard to get that kind of breakfast except in hotels. The morning meal I saw most Japanese eating in those years was bacon or sausage and eggs, white toast with butter, or cereal and milk, and coffee.

Such radical changes in eating habits can affect the health of populations very quickly, even over a few years. Between 1999 and 2002, I made three trips to Okinawa to collect information on healthy aging for a book I was writing. Okinawa had the highest concentration of centenarians in the world, the greatest rates of longevity, and unusual numbers of very old people in good health. I found the traditional Okinawan diet (different from that of the rest of Japan) most interesting. It included a great variety and abundance of land and sea vegetables, fruits, unusual herbs and spices, fish, tofu, and pork (long simmered to remove fat). But it seemed risky to me to attribute Okinawan health and longevity to diet alone. People there are genetically distinct, are more physically active throughout life than we are, and enjoy clean air and water. Okinawan culture also values aging; the oldest members of the community are considered living treasures and included in all community activities.

Nevertheless, within a few years of my last visit, Okinawan longevity plummeted, especially among men. Experts attributed the change mostly to changed eating habits, in particular, the sudden popularity of American-type fast food (Onishi 2004).

Research on nutrition and health has come a long way since the simplistic view of high intake of dietary fat as the main risk factor for disease in general and heart disease in particular. It is now clear that the typical Western diet is unhealthy both because of what it does not provide as well as because of what it does. We know that there are good fats and bad fats; some types of fat are strongly heart protective. We know that carbohydrate foods differ in how quickly they digest and raise blood sugar; those with the highest glycemic load can be very unhealthy for the many genetically susceptible people in our population. We have confirmed the protective effects of key micronutrients on cardiovascular health and have identified many protective phytonutrients in fruits, vegetables, herbs, spices, and beverages. And the new view of atherosclerosis and coronary heart disease as an inflammatory disorder makes it a priority to evaluate the influence of dietary choices on the inflammatory process (Fito et al. 2007; Lichtenstein et al. 2006).

With this broader knowledge, we can easily see why the mainstream North American diet promotes obesity, insulin resistance, and cardiovascular disease:

- It provides too much of the unhealthy fats: saturated fat (especially from beef, cheese, and other full-fat dairy products); polyunsaturated vegetable oils (which are pro-inflammatory); and chemically altered fats, including trans and partially hydrogenated ones (which are atherogenic and pro-inflammatory) (Simopoulos and Robinson 1999; Weil 2001). It also provides excessive amounts of pro-inflammatory omega-6 fatty acids, mostly from refined soybean oil, a ubiquitous, cheap ingredient found in many processed foods (Simopoulos 1999).
- It is full of high-glycemic-load carbohydrate foods (made from flour, other refined starches, sugar, and high-fructose corn syrup) that promote insulin resistance in many people and, by causing spikes in blood sugar, promote glycation reactions that result in pro-inflammatory end products (de Groof 2003).

- It is top-heavy in animal foods, especially beef. Diets high in animal foods correlate with increased cardiovascular risk and other long-term health risks (Menotti et al. 1999).
- It is full of refined, processed, and manufactured foods new to human diets. These foods contain numerous additives, artificial ingredients, and ingredients altered from their natural forms. Introduction of refined, processed, and manufactured foods in diverse populations throughout the world is associated with a rapid increase of diseases common in our society, including cardiovascular disease.
- It is deficient in health-protective fats, especially the antiinflammatory, anti-thrombotic omega-3 fatty acids, which are mostly found in oily fish (Harper and Jacobson 2001; Psota, Gebauer, and Kris-Etherton 2006).
- It is deficient in fruits and vegetables, the main dietary sources of protective antioxidants and phytonutrients (Heber 2002).
- It is often deficient in protective micronutrients, such as folate and other B-vitamins that regulate homocysteine metabolism (Bonaa et al. 2006; Joshipura et al. 2001), vitamin D (Scragg et al. 1990; Wang et al. 2008), and magnesium (Ohira et al. 2009).

Proposed heart-healthy diets of recent years have not addressed all of these problems and are overly restrictive, making long-term adherence difficult except for highly motivated patients. Ultra-low-fat diets may worsen omega-3 fatty acid deficiency and fail to lower glycemic load. Ultra-low-carbohydrate diets may be high in animal foods and unhealthy fats and low in protective phytonutrients and micronutrients. Calorie-restricted diets may include processed foods and worsen deficiencies of essential fatty acids. All of these diets can reduce risk of cardiovascular disease; recent research shows no significant advantage to any one of them (Dansiger et al. 2005). But all may fail to promote optimum long-term health, and their restrictive nature makes it likely that people will not stick to them.

A more realistic strategy is to design a nutritional program that addresses all the problems of the mainstream diet without denying people the pleasures of eating. Very low-fat foods tend to be tasteless and uninteresting. Carbohydrate foods are comfort foods for many. Vegetables need to be prepared in ways that make them appetizing.

Using the Mediterranean diet as a template for such a nutritional program is a sensible starting point. A composite of the traditional diets of Italy, Greece, Crete, parts of Spain, the Middle East, and North Africa, the Mediterranean diet is high in fish but low in red meat, high in low-to-moderate glycemic load carbohydrates, low in sugar, rich in vegetables and fruit, and liberal in the use of olive oil. Absent are the refined, processed, and manufactured foods that North Americans consume in such high quantities. Heart health (and general health) of Mediterranean peoples who eat this way is superior to that of North Americans (de Lorgeril 1999; de Lorgeril et al. 1994).

It is important to note, however, that the traditional Mediterranean diet, like the traditional Japanese diet, is rapidly going out of fashion, as fast food and processed food become increasingly available and popular throughout the region. In fact, it may only be in remote areas today that people eat the way their grandparents did.

However, a great advantage of the Mediterranean diet is that it appeals to people all over the world and can be adapted to local circumstances. Some descriptions of it in words or pictures fail to distinguish between truly whole-grain foods and those made with pulverized grains (flour), which have a much higher glycemic impact. (This is an important point. Many people think that whole wheat bread is a whole-grain product, and the Food and Drug Administration allows it to be so labeled. In fact, when grains are milled into flour, whether or not they retain the germ and some bran, the starch in them is reduced to tiny particles with a very large collective surface area available for enzymatic conversion to glucose. All food products made from pulverized grains have much higher glycemic loads than whole or cracked grains that are parched, boiled, or steamed.) Also, I think the antiinflammatory power of the Mediterranean diet can be improved with a few tweaks and additions.

The antiinflammatory diet I recommend is a key strategy for healthy aging, intended to increase the likelihood of compression of morbidity in the later years of life. My specific recommendations follow.

The Antiinflammatory Diet

GENERAL

- Aim for variety.
- Include as much fresh food as possible.
- Minimize consumption of processed foods and fast food.
- Eat an abundance of fruits and vegetables.

CALORIC INTAKE

- Most adults need to consume between 2,000 and 3,000 calories a day.
- Women and smaller and less active people need fewer calories.

- Men and bigger and more active people need more calories.
- If you are eating the appropriate number of calories for your level of activity your weight should not fluctuate greatly.
- The distribution of calories you take in should be as follows: 40 to 50 percent from carbohydrates, 30 percent from fat, and 20 to 30 percent from protein.
- Try to include carbohydrates, fat, and protein at each meal.

CARBOHYDRATES

- On a 2,000-calorie-a-day diet, adult women should eat about 160 to 200 grams of carbohydrates a day.
- Adult men should eat about 240 to 300 grams of carbohydrates a day.
- The majority of carbohydrates eaten should be in the form of less-refined, less-processed foods with low glycemic loads.
- Reduce consumption of foods made with flour and sugar, especially bread and most packaged snack foods (including chips and pretzels).
- Eat more whole grains (not whole-wheat-flour products), beans, winter squashes, and sweet potatoes.
- Cook pasta al dente and eat it in moderation.
- Avoid products made with high-fructose corn syrup.

FAT

- On a 2,000-calorie-a-day diet, 600 of those calories can come from fat–that is, about 67 grams. This should be in a ratio of 1:2:1 of saturated to monounsaturated to polyunsaturated fat.
- Reduce intake of saturated fat by eating less butter, cream, cheese, and other full-fat dairy products, as well as chicken with the skin on, fatty meats, and products made with palm kernel oils.
- Use extra-virgin olive oil as a primary cooking oil. If you want a neutral-tasting oil, use expeller-pressed organic canola oil. High-oleic versions of sunflower and safflower oil are acceptable also, preferably non-GMO (genetically modified organism) versions.
- Avoid regular safflower and sunflower oils, corn oil, cottonseed oil, and mixed vegetable oils.
- Strictly avoid margarine, vegetable shortening, and all products listing them as ingredients. Strictly avoid all products made with partially hydrogenated oils of any kind. Avoid products made with refined soybean oil.

- Include in your diet avocados and nuts–especially walnuts, cashews, and almonds and nut butters made from them.
- To ensure appropriate intake of omega-3 fatty acids, eat salmon (preferably fresh or frozen wild or canned sockeye), sardines packed in water or olive oil, herring, black cod (sablefish, butterfish), omega-3 fortified eggs, hemp seeds, flaxseeds (preferably freshly ground), and walnuts, or take a fish oil supplement (2-3 grams a day).

PROTEIN

- On a 2,000-calorie-a-day diet, daily intake of protein should be between 80 and 120 grams. Eat less protein if you have liver or kidney problems, allergies, or autoimmune disease.
- Decrease consumption of animal protein, except for fish and dairy products.
- Eat more vegetable protein, especially from beans in general and soybeans in particular. Become familiar with the range of soy foods available to find ones you like.

FIBER

- Try to eat 40 grams of fiber a day. You can achieve this by increasing consumption of fruit (especially berries), vegetables (especially beans), and whole grains.
- Ready-made cereals can be good sources of fiber, but read labels to make sure they give you at least 4, and preferably 5, grams of bran per one-ounce serving.

PHYTONUTRIENTS

- To get maximum natural protection against age-related diseases, including cardiovascular disease, cancer, and neurodegenerative disease, as well as against environmental toxicity, eat a variety of fruits, vegetables, and mushrooms.
- Choose fruits and vegetables from all parts of the color spectrum, especially berries, tomatoes, orange and yellow fruits, and dark leafy greens.
- Choose organic produce whenever possible. Learn which conventionally grown crops are most likely to carry pesticide residues (see www.foodnews.org) and avoid them.

- Eat cruciferous (cabbage-family) vegetables regularly.
- Include whole soy foods in your diet (such as edamame, soy nuts, soy milk, tofu, and tempeh).
- Drink tea instead of coffee, especially good-quality white, green, or oolong tea.
- If you drink alcohol, use red wine preferentially and in moderation.
- Enjoy plain dark chocolate (with a minimum cocoa content of 70 percent) in moderation.

VITAMINS AND MINERALS

- The best way to obtain all of your daily vitamins, minerals, and micronutrients is by eating a diet high in fresh foods with an abundance of fruits and vegetables.
- In addition, supplement your diet with the following antioxidant cocktail:
  - Vitamin C: 200 milligrams a day
  - Vitamin E: 400 International Units IU of natural mixed tocopherols (d-alpha-tocopherol with other tocopherols, or, better, a minimum of 80 milligrams of natural mixed tocopherols and tocotrienols)
  - Selenium: 200 micrograms of an organic (yeast-bound) form
  - Mixed carotenoids: 10,000 to 15,000 IU daily.
- In addition, take daily multivitamin–multimineral supplements that provide at least 400 micrograms of folic acid. They should contain no iron (unless you are female and having regular menstrual periods) and no preformed vitamin A (retinol).
- Take 2,000 IU a day of vitamin D with your largest meal.
- Women may take supplemental calcium, preferably as calcium citrate, 500 to 700 milligrams a day, depending on their dietary intake of this mineral; men should avoid supplemental calcium.

WATER

- Try to drink six to eight glasses of pure water a day or drinks that are mostly water (tea, very diluted fruit juice, sparkling water with lemon).
- Use bottled water or get a home water purifier if you tap water tastes of chlorine or other contaminants, or if you live in an area where the water is known or suspected to be contaminated.

The following chart offers practical suggestions for how to incorporate appropriate amounts of heart-healthy foods into your diet.

Because chronic, inappropriate inflammation appears to be the common root of much age-related disease, this kind of diet promotes optimum health at any age and broadly reduces risk of disease, including cardiovascular disease. It avoids the problems of restrictive diets, allowing for much variety and pleasure in eating. It takes account of the most current findings of research on nutrition and health. It is the best corrective remedy for the dietary habits that now prevail in North America and are rapidly spreading to other parts of the world, habits that undermine health in general and heart health in particular.

Healthy Sweets

How much: Sparingly
Healthy choices: Unsweetened dried fruit, dark chocolate, fruit sorbet
Why: Dark chocolate provides polyphenols with antioxidant activity. Choose dark chocolate with at least 70 percent pure cocoa and have an ounce a few times a week. Fruit sorbet is a better option than other frozen desserts.

Red Wine

How much: Optional, no more than 1–2 glasses per day
Healthy choices: Organic red wine
Why: Red wine has beneficial antioxidant activity. Limit intake to no more than 1–2 servings per day. If you do not drink alcohol, do not start.

Tea

How much: 2–4 cups per day
Healthy choices: White, green, oolong teas
Why: Tea is rich in catechins, which are antioxidant compounds that reduce inflammation. Purchase high-quality tea and learn how to correctly brew it for maximum taste and health benefits.

Healthy Herbs & Spices

How much: Unlimited amounts
Healthy choices: Turmeric, curry powder (which contains turmeric), ginger and garlic (dried and fresh), chili peppers, basil, cinnamon, rosemary, thyme
Why:Use these herbs and spices generously to season foods. Turmeric and ginger are powerful, natural, antiinflammatory agents.

Other Sources of Protein

How much: 1–2 servings a week (one portion is equal to 1 ounce of cheese, 1 eight-ounce serving of dairy, 1 egg, or 3 ounces cooked poultry or skinless meat)

Healthy choices: Natural cheeses, natural yogurt, omega-3 enriched eggs, skinless poultry, grass-fed lean meats
Why: In general, try to reduce consumption of animal foods. If you eat chicken, choose organic, cage-free chicken and remove the skin and associated fat. Use organic dairy products moderately, especially yogurt and natural cheeses such as Emmental (Swiss), Jarlsberg, and true Parmesan. If you eat eggs, choose omega-3 enriched eggs (made by feeding hens a flax-meal-enriched diet), or organic eggs from free-range chickens.

Cooked Asian Mushrooms

How much: Unlimited amounts
Healthy choices: Shiitake, enokidake, maitake, and oyster mushrooms (and wild mushrooms if available)
Why: These mushrooms contain compounds that enhance immune function. Never eat mushrooms raw, and minimize consumption of common commercial button mushrooms (including crimini and portobello).

Whole Soy Foods

How much: 1–2 servings per day (one serving is equal to one-half cup tofu or tempeh, 1 cup soymilk, one-half cup cooked edamame, 1 ounce of soynuts)
Healthy choices: Tofu, tempeh, edamame, soy nuts, soymilk
Why: Soy foods contain isoflavones that have antioxidant activity and are protective against cancer. Choose whole soy foods over fractionated foods, such as isolated soy protein powders and imitation meats made with soy isolate.

Fish & Seafood

How much: 2–6 servings per week (one serving is equal to 4 ounces of fish or seafood)
Healthy choices: Wild Alaskan salmon (especially sockeye), herring, sardines, and black cod (sablefish)
Why: These fish are rich in omega-3 fats, which are strongly antiinflammatory. If you choose not to eat fish, take a molecularly distilled fish oil supplement, 2–3 grams per day.

Healthy Fats

How much: 5–7 servings per day (one serving is equal to 1 teaspoon of oil, 2 walnuts, 1 tablespoon of flaxseed, or 1 ounce of avocado)
Healthy choices: For cooking, use extra-virgin olive oil and expeller-pressed organic canola oil. Other sources of healthy fats include nuts (especially walnuts), avocados, and seeds (including hemp seeds and freshly ground flaxseed). Omega-3 fats are also found in cold-water fish, omega-3 enriched

eggs, and whole soy foods. High-oleic sunflower or safflower oils may also be used, as well as walnut and hazelnut oils in salads and dark roasted sesame oil as a flavoring for soups and stir-fries.

Why: Healthy fats are those rich in either monounsaturated or omega-3 fats. Extra-virgin olive oil is rich in polyphenols with antioxidant activity, and canola oil contains a small fraction of omega-3 fatty acids.

Whole & Cracked Grains

How much: 3–5 servings a day (one serving is equal to about one-half cup cooked grains)

Healthy choices: Brown rice, basmati rice, wild rice, buckwheat, groats, barley, quinoa, steel-cut oats

Why: Whole grains digest slowly, reducing frequency of spikes in blood sugar that promote inflammation. "Whole grains" means grains that are intact or in a few large pieces, not whole wheat bread or other products made from flour.

Pasta (al dente)

How much: 2–3 servings per week (one serving is equal to about one-half cup cooked pasta)

Healthy choices: Organic pasta, rice noodles, bean thread noodles, and part whole wheat and buckwheat noodles, such as Japanese udon and soba

Why: Pasta cooked al dente (when it is slightly firm rather than soft, and has "tooth" to it) has a lower glycemic index than fully cooked pasta. Low-glycemic-load carbohydrates should be the bulk of your carbohydrate intake, to help minimize spikes in blood glucose levels.

Beans & Legumes

How much: 1–2 servings per day (one serving is equal to one-half cup cooked beans or legumes)

Healthy choices: Beans like Anasazi, adzuki, and black, as well as chickpeas, black-eyed peas and lentils

Why: Beans are rich in folic acid, magnesium, potassium, and soluble fiber. They are a low-glycemic-load food. Eat them well cooked, either whole or pureed into spreads like hummus.

Vegetables

How much: 4–5 servings per day minimum (one serving is equal to 2 cups salad greens, or one-half cup vegetables cooked, raw, or juiced)

Healthy choices: Lightly cooked dark leafy greens (spinach, collard greens, kale, Swiss chard), cruciferous vegetables (broccoli, cabbage, Brussels sprouts, kale, bok choy, and cauliflower), carrots, beets, onions, peas, squashes, sea vegetables, and washed raw salad greens

Why: Vegetables are rich in flavonoids and carotenoids, with both antioxidant and antiinflammatory activity. Go for a wide range of colors, eat them both raw and cooked, and chooseorganic when possible.

Fruits

How much: 3–4 servings per day (one serving is equal to 1 medium-sized piece of fruit, one-half cup chopped fruit, or one-quarter cup of dried fruit)
Healthy choices: Raspberries, blueberries, strawberries, peaches, nectarines, oranges, pink grapefruit, red grapes, plums, pomegranates, blackberries, cherries, apples, and pears—all are lower in glycemic load than most tropical fruits
Why: Fruits are rich in flavonoids and carotenoids, with both antioxidant and antiinflammatory activity. Go for a wide range of colors, choose fruit that is fresh and in-season or frozen, and buy organic when possible.

Supplements

Recent research has questioned the value of "vitamin therapy" with supplemental antioxidants (vitamin E, vitamin C, beta-carotene, and selenium) for improving serum cholesterol levels or existing coronary artery disease (Brown et al. 2001). Most studies have used d-alpha-tocopherol, not the full complex of tocopherols and tocotrienols that occur in natural vitamin E, and they have used isolated beta-carotene, not a complex of carotenoids more representative of the family of pigments found in many fruits and vegetables. I recommend the above forms and doses of vitamins C and E, mixed carotenoids, and selenium for general health-protective effects, especially because daily consumption of fruits and vegetables is generally low in much of the North American population.

REFERENCES

Beaglehole, R., P. Magnus. 2002. The search for new risk factors for coronary heart disease: occupational therapy for epidemiologists? *Int J Epidemiol* 32: 1177–22.

Bonaa, K., L. Njolstad, P. Ueland, H. Schirmer, A. Tverdal, T. Steigen, H. Wang, J. Nordrehaug, E. Arnesen, K. Rasmussen. 2006. Homocysteine lowering and cardiovascular events after myocardial infarction. *N Engl J Med* 354: 1578–88.

Brown, B., Z. Zhao, A. Chait., L. Fisher, M. Cheung, J. Morse, A. Dowdy, E. Marino, E. Bolson, P. Alaupovic, J. Frohlich, J. Albers. 2001. Simvastatin and niacin, antioxidant vitamins, or the combination for the prevention of coronary disease. *New Eng J Med* 345: 1583–92.

Dansiger, M., J. Gleason, J. Griffith, H. Selker, E. Schaefe. 2005. Comparison of the Atkins, Ornish, Weight Watchers, and Zone diets for weight loss and heart disease risk reduction: a randomized trial. *JAMA* 293: 43–53.

de groof, R. Remodeling of age- and diabetes-related changes in extracellular matrix. In *Proceedings of the 10th International Association of Biomedical Gerontology.* New York: New York Academy of Sciences, 2003.

de lorgeril, M. 1999. Mediterranean diet, traditional risk factors, and the rate of cardiovascular complications after myocardial infarction: final report of the Lyon diet heart study. *Circulation* 99: 779–85.

de Lorgeril, M., S. Renaud, N. Mamelle, P. Salen, J. Martin, I. Monjaud, J. Guidollet, P. Touboul, J. Delaye. 1994. Mediterranean alpha-linolenic-acid-rich diet in secondary prevention of coronary heart disease. *Lancet* 343: 1454–9.

Fito, M., Guxens, M., Corella, D., Saez, G., Estruch, R., De La Torre, R., Frances, F., Cabezas, C., Lopez-Sabater Mdel, C., Marrugat, J., Garcia-Arellano, A., Aros, F., Ruiz-Gutierrez, V., Ros, E., Salas-Salvado, J., Fiol, M., Sola, R. & Covas, M. I. 2007. Effect of a traditional Mediterranean diet on lipoprotein oxidation: a randomized controlled trial. *Arch Intern Med,* 167, 1195–203.

Harper, C., and T. Jacobson. 2001. The fats of life: The role of omega-3 fatty acids in the prevention of coronary heart disease. *Arch Intern Med* 161: 2185–92.

Heber, D. 2002. *What color is your diet?* New York: Regan.

Joshipura, K., F. Hu, J. Manson, M. Stampfer, E. Rimm, F. Speizer, G. Colditz, A. Ascherio, B. Rosner, D. Spiegelman, and W. Willett. 2001. The effect of fruit and vegetable intake on risk for coronary heart disease. *Arch Intern Med* 134: 1106–14.

Lichtenstein, A. H., Appel, L. J., Brands, M., Carnethon, M., Daniels, S., Frankch, H. A., Franklin, B., Kris-Etherton, P., Harris, W. S., Howard, B., Karanja, N., Lefevre, M., Rudel, L., Sacks, F., Van Horn, L., Winston, M. & Wylie-Rosett, J. 2006. Diet and lifestyle recommendations revision 2006: a scientific statement from the American Heart Association Nutrition Committee. *Circulation,* 114, 82–96.

Malmros, H. 1980. Diet, lipids, and atherosclerosis. *Acta Med Scandinavica* 207(3): 145–9.

Menotti, A., D. Kromhout, H. Blackburn, F. Fidanza, R. Buzina, and A. Nissinen. 1999. Food intake patterns and 25–year mortality from coronary heart disease: cross-cultural correlations in the seven countries study. *European J Epidemiol* 15: 507–15.

Ohira, T., J. Peacock, H. Iso, L. Chambless, W. Rosamond, and A. Folsom. 2009. Serum and dietary magnesium and risk of ischemic stroke-the atherosclerosis risk in communities study. *Am J Epidemiol* 169: 1437–44.

Onishi, N. 2004. On U.S. fast foods, Okinawans are supersized. *New York Times,* March 30, A–1.

Ornish, D. (1990) *Dr. Dean Ornish's program for reversing heart disease: the only system scientifically proven to reverse heart disease without drugs or surgery.* New York: Random House.

Psota, T., S. Gebauer, and P. Kris-Etherton. 2006. Omega-3 fatty acid intake and cardiovascular risk. *Am J Cardiol* 98: 3–18.

Scragg, R., R. Jackson, I. Holdaway, T. Lim, and R. Beaglehole. 1990. Myocardial infarction is inversely associated with plasma 25-hydroxyvitamin D3 levels: a community-based study. *Int J Epidemiol* 19: 559–63.

Simopoulos, A. 1999. Essential fatty acids in health and chronic disease. *Am J Clin Nutr* 70(3 suppl): 560S–569S.

Simopoulos, A., and J. Robinson. 1999. *The Omega diet: The lifesaving nutritional program based on the diet of the island of Crete.* New York: HarperPerennial.

Wang, T., M. Pencina, S. Booth, P. Jacques, E. Ingelsson, K. Lanier, E. Benjamin, R. D'agostino, M. Wolf, and R. Vasan. 2008. Vitamin D deficiency and risk of cardiovascular disease. *Circulation* 117: 503–11.

Weil, A. 2001. *Eating well for optimum health: The essential guide to bringing health and pleasure back to eating.* New York: Quill.

2

Exercise

CRAIG S. SMITH

KEY CONCEPTS

- Physical inactivity is one of the most prevalent modifiable risk factors for coronary artery disease.
- Regular exercise induces physiologic changes in multiple organ systems that allow for greater exertional capacity across all age groups.
- Aerobic training has favorable effects upon cardiovascular risk factors including hypertension, diabetes mellitus, cholesterol levels, and blood clotting factors. Resistance training appears to have beneficial effects as well.
- An exercise prescription should be tailored to maximize compliance and modified, as needed, based on cardiac status and other medical conditions.

■

Introduction

It has long been recognized, and promoted, that regular physical activity is associated with improved personal longevity and health. In recent decades, this belief has been reinforced by an increasing body of evidence in the scientific literature demonstrating a wide range of health benefits linked to physical fitness, regardless of age, place of origin, or gender. The cumulative effect of this evidence has led to a heightened awareness in both the medical profession and the general public of the importance of regular physical activity as both a preventive and therapeutic tool. While there have been formal recommendations and calls to action for increased physical activity by the surgeon general and various medical organizations, many individuals have embarked on exercise regimens on their own, as evidenced by the increasing number of individuals who report regular physical activity in their lives (Caspersen 2000; Morbidity and Mortality Weekly Report 2008). Despite the apparent acceptance by the public and the medical profession of the importance of physical activity, more than 60 percent of Americans do not achieve recommended activity levels, and one-quarter of the population remains sedentary, reporting little to no activity (Jones et al. 1998).

In the United States, over 250,000 deaths per year are attributed solely to a sedentary lifestyle, most of which are due to complications of cardiovascular disease and type 2 diabetes mellitus (Pate et al. 1995). This represents approximately 12 percent of all deaths per year. The lack of physical activity is associated with a doubling of the risk for coronary events, the largest cause of mortality in the population (Powell and Blair 1994). As such, a sedentary lifestyle represents the most prevalent modifiable risk factor for mortality in the population at large, and its elimination accrues health benefits for the individual on par with smoking cessation, treatment of high blood pressure, and reduction of obesity (Miller, Balady, and Fletcher 1997).

The wide range of health benefits derived from physical activity and exercise is likely reflective of the multitude of body systems involved, and the scope of body traits and functions encompassing the concept of physical fitness. These include cardiopulmonary endurance, skeletal muscle power and endurance, speed, flexibility, body composition, and balance. Ironically, while the multifaceted nature of exercise is likely responsible for its varied benefits, it also makes its study more difficult. Randomized trials to evaluate the effects of exercise are often plagued with noncompliance to exercise regimens, "drop-in" of controls who perform exercise (and the unethical stance of asking them not to), and inadequate subject numbers to account for the multitude of patient factors and the varied types of exercise performed to allow statistically significant conclusions. As a result, most of the scientific literature is based on observational studies, which are subject to bias due to confounding variables such as adoption of a heart-healthy diet, increased medical care, and alterations in other behaviors that may have health benefits above and beyond the performance of exercise alone. Nevertheless, the preponderance of evidence strongly favors the adoption of regular exercise in improving overall health–and particularly cardiovascular health.

Physiology

Exercise places a considerable demand upon the heart which, in turn, undergoes dramatic physiologic changes to accommodate the body's needs. Despite massive increases (up to 50x) in skeletal muscle metabolism and work performed with even moderate physical activity, oxygen delivery to peripheral tissue and acid-base balance remain remarkably stable during exercise. This is made possible by a complex and tight coupling of the neuromuscular, peripheral muscles/vasculature, respiratory, and cardiac systems to ensure that the metabolic needs of exercising muscle are met. As a result of such multisystem interaction, a large increase in cardiac output occurs that is proportional to the increased metabolic demands on the body. Due to the fact that so many systems are involved in the exercise response, evaluation of exercise tolerance via multiparameter exercise testing is an invaluable tool in both diagnosis and prognosis for a number of health conditions. An adequate response to exercise testing will, in most cases, rule out any serious pathology within the cardiopulmonary and neuromuscular systems, although compensatory responses can occur for more mild disease.

The amount of physical exercise performed can be estimated by a number of parameters. The most common include directly measuring the amount of work performed (in watts), or by assessing how much metabolic fuel (O_2) is consumed in the process. Directly measuring work performed (watts) to assess exercise capacity/tolerance can be misleading due to the fact that a number of factors (most commonly obesity) may increase the work of exercise, but not reflect the condition of the cardiopulmonary systems. As a result, exercise capacity is most often assessed by oxygen consumption. This is done either by directly measuring consumption, generating a maximum amount of oxygen uptake (or VO_2 max), or is estimated by clinical history. The units used to estimate the metabolic cost of physical activity are referred to as metabolic equivalents (or METs). A single MET is defined as the amount of oxygen consumed (approximately 3.5ml O_2/kg/min) by an average adult at rest. This clinical estimation correlates well with measured VO_2 across a broad array of activities and is highly predictive of exercise capacity. The metabolic equivalents of various common activities are listed in Table 2.1 (Pate, 1995). METs perform by an individual in his or her daily life is an important tool in formulating an effective exercise program as well as screening for general cardiovascular health.

PERIPHERAL MUSCLE AND VASCULATURE

The peripheral, or skeletal, muscles performing the work of exercise are specialized and excel in various types of work. Their efficiency and metabolism greatly influence the demand placed on the heart to supply the oxygen and other nutrients required for exertion. Muscle fibers are clustered into groups of homogenous muscle units, all of which are innervated by a single motor

Table 2.1. Examples of Common Physical Activities for Healthy US Adults by Intensity of Effort Required in MET Scores and Kilocalories per Minute

LIGHT	MODERATE	HARD/VIGOROUS
< 3 METs or <4 kcal/min	3–6 METs or 4–7 kcal/min	6 METs or > 7 kcal/min
Walking slowly/strolling (1–2 mph)	Walking briskly (3–4 mph)	Walking briskly uphill or with a load
Cycling, stationary (<50 W)	Cycling for pleasure or transportation (< 10 mph)	Cycling, fast or racing (>10 mph)
Swimming, slow treading	Swimming, moderate effort	Swimming, fast treading or crawl
Stretching exercises/yoga	General calisthenics	Cross-country skiing/ cardio machine
***	Racket sports/table tennis	Singles tennis/ racquetball
Golf, power cart	Golf, pulling cart/carrying clubs	***
Bowling	***	***
Fishing, sitting	Fishing, standing/casting	Fishing in stream
Boating, power	Canoeing, leisurely (up to 4 mph)	Canoeing, rapid (>4 mph)
Home care, carpet sweeping	Home care, general cleaning	Moving furniture
Mowing lawn, riding mower	Mowing lawn, power mower	Mowing lawn, hand push mower
Home repair, carpentry	Home repair, painting	***

Pate et al. 1995. Physical activity and public health—a recommendation from the Centers for Disease Control and prevention and the American College of Sports Medicine. *JAMA* 273: 402–407.

neuron and can be one of two types: red or "slow" fibers (twitch type 1) and white or "fast" fibers (twitch type 2). Metabolically, the muscle types are distinct, allowing for specialization. Fatigue-resistant type 1 fibers have a high oxidative (oxygen-using) capacity, which is best suited for endurance exercise. Type 2 fibers have a high glycolytic (glucose-using) capacity and best suited for burst activity with heavy loads, but are prone to fatigue. The relative amount of each muscle type in the body is genetically predetermined and cannot be altered with exercise training. However, regular exercise can increase blood supply to muscle via recruitment of capillary networks, as well as increase the mitochondria in muscle fibers, leading to greater capacity of substrate utilization and efficiency (Terjung, 1995).

The energy "currency" of muscle contraction are high-energy phosphates, generated from the hydrolysis of adenosine triphosphate (ATP). ATP is produced primarily through pathways that require either glucose (anaerobic) or oxygen (aerobic). Despite massive turnover and relatively small ATP stores in the cell, the concentration of ATP remains remarkably constant during exercise. This is due to a redundancy and overlap in the three primary energy sources of muscle tissue: the phosphocreatine shuttle, anaerobic glycolysis, and oxidative phosphorylation.

Phosphocreatine (PCr) is a small particle that serves as a high-energy phosphate reservoir near actin-myosin complexes (responsible for muscle contraction) and quickly replenishes supplies of ATP and reduces concentration of ADP locally, to allow for continued muscle contraction. This is accomplished by creatine kinase:

$$PCr + ADP \rightarrow Cr + ATP \leftrightarrow ADP + Pi$$

When ATP is used for muscle contraction, PCr "donates" a high-energy phosphate to keep ATP concentration high near the muscle. This rapid availability of phosphate near the actin-myosin complex serves as the first energy "buffer" for muscle and is particularly useful for bursts of activity. The use of creatine as an oral supplement has been shown to improve muscle performance for short intense activities, but not for endurance work. Whether the use of creatine supplementation helps patients with heart failure—who are unable to provide enough blood flow to meet the energy demands of peripheral muscle—remains uncertain.

Anaerobic glycolysis is the process in which glucose is utilized to produce ATP, ultimately yielding lactate. This occurs when the energy requirement of muscle outstrips its oxygen supply. It is a particularly useful pathway during short intense exercise, as the speed at which ATP is produced is 100 times that of oxidative phosphorylation (but yields less ATP per molecule).

Oxygen-dependent *oxidative phosphorylation* of glycogen and free fatty acids is the most efficient, and largest, source of intracellular ATP. With exercise training, skeletal muscle is able to increasingly utilize fat as a substrate for oxidation, prolonging the duration and amount of work performed until glycogen stores are utilized. Peripheral muscle fatigue during endurance activity is not limited by the availability of high energy phosphates, but is instead triggered by the depletion of glycogen stores and the rise of blood lactate concentration. The threshold of exertion at which this occurs is called the *lactate threshold,* and is not due to lack of oxygen delivery to muscles, but rather to accumulation of lactate (via pyruvate) which exceeds the muscle capacity to process this byproduct through the Krebs cycle (Graham and Saltin 1989; Putman et al. 1995; Stainsby et al. 1989). Lactate threshold is a powerful predictor of cardiovascular health, and a clinically useful tool in evaluation and prognosis of patients with cardiovascular disease, particularly in cases of heart failure, where it is often used to determine cardiac transplant status (Sue and Hansen 1984; Wasserman and McIlroy 1964). While habitual exercise cannot increase the type of muscle cells present, it can substantially increase both the maximum work and the lactate threshold in normal individuals and those with cardiopulmonary disease. For optimal improvement in cardiovascular fitness to occur, exercise intensity should approach the lactate threshold.

Peripheral circulation plays a central role in directing the increased cardiac output to nutrient-starved exercising skeletal muscle, and thus in maintaining the physiological homeostasis required for continued activity. While cardiac output may increase 5-fold with vigorous exercise, the rise in mean systemic blood pressure is far less, due to the reduction of systemic vascular resistance (SVR). This drop in vascular resistance is mediated through selective constriction and dilation of vascular beds, which in turn are mediated by the nervous system. With exercise, parasympathetic activity is withdrawn and plasma catecholamines rise, as a result of sympathetic activity. Vasoconstriction occurs in the majority of the body's vascular beds, with the exception of skeletal muscle that undergoes nitric-oxide mediated vasodilation. At maximal exercise, skeletal muscle can receive upwards of 90 percent of systemic blood flow, compared with one-fifth of cardiac output at rest (Wade and Bishop 1962). Similarly, metabolically inactive organs, such as the GI tract, can see reductions of cardiac output of up to 90 percent of their resting levels (less than 1 percent of total blood flow at peak exercise). This preferential shunting of cardiac output can be augmented by repeated training (Koller et al. 1995). Unlike skeletal muscle, the pulmonary circulatory system receives virtually all of the cardiac output and shunting is *decreased* during exercise. However, a similar NO-mediated vasodilatory mechanism occurs within the pulmonary vasculature. This allows for accommodation of the increase in cardiac output without a subsequent rise in pulmonic pressures, aiding the return of peripheral deoxygenated blood to the heart.

PULMONARY CONTRIBUTION TO EXERCISE TOLERANCE

Despite a nearly 15-fold increase in whole body oxygen uptake and a 10-fold increase in minute ventilation with intense exercise, systemic arterial oxygen content remains remarkably stable even with extreme exertion. The partial pressure of oxygen (and its diffusion across the alveolar-capillary membrane) is maintained in spite of the increased extraction by a number of compensatory mechanisms. These include an increase in breathing rate (minute ventilation), more efficient elimination of CO_2 during exercise, a reduction in low ventilation/low perfusion areas of the lung due to larger volume breaths, and greater cardiac output into the lung vasculature (Jones, 1984). These respiratory mechanisms are typically more than sufficient to maintain physiologic homeostasis at prolonged peak exercise. It is exceedingly rare that either oxygen diffusion or pulmonary mechanics are the limiting factors to maximum exert ional tolerance. For the vast majority, maximal exercise capacity and cardiovascular fitness are limited by factors affecting cardiac output and function.

CARDIAC PHYSIOLOGY

Cardiac output, the major determinant of exercise capacity, is increased by alterations in both heart rate and the stroke volume of the heart, and increases by 5ml/min for every 1ml/min increase in oxygen consumption. Habitual exercise may increase the maximum cardiac output attained (approximately 5 times the resting output), but it does not alter the slope of the relationship of CO to VO_2. The relationship between VO_2 and heart rate is linear, however, with the near instantaneous increase in heart rate at the beginning of exercise due to vagal tone withdrawal. Later increases in heart rate are mediated through sympathetic responses triggered by pulmonary stretch receptors and increased circulating catecholamines. At extremely high levels of exertion, heart rate contributes proportionally more to changes in CO than stroke volume of the heart; however, both age and nutritional factors determine the maximum heart rate that is obtainable. An accurate predictor of maximal heart rate in adults is:

Max HR= 208 – 0.7(age) (Tanaka, Monahan, and Deals 2001)

Stroke volume, on the other hand, increases in a hyperbolic fashion with exercise (Blomqvist and Saltin 1983) by two mechanisms: changes in the contractility of heart muscle and increases in left ventricular end-diastolic volume (LVEDP). Diastolic volume can increase up to 40 percent during exercise, increasing cardiac output via the Frank-Starling principle. The augmentation of venous return to the heart during exertion is accomplished through greater negative intrathoracic pressures generated by increased respiratory effort, and increased venous flow via the pumping of limbs and venoconstriction. Changes to cardiac contractility are not related to venous return and filling characteristics per se, but are reflective of a more intrinsic forceful contraction due to neurohormonal effects, which results in greater emptying of the left ventricle (ionotropy).

The body's response to intensive exercise requires a highly coordinated and tightly coupled biofeedback across many organ systems. While maximal cardiac output usually limits aerobic capacity, habitual exercise and physical activity increases the capacity and efficiency of almost all systems involved in this integrated response.

Exercise Benefits and Prevention of CV Disease

Coronary heart disease (CHD) remains the leading killer of both men and women in most developed areas of the world, and in the United States it exceeds the number of deaths of the next seven causes combined (American Heart Association 2002; Yusuf et al. 2001). Because CHD is often fatal, and over one-half of individuals who die suddenly from CHD have no prior symptoms, it is imperative to identify strategies to reduce the risk of CHD in the general population. A sedentary lifestyle carries a risk for development of CHD on par with the more traditionally recognized factors of cigarette smoking, hypertension, and hypercholesterolemia (Fletcher et al. 1996). Physical inactivity has now been recognized by the American Heart Association as one of the four modifiable risk factors for CHD (Fletcher et al. 1996). While the benefits of habitual exercise appear to apply to both the general population and individuals with established coronary heart disease, it has been more difficult to demonstrate the cardioprotective effects of exercise in the general population due to lower event rates when compared to individuals with established cardiovascular disease.

Despite these limitations, there exists an abundance of evidence to recommend exercise training to the general population on its own merits. Short- and long-term aerobic exercise is associated with increased quality of life for both physical and psychological attributes. In addition to reductions in body weight and fat content, exercise is beneficial in prevention and management of musculoskeletal injuries and disorders (Braith and Stewart 2006). Regular exercise is also associated with reduced prevalence and severity of stress, anxiety and depression (Martin et al. 2009; Martinsen, Medhus, and Sandvik 1985; Warburton, Gledhill, and Quinney 2001).

The physiological changes in the heart induced with exercise may be intrinsically cardioprotective, but may also favorably modify other risk factors for disease. When combined with a smoking cessation program, exercise facilitates short- and long-term smoking cessation and attenuates the weight gain often seen after cessation (Marcus et al. 1999; Shepard and Shek 1999). These diverse benefits of exercise translate into more cost-effective health care, with reductions of over $300 per year in direct medical costs for individuals with regular physical activity and, approximately $5000 per year of life saved in individuals with known coronary heart disease (Ades, Pashkow, and Nestor 1997; Pratt, Macera, and Wang 2000).

Improvement in exercise capacity is the most consistent benefit seen with regular exercise (Wenger et al. 1995). As cardiac output is the major determinant of exercise capacity, it is not surprising that many of the structural and functional changes that occur with endurance training augment stroke volume in particular. These changes include alterations that directly affect cardiac functioning (central adaptations) or improve peripheral oxygenation extraction for any given CO (peripheral adaption). The latter is likely due to the increase in skeletal muscle capillary networks seen with exercise. A 1–5 month regimen of aerobic exercise performed at 50–80 percent of maximal heart rate for 30 minutes 3–5 times weekly is frequently used in the literature to elicit exercise-induced physiological changes, and will often result in an increase in exercise capacity upwards of 30 percent.

PHYSIOLOGIC CHANGES WITH EXERCISE

Increase in stroke volume is the predominant change in cardiac output with exercise, and occurs across all levels of physical activity. A large part of the increased volume occurs primarily due to increased preload as a result of increases in diastolic and plasma volume (Green, Jones, and Painter 1990; Rerych et al. 1980; Seals et al. 1994). Considerable enlargement of the ventricle can occur in elite athletes to accommodate a larger stroke volume, but is not associated with the abnormalities in ventricular function seen with dilated cardiomyopathies (Pelliccia et al. 1999; Pluim et al. 2000). Cardiac muscle hypertrophies resulting in greater cardiac mass and, likely, greater contractility.

The other determinant of cardiac output—heart rate—is lowered at rest and with mild exertion due to increased vagal tone, but is augmented at peak exercise levels. As a consequence, there is greater baroreflex sensitivity and heart rate variability in physically fit individuals. Endothelial function is also improved with training, increasing vasodilatory responses at higher cardiac outputs and improving blood flow to areas of greater metabolic demand. Coronary arteries in endurance athletes are similar in size to age-matched sedentary controls, but exhibit 200 percent greater vasodilatory response to nitroglycerin (Currens and White 1961; Haskell et al. 1993). It is believed the short, repetitive increases in pressure and shear stress seen with exertion create a favorable milieu for the release of the vasodilators nitric oxide and prostacy-clin from vascular endothelium, as opposed to prolonged periods of exposure, as seen with chronic hypertension (Niebauer and Cooke 1996).

EXERCISE BENEFITS

Early studies demonstrating the benefits of physical activity were observational in nature and found lowered rates of total mortality and cardiovascular events in active individuals (Morris et al. 1953; Taylor et al. 1962). Many of these early studies compared individuals with physically demanding jobs with their more sedentary peers. As rates of leisure-time physical activity in the general popu-lation grew, more recent studies have relied on estimates of energy expenditure from activity questionnaires. Almost all have shown a strong inverse relation-ship between habitual physical activity and rates of cardiovascular disease and death, regardless of gender, age or origin. The best known of these studies is the Harvard Alumni Study, which was a retrospective analysis of self-reported physical activity over 12 years in 10,269 men. Men who were physically active at baseline (defined as total physical activity of >2000 kcal a week and includ-ing home repair, yard work, or exercise for 30 minutes/day on most days of the week) had a 25 percent lower risk of death from any cause and a 36 percent reduction in cardiovascular death when compared to their sedentary controls (Paffenbarger et al. 1986; Paffenbarger et al. 1993; Sesso, Paffenbarger, and Lee 2000). Data from the MR FIT Trial (Multiple Risk Factor Intervention Trial) yielded similar results where moderately active men (leisure time activi-ties of 224kcal/day) had 70 percent of the overall deaths and 63 percent of the deaths from cardiovascular causes when compared to inactive men (Leon et al. 1987). In a metanalysis of over 40 studies, the relative risk of developing coronary artery disease was 1.9 in sedentary individuals, on par with the risk seen with other coronary risk factors, such as smoking and high cholesterol (Powell et al. 1987). Instead of subjective questionnaires, the use of objective and quantitative measures to evaluate energy expenditure may correlate more strongly with cardiovascular risk. Energy expenditure as measured by radio-isotope-labeled water was more predictive of reductions in overall mortality in an elderly population (70–82 years of age) over 6 years than self-reported exercise levels (Manini et al. 2006). Individuals in the highest measured activ-ity level had a hazard ratio of 0.3 for all causes of mortality when compared to the lowest activity group. Similar findings were found when comparing activity levels based on metabolic equivalents (METs) in a large analysis com-prising over 100,000 participants (Kodama et al. 2009).

The cardioprotection conferred by physical activity (self-reported or objective) appears to be a graded response to the duration of activity and occurs regardless of the presence of cardiovascular disease. The Framingham Heart Study demonstrated an increase of life expectancy at all levels of activity in those with and without cardiovascular disease, with the greatest gains seen in those individuals (men or women) in the highest tertile of activity (see Figure 2.1). (Franco et al. 2005). In the Nurses's Health Study (women between 40 and 65 years of age), age-adjusted relative risk of coronary events decreased across increasing quintile groups of energy expenditure (0.88–0.66) (Manson et al. 1999). In men and women, distance of daily walking was strongly correlated with lower mortality rates (Hakim et al. 1998; Lee et al. 2001). This graded cardioprotective effect of exercise is also well demonstrated in the Finnish Twin Cohort study. In almost 8000 same-sex pairs of twins, the odds ratio for death was 0.44 in regular vigorous exercisers as compared to 0.66 in those who only occasionally exercised (Kujala et al. 1998).

Intensity of exercise, in addition to duration, appears to play an important role in both identifying cardiovascular risk and accruing the cardiovascular

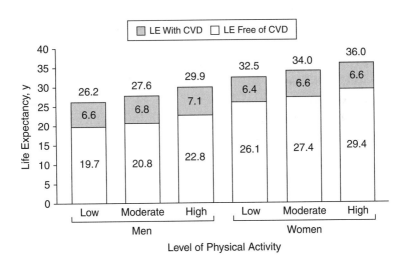

FIGURE 2.1. Effect of physical activity level on life expectancy (LE) at age 50 years. All LEs have been calculated with hazard ratios adjusted for age, sex, smoking, examination at start of follow-up period, and any comorbidity (cancer, left ventricular hypertrophy, arthritis, diabetes, ankle edema, or pulmonary disease). CVD indicates cardiovascular disease.

Franco et al. 2005. Effects of physical activity on life expectancy with cardiovascular disease. *Archives of Internal Medicine* 165: 2355.

benefit of exercise. Separately, both regular and high-intensity activity are cardioprotective, but the addition of vigorous exercise to moderate activity (defined as 30 minutes of activity most days a week) confers an additional reduction in cardiovascular risk across gender, ethnicity, and body mass index of upwards of 50 percent. (Leitzman et al. 2007; Manson 1999). Even the perception of intense exercise appears to have cardioprotective benefits. Over a 5-year follow-up period in 7337 men (mean age 66 years), participants who perceived their exercise to be of moderate to high intensity had a substantially lower (RR of 0.66-0.72) risk of coronary heart disease when compared to their peers who felt their exercise intensity was weak. This protection was observed even in individuals whose actual exercise did not meet current recommendations for either intensity or duration (Lee et al. 2003).

The degree of cardiovascular fitness, as defined by both the duration and maximal oxygen uptake during exercise performance, is associated with reduced rates of overall and cardiac mortality and morbidity (Blair et al. 1989; Ekelund et al. 1988; Powell et al. 1987). In 3043 participants in the Framingham Heart Study, greater exercise capacity on a treadmill was predictive of a lower coronary risk over an 18-year follow-up, with an incremental decrease in risk seen with each MET achieved (Balady et al. 2004). In middle-aged men, metabolic equivalents were the strongest predictor of mortality regardless of the presence or absence of cardiovascular disease, with each MET conferring a 12 percent reduction in mortality (Myers et al. 2002).

Exercise-induced ST segment deviation was not predictive of cardiovascular death in women, whereas total exercise capacity and heart rate recovery were strongly correlated and those below the median for both measures had a hazard ratio for death of 3.5 (Mora, et al. 2003). In trials involving both genders, the least exercise-conditioned participants (as measured by treadmill exercise performance) had 8-fold higher rates of cardiovascular death compared to the best conditioned participants (Blair et al. 1995; Ekelund et al. 1988).

The observational nature of these studies does subject the conclusions to selection bias. Higher activity and exercise levels may be achieved only by healthier individuals, and the observed reductions in mortality rates may be attributable not to cardioprotective effects of exercise, but rather reflect the fact that healthier individuals live longer. Arguing against this criticism are several randomized animal models which demonstrate reductions in coronary atherosclerosis with exercise (Kramsch et al. 1981), in addition to several "crossover" observational studies in humans. In one such study, exercise capacity was assessed in nearly 10,000 men (mean age 43) across 5 years. Those subjects who remained unfit throughout the observational period had a threefold higher rate of death than their fit colleagues. Initially unfit subjects who

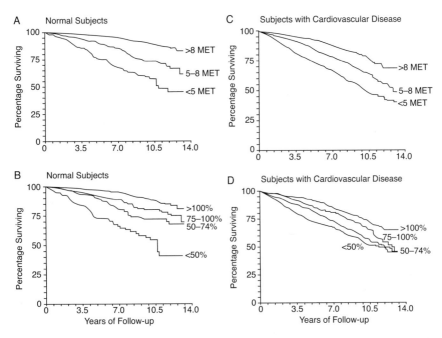

FIGURE 2.2. Survival Curves for Normal Subjects Stratified According to Peak Exercise Capacity (Panel A) and According to the Percentage of Age-Predicted Exercise Capacity Achieved (Panel B) and Survival Curves for Subjects with Cardiovascular Disease Stratified According to Peak Exercise Capacity (Panel C) and According to the Percentage of Age-Predicted Exercise Capacity Achieved (Panel D).

Myers et al. 2002. Exercise capacity and mortality among men referred for exercise testing. *NEJM* 346: 793. Reprinted with permission.

became exercise-trained by the end of the study, however had reductions of 44 percent and 52 percent in all causes and cardiac mortality (Blair et al. 1995). Another study found similar reductions in previously inactive men who underwent exercise training (Paffenbarger, 1993). While there is not conclusive evidence that withdrawal of activity increases cardiac risk, the Harvard Alumni Study found physically fit individuals who became inactive over time had the same risk of death as those who remained inactive throughout their lives (Paffenbarger et al. 1986). Although a large randomized, controlled trial to demonstrate the cardioprotective effects of exercise will not likely be performed due to the necessary size, cost, and compliance issues, the multitude of epidemiological studies (in addition to the plausible biological mechanisms) have led the American Heart Association to conclude that physical activity reduces the risk of coronary artery disease (Thompson et al. 2003)

Exercise and Cardiovascular Risk Factors

Given the complex interactions of established risk factors on cardiovascular morbidity and mortality, measuring the direct impact of exercise on cardiac risk predictors is difficult. Weight loss associated with regular exercise can directly affect other risk factors such as hypertension and insulin resistance independent of the potential benefit of exercise. Nevertheless, similar to overall cardiac risk, enough evidence exists to support the claim that regular physical activity has a favorable effect on a number of cardiac risk factors, including hypertension, diabetes/insulin resistance, and obesity. In general, the reduction of cardiac risk factors achieved with exercise is less than that of pharmacologic intervention. However, the magnitude of reduction with exercise may be enough to obviate the need for further intervention in patients at risk. Type of exercise regimen, concomitant weight loss, and dietary modifications all add to the variable effect that exercise confers on an individual's cardiovascular risk profile.

HYPERTENSION

Distinct from other risk factors, beneficial effects on hypertension are seen in both acute and long-term exposure to exercise. Immediately at the end of exercise, reductions in cardiac output and heart rate are seen from a simultaneous increase in vagal tone and removal of sympathetic stimulation. Due to persistent vasodilatory responses in the muscle vascular bed, systemic vascular resistance remains low for up to 12 hours after intense activity, with eventual normalization of blood pressure by baroreceptor reflexes (Pescatello et al. 1991). Over 40 randomized trials have demonstrated a reduction in resting blood pressure and some have shown a decreased incidence of hypertension with long-term aerobic exercise (Arroll and Beaglehole 1992; Seals and Hagberg 1984). The baseline resting blood pressure appears to be an important mediator of the magnitude of the exercise effect. Normotensive subjects, on average, will decrease systolic and diastolic blood pressure by 2.6 and 1.8mmHg, respectively. Hypertensive subjects demonstrate greater reduction, with mean systolic and diastolic reductions of 7.4mmHg and 5.8mmHg (Fagard, 2001). The magnitude of exercise effect on blood pressure (up to 15mmHg in some studies) suggests the initiation of regular aerobic regimen may be the sole intervention required for mildly hypertensive patients. Conversely, lack of exercise is a risk factor for the development of hypertension (Blair et al. 1984).

Maintenance of blood pressure reduction is also dependent on the continuation of exercise, with regression to pre-exercise BP seen with discontinuation of regular exercise (Somers et al. 1991).

Unlike other cardiovascular benefits derived from exercise, reductions in blood pressure are not dependent upon the frequency of exercise, but rather the intensity. Blood pressure was as reduced in hypertensive subjects in one study with 60 minutes/week of moderately intense exercise (50 percent max VO2) as it was with subjects who performed double the frequency and duration of exercise (Ishikawa-Takata, Ohta, and Tanaka 2003). The lack of correlation between time spent exercising and reduction in blood pressure suggests a threshold effect on blood pressure and a flat dose-response curve with regards to exercise frequency. One proposed mechanism for reduction of blood pressure by aerobic exercise is the augmentation of endothelium-dependent vasodilation by nitric oxide, which occurs when moderate intensity exercise is undertaken. Due to the effects of nitric oxide, systemic vascular resistance is reduced with aerobic exercise, resulting in isolated elevation of systolic blood pressure during exercise. An exaggerated blood pressure response to aerobic exercise (defined as BP> 210mmHg in men and >190mmHg in women) may reflect abnormalities in cardiovascular regulatory mechanisms and can predict increases risks of left ventricular hypertrophy, coronary artery disease and cardiovascular morbidity (Mundal et al. 1996; McHam et al. 1999).

In contrast to aerobic exercise, resistance training (or pure isometric exercise) has historically not been considered beneficial in controlling hypertension. This has been in part due to the acute rise in systolic and diastolic blood pressure seen in strength training (as high as 230–330/170–250 mmHg) (Morales et al. 1991). Unlike aerobic training, vascular resistance increases in strength training due in part to mechanical compression of the skeletal muscle vascular beds. While some long-term strength training protocols have resulted in reductions of systolic and diastolic BP, these have been modest at best. The recent adoption of circuit training, which involves moving quickly between higher repetition and lower resistance exercises, adds a component of aerobic training to the workout and may result in improved blood pressure effects. Several programs including resistance training to aerobic exercise regimens have shown favorable reductions in both resting systolic and diastolic BP (Cornelissen and Fagard 2005; Kelly and Kelly 2000). This, and the fact that resistance training is correlated with improved glycemic control (as evidenced by reduced HbA1c) and a reduction in total body fat mass, has led the American Heart Association and the American College of Sports Medicine to endorse resistance training as a complement to aerobic exercise in the treatment of hypertension.

LIPIDS

Regular aerobic exercise has favorable effects on lipid profiles, but the effect is modest as assessed by standard serological assays. While early observational studies showed significant lipid differences in runners as compared to their sedentary peers, confounding variables of a heart-healthy diet and lifestyle, body weight, and comorbidities made any causal relationship difficult to confirm (Wood et al. 1976; Wood et al. 1988; Williams et al. 1986). Subsequently, randomized trials have found a definite beneficial effect of exercise, albeit more it is modest than original cross-sectional studies had suggested. A metaanalysis of 52 trials of at least 12 weeks of exercise training showed reductions in triglyceride and LDL-C concentrations of 3.7 percent and 5 percent, with an increase in HDL-C of 4.6 percent (Leon and Sanchez 2001a; Leon and Sanchez 2001b). In comparison to the effects of exercise on hypertension, exercise intensity *and* duration mediate the effect on lipoproteins, with duration of exercise contributing more (King 1995 et al.; Kokkinos et al. 1995). In addition, there is a graded dose–response in modifying lipoproteins with regards to exercise duration. In a randomized trial involving men and women, frequent low-intensity exercise was associated with significantly higher HDL levels than higher intensity, less frequent exercise (King et al. 1995). Another randomized study comparing frequency of high intensity regimens found only a significant decrease in very-low-density lipoprotein and increase in HDL with more frequent exercise (Kraus et al. 2002). This effect was independent of change in body weight.

Several studies have also suggested gender plays a role in exercise effects on lipoproteins (Stefanick et al. 1998; Wood et al. 1991). Gender-specific changes in lipid profiles were seen in several studies where men and women were randomized to diet alone, diet with exercise (moderate intensity), or controls. While weight loss occurs in both genders and both intervention groups, diet alone did not change HDL levels compared with controls, and actually caused a decrease in HDL concentrations in women (Wood et al. 1991). An AHA, step-2 diet alone was not found to reduce total cholesterol or LDL, but when added to exercise produced significant decreases in both (Stefanick et al. 1998). Diet with exercise does appear to significantly raise HDL in men, but not in women (Wood et al. 1991). These results highlight the importance of including regular exercise into any dietary intervention, and in the difficulty in isolating the effects of both due to differences in baseline lipid profiles, body mass, and the broad variability of diet and exercise programs.

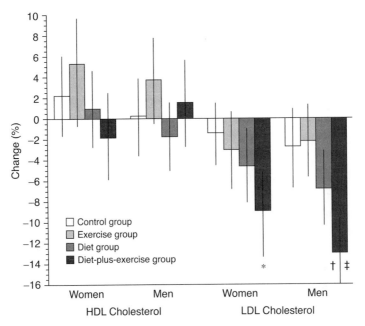

FIGURE 2.3. **Mean Changes in Plasma HDL Cholesterol and LDL Cholesterol Levels in the Study Groups at 1Year.** The vertical lines represent 95 percent confidence intervals. Significance levels, after Bonferroni's adjustment for the six pairwise comparisons, are indicated as follows: the asterisk denotes P<0.05 for the comparison with the control group, the dagger P<0.001 for the comparison with the control group, and the double dagger P<0.001 for the comparison with the exercise group.

Stefanick et al. 1998. Effects of diet and exercise in men and postmenopausal women with low levels of HDL cholesterol and high levels of LDL cholesterol. *NEJM* 339: 12. Reprinted with permission.

Alterations in the activity of enzymes involved in lipid metabolism likely mediate the effect of exercise on lipid profiles. Accompanying the absolute increase in HDL levels with exercise is a shift to the larger, more cardioprotective HDL2 particle from the smaller HDL3. Exercise increases lipoprotein lipase (LPL) activity, resulting in greater breakdown of triglyceride-rich particles generating greater HDL2,while decreases in hepatic triglyceride lipase (HTGL) reduce catabolism of the HDL2 particle leading to higher concentrations (Seip et al. 1993). Exercise also alters the chemical composition of LDL particles, causing a shift toward the larger LDL subtypes which are less atherogenic (Houmard et al. 1994). The shift toward more cardioprotective subtypes of both LDL and HDL would not be seen on most lipid assays obtained in clinical practice, and thus, the modest absolute concentrations of lipid changes observed with exercise may underestimate the true benefit derived from exercise.

DIABETES MELLITUS

Insulin resistance, glucose intolerance, and diabetes mellitus are powerful mediators of cardiovascular risk and often precede the clinical onset of clinically apparent disease. Habitual physical activity has been shown to favorably affect insulin resistance, glucose intolerance, postprandial hyperglycemia, and hepatic glucose output resulting in HbA1C reductions of up to 1 percent and reduced use of diabetic medications (Thompson et al. 2001). Perhaps due to the diverse nature of the benefits associated with exercise, large cohort studies have demonstrated that the substantial lowering of cardiovascular morbidity in diabetics is greater than would be expected from glucose lowering alone (Sigal et al. 2007). In type 2 diabetic patients, there is an incremental benefit to both duration and pace of aerobic exercise independent of age, gender, body mass, and severity of diabetes (Tanasescu et al. 2003). One analysis concluded that two hours of walking per week could prevent one death for every 61 diabetic adults (Gregg et al. 2003). As with cardiovascular risk in the general population, cardiovascular fitness, as defined by exercise capacity, is highly predictive of all-cause and cardiac mortality rates in type 2 diabetic patients (Wei et al. 2003).

Regular compliance with an exercise regimen leads to more efficient energy utilization by skeletal muscles. In addition to the aforementioned increase in skeletal muscle blood flow and mitochrondria found in exercise-trained individuals, there is an upregulation of the insulin-responsive glucose transporter, GLUT 4, on skeletal muscle cells (Rodnick et al. 1990). GLUT 4 promotes glucose uptake from the blood into muscles, and is likely the mediator of increased insulin sensitivity seen with exercise. The ability of resistance training to increase skeletal muscle mass allows it to play an important role in regulating glucose metabolism. A comprehensive resistance training program has the capacity to recruit equal, if not greater, muscle mass over extended periods of time when compared with aerobic training. Resistance training has been demonstrated to favorably influence insulin responses to glucose loads in both diabetic and normal subjects in men and women across the full age spectrum (Miller et al. 1994; Smutok et al. 1993). Several studies have randomized diabetic patients to aerobic, resistance, or combined exercise programs. Improved HgA1c or insulin sensitivity were observed in all groups that performed exercise, with the most favorable results associated with combined aerobic and resistance regimens (Cuff, 2003; Sigal, 2007; Snowling and Hopkins 2006).

In the acute response to exercise, diabetes may exhibit more volatility in blood glucose, particularly in insulin-dependent diabetics. In the presence of an exogenous source of insulin (i.e., insulin injections), exercise-induced catecholamine responses may paradoxically elevate serum glucose (in poorly controlled diabetics) or precipitously drop serum glucose if exercise is unusually vigorous (tightly controlled diabetics). Oral and diet-controlled type 2 diabetics experience less variability in serum glucose with exercise, but serum glucose can be lowered if medications and meals are taken prior to vigorous exercise (Poirier et al. 2000). There is conclusive evidence, however, that the long-term physiologic changes induced with exercise training are beneficial in glycemic control and are present even in the absence of weight loss (Duncan et al. 2003).

Several studies are suggestive that regular exercise may prevent the development of type 2 diabetes mellitus, likely through increased insulin sensitivity (Helmrich et al. 1991; Lynch et al. 1996). Physical activity at the level of brisk walking (5.5 METs) for at least 40 minutes per week appears to be protective (Lynch et al. 1996).

Due to the high incidence of occult vascular disease in long-standing diabetics, it is recommended that anyone over the age of 35 with diabetes of 10 years duration undergo a complete physical examination prior to starting an exercise regimen. In sedentary subjects, the risk of myocardial infarction is increased with the adoption of vigorous exercise (Willich et al. 1993). As diabetes is often associated with a sedentary lifestyle (upwards of 60 percent prevalence in one survey) and obesity, strong consideration should be given to performing an exercise stress test prior to the initiation of an exercise program. Unfortunately, there are presently no randomized trials or large cohort studies that have looked at the utility of exercise stress testing in diabetics prior to starting regular physical activity (Nelson, Reiber, and Boyko 2002). In a recent statement, the American Diabetic Association (ADA) recommended an exercise stress test be performed in individuals who meet the any of the following criteria (Sigal et al. 2004):

- Age >40 years, with or without CVD risk factors other than diabetes
- Age >30 years and
  - Diabetes of >10 years duration
  - Hypertension
  - Cigarette Smoking
  - Dyslipidemia
  - Secondary complications of diabetes (retinopathy, nephropathy-including microalbuminuria)
- Known coronary artery disease, peripheral vascular disease
- Autonomic neuropathy
- Advanced nephropathy with renal failure.

The presence of diabetic complications should be considered before an exercise regimen is prescribed. Patients with peripheral neuropathy should avoid long durations of weight-bearing exercise (running) that may precipitate or exacerbate foot ulcers. Similarly, high-intensity resistance training should be discouraged in individuals with retinopathy, given the elevation of both systolic and diastolic blood pressure that occurs (as above). Diabetics should be instructed to carefully monitor their blood glucose before, during, and after exercise so that any changes can be anticipated in subsequent sessions. With exercise, insulin requirements will be expected to be reduced by 30 percent. The depletion of muscle glycogen with prolonged exercise may result in hypoglycemia. Carbohydrate-rich foods or energy supplements should be available and taken with aerobic exercise of long-duration (1 hour), both during the exercise and for several hours afterwards.

Currently, the American Diabetic Association recommends implementing a goal-based exercise protocol for diabetic patients (Sigal et al. 2004):

- For reduction of CVD, improved glycemic control and weight maintenance: 150min/wk of moderate-intensity aerobic exercise (50–70 percent max HR) *or* 90min/wk of vigorous exercise (>70 percent max HR). This should be done at least 3 days/wk with never more than 2 consecutive days off.
- For greater CVD reduction: ≥4hrs/wk of moderate to vigorous aerobic and/or resistance exercise
- For long-term weight loss and maintenance: 7hrs/wk of aerobic exercise.

When resistance training is added, the ADA recommends three sessions per week, performing large muscle group exercises. Resistance training should include 3 sets with 8–10 repetitions of a weight that produces near failure at the last repetition (Sigal et al. 2004).

HEMOSTATIC EFFECTS

The intrinsic clotting mechanism plays a substantial role in the pathogenesis of cardiovascular disease. There is significant evidence that exercise conditioning has a favorable effect on the body's fibrinolytic system. In one study, platelets exhibited less adhesion and aggregation after eight weeks of performing moderate-intensity exercise when compared to sedentary peers, and return to baseline levels with cessation of regular exercise (Wang, Jen, and Chen, 1995). It remains controversial whether or not exercise reduces whole blood viscosity, with disparate results seen in the medical literature. Nevertheless, regular physical activity does appear to influence hemostatic factors that mediate vascular thrombosis, and is a recommended therapy for patients with both cardiac and peripheral vascular disease.

EXERCISE IN SELECTED POPULATIONS

Women

In the United States, one woman dies every minute from cardiovascular disease (Mosca et al. 2004). Despite this, only 7 of the 43 studies of exercise and primary prevention of cardiovascular events have included women (Manson et al. 2002). Thankfully, several of these studies, most notably the Nurse's Health Study and the Women's Health Initiative Observational Study, were of considerable size (over 70,000 subjects each) to allow for definite conclusions regarding the protective effect of physical activity and cardiovascular risk. The available evidence suggests that women derive similar cardioprotective effects from exercise as men. In women with or without cardiovascular disease, physiologic changes with exercise occur on par with men, resulting in increases up to 20–30 percent of VO2 max with training (Cannistra et al. 1992; Spina et al. 1993). In addition to physiologic changes, clinical outcomes are also similarly improved in women, despite the lack of improvement in lipid profiles as seen with men (as above). All cause mortality is increased 5-fold in the least conditioned women, and cardiovascular risk is reduced by 30–50 percent with exercise in both genders. Cardiovascular benefit appears to be independent of age and ethnicity in postmenopausal women, and can be obtained with both moderate and vigorous exertion (Manson et al. 2002).

The Young

While physical activity in children is difficult to quantify, over the last several decades children have been spending more time in sedentary activities, and the prevalence of childhood obesity is increasing (Ross and Gilbert 1985; Ross and Pate 1987; Dietz and Gortmaker 1985). Cardiovascular events in children remain rare, but exercise habits in childhood have been shown to mirror activity levels as an adult (Kuh and Cooper 1992). A majority of 12-year-old children will have developed one modifiable cardiovascular risk factor (Riddoch and Boreham 1995). The efficacy of direct intervention on childhood risk factors remains controversial, but there is evidence that school-based programs can reduce the sedentary behavior patterns observed with advancing age (Kelder, Perry, and Klepp 1993).

Participation in organized team sports is highest in adolescence and young adulthood. While cardiac events remain low in this age group, the sudden deaths of young competitive athletes are tragic and often due to unsuspected cardiovascular disease. Both in the United States and Europe, the incidence of sudden death in young athletes appears to be increasing (Maron, 2003). The majority of deaths that occur in U.S. athletes under the age of 35 are due to congenital or acquired cardiac malformation, as opposed to coronary artery disease in older individuals. Most of these deaths are due to hypertrophic cardiomyopathy or coronary anomalies, and occur in sports with intense bursts of activity, such as football or basketball. The combined prevalence of all of these disease states in young athletes is approximately 0.3 percent, with the

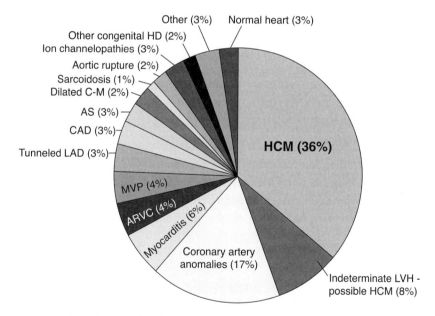

FIGURE 2.4. Distribution of cardiovascular causes of sudden death in 1435 young competitive athletes. From the Minneapolis Heart Institute Foundation Registry, 1980 to 2005. ARVC indicates arrhythmogenic right ventricular cardiomyopathy; AS, aortic stenosis; CAD, coronary artery disease; C-M, cardiomyopathy; HD, heart disease; LAD, left anterior descending; LVH, left ventricular hypertrophy; and MVP, mitral valve prolapse.

Maron, B. J. et al. 2007 (Update). Recommendations and considerations related to preparticipation screening for cardiovascular abnormalities in competitive athletes. Reprinted by permission from *Circulation* 2007; 115:1643–1655. Copyright 2007 American Heart Association.

most common condition, hypertrophic cardiomyopathy, present in 1:500 people in the general population (Maron 2003; Maron et al. 2007). The overall occurrence of sudden death in high school athletes is estimated at 1:200,000 per year (Maron 2003; Maron et al. 2007).

The sheer numbers of young competitive athletes (approximately 10 million), combined with the low prevalence of disease, makes the adoption of a universal screening strategy for elevated cardiovascular risk difficult in this population. At present, the American Heart Association recommends a personal and family history in addition to a physical examination before participation in competitive sports as an effective screen for cardiovascular disease (Maron et al. 2007). The recommendations highlight 12 items in the pre-participation screening. A positive value of 1 of the 12 items may be judged sufficient to

Table 2.2. The 12-Element AHA Recommendations for Pre-Participation Cardiovascular Screening of Competitive Athletes

Medical history*

Personal history

    1. Exertional chest pain/discomfort

    2. Unexplained syncope/near-syncope[†]

    3. Excessive exertional and unexplained dyspnea/fatigue, associated with exercise

    4. Prior recognition of a heart murmur

    5. Elevated systemic blood pressure

Family history

    6. Premature death (sudden and unexpected, or otherwise) before age 50 years due to heart disease, in ≥1 relative

    7. Disability from heart disease in a close relative <50 years of age

    8. Specific knowledge of certain cardiac conditions in family members: hypertrophic or dilated cardiomyopathy, long-QT syndrome or other ion channelopathies, Marfan syndrome, or clinically important arrhythmias

Physical examination

    9. Heart murmur[‡]

   10. Femoral pulses to exclude aortic coarctation

   11. Physical stigmata of Marfan syndrome

   12. Brachial artery blood pressure (sitting position)[§]

* Parental verification is recommended for high school and middle school athletes.

[†] Judged not to be neurocardiogenic (vasovagal); of particular concern when related to exertion.

[‡] Auscultation should be performed in both supine and standing positions (or with Valsalva maneuver), specifically to identify murmurs of dynamic left ventricular outflow tract obstruction.

[§] Preferably taken in both arms.

Maron, B. J., et al. 2007. Recommendations and considerations related to preparticipation screening for cardiovascular abnormalities in competitive athletes: 2007 Update. Reprinted by permission from *Circulation* 2007; 115: 1643–1655. Copyright 2007 American Heart Association.

warrant further cardiac evaluation. The use of a routine screening ECG, while recommended by the European Society of Cardiology and the International Olympic Committee, has not been universally accepted, and at present, is left up to the discretion of the practitioner. Possibly due to physiologic changes of exercise on the heart, ECG abnormalities can occur in up to 40 percent of well-conditioned athletes (Maron et al. 2007). Furthermore, exercise-induced cardiac enlargement can often mimic hypertrophic cardiomyopathy on echo-cardiograms, making it difficult to distinguish between an adaptive physiologic response and a life-threatening cardiac condition. At present, a targeted and complete personal and family history, combined with a thorough physical examination, appear to be the most practical screening strategy for young adults prior to initiation of competitive sports.

The Elderly

Age-related changes in cardiovascular physiology likely contribute to the greater incidence of and worse prognosis for cardiovascular disease in individuals over the age of 70. Reductions in maximum heart rate, stroke volume reserve, and VO2 max are accompanied by increases in central artery stiffness, left ventricu-lar mass, and impaired diastolic filling (Gerstenblith, Lakatta, and Weisfeldt 1976). Exercise training attenuates some of these changes, with less aortic stiff-ness, improved ventricular filling, increased nitric-oxide mediated vasodilation, and a slower rate of decline in exercise capacity seen with regular activity (Ehsani et al. 1991; Forman et al. 1992; Vaitkevicius et al. 1993). It is important to note that no adverse outcomes have been reported in older subjects enrolled in exercise programs. Both older men and women demonstrate improvement in exercise capacity with training even in the presence of CVD, and have 25 to 50 percent lower risk of death with regular exercise (Blair et al. 1995; Miller, Balady, and Fletcher 1997; Paffenbarger, 1993). In addition to cardiovascular protection, aerobic and/or resistance exercise has been associated with reduced cognitive decline, physical disability, and prolonged autonomy (Miller, Balady, and Fletcher 1997). For these reasons, older individuals of both genders should be strongly encouraged to incorporate exercise into their daily regimen.

The Prescription of Exercise

For the beneficial effects of exercise to be maintained, physical activity needs to be a permanent lifestyle behavior. The recommendation of a health care provider and an exercise prescription can be powerful motivating factors for change, but lasting change is difficult to achieve for most patients. Long-term compliance with exercise programs in patients enrolled in studies is often a discouragingly low 20 to 50 percent, even at one year of follow up (Schneider et al.1992; Simons-Morton et al.1998). Poor long-term compliance, in addition to financial and time constraints, makes physical activity counseling difficult to incorporate into an active medical practice. In addition, many health care providers feel they lack training to provide specific recommendations and to implement counseling in a cost-effective manner. The Centers for Disease Control developed Project PACE: Physician-Based Assessment and Counseling for Exercise in an attempt to address some of these issues (Patrick et al. 1996). This system is a tool designed to help providers utilize paramedical personnel to efficiently introduce physical activity counseling into practice.

Factors that have been identified to positively influence adherence to an exercise recommendation are continued intervention/counseling, multiple contacts, supervised activity, and utilization of behavioral approaches (Fletcher et al. 2001). The latter includes a selection of exercises that are enjoyable to the patient. These should incorporate activities in which the person feels both comfortable and safe. Realistic goals, a social support network, and feedback are essential components. Health care providers themselves should personally engage in regular exercise—not just to set an example, but to offer insight into identifying barriers that arise when attempting to maintain an exercise program. One approach that appears to aid adherence to exercise is the recommendation that exercise start slowly and gradually increase to meet the target level. Shorter duration, less intense, and less frequent exercise is safer and more realistic for previously sedentary individuals to achieve. Exercise programs that begin immediately with high intensity activity are associated with higher dropout rates (Schneider et al. 1992). Successful implementation of effective exercise programs in the health care setting will not only require improved education of providers, but changes in health care policy and reimbursement as well.

RISKS

The benefits of exercise far outweigh the potential risks, but consideration should be given to individualize recommendations in an effort to avoid potential harm. The most common risk of exercise is musculoskeletal injury, typically from overuse. As up to one-third of injured adults fail to return to exercise within a year (Hootman et al. 2002), proven prophylactic strategies such as gradual initiation of exercise, supervised activity, and stretching are of tantamount importance. Intensity and nature of impact correlate more closely with musculoskeletal injury than duration and should be adjusted accordingly. Rare, but potentially catastrophic, risks of exercise include cardiac arrhythmia, myocardial infarction and sudden cardiac death.

Unlike younger athletes, occult coronary artery disease is the overwhelming cause of exercise-related deaths in individuals over 40. Performance of high-intensity exercise appears to increase the incidence of sudden death. In the Physician's Health Study, the *relative risk* of sudden death in men was 16.9 up to 30 minutes after exercise when compared with other time periods (Albert et al. 2000). This increase is also observed in women. However, the *absolute* risk remains exceedingly low during any given episode of vigorous exertion and has been estimated at 1 per 1.5 million episodes of exercise (Albert et al. 2000). Fatality rates observed in health clubs have been estimated at 1 case per approximately 900,000 person-hours (Vander, Franklin, and Rubenfire 1982). Furthermore, while the chance of sudden death is increased with intensive exercise, this risk is attenuated with the performance of habitual exercise. In sum, the absolute risk of death for intensive-trained individuals is lower than their sedentary peers (Whang et al. 2006). Unaccustomed rigorous activity in sedentary adults confers the greatest risk of sudden cardiac death. The likely mechanisms of cardiac arrest with exercise include myocardial infarction from a ruptured cholesterol plaque, or cardiac arrhythmia.

Similar to sudden death, myocardial infarctions are more likely to occur with exercise, but are less likely to occur in individuals who exercise regularly. Intense exercise in conditioned individuals confers a risk of myocardial infarction 2.4 times the baseline level, compared to over 100 times the risk in sedentary persons (Mittleman et al. 1993). While still rare, heart attacks occur up to seven times more frequently than sudden death during exercise. Physical activity of ≥6 METs within one hour is reported in up to 7 percent of patients with myocardial infarction (Willich et al. 1993). Nevertheless, the ability of exercise to reduce cardiovascular events has been demonstrated in symptomatic and asymptomatic coronary patients as well as healthy individuals, and should be encouraged in all individuals.

Both ventricular and atrial arrhythmias are also more likely to occur during exercise, and are much more common in individuals with prior arrhythmia or structural heart disease. Regular exercise reduces the incidence of arrhythmia, likely due to increased vagal tone and reduction of sympathetic nerve stimulation. Of note, this is distinct from arrhythmias observed during diagnostic cardiac exercise testing, whose significance for predicting flow-limiting coronary disease is well documented.

PRE-EXERCISE EVALUATION

Medical screening prior to the initiation of an exercise program ensures the lowest possible risk of injury or death during exercise. The presence of significant medical comorbidities would likely necessitate further testing and possibly specialist consultation prior to starting exercise under close supervision. For individuals with known or suspected cardiovascular disease, the American Heart Association has published recommendations for secondary prevention, which include enrollment in cardiovascular rehabilitation programs (Fletcher et al. 2001). While all individuals derive benefit from exercise training, the purpose of the medical evaluation is to help guide the level of supervision and monitoring required during exercise and the individualization needed in the exercise prescription.

A fitness facility, not a health care provider's office, may be the site of initial contact where an evaluation should be performed. The American College of Sports Medicine/AHA (among others) has published pre-participation screening questionnaires which will prompt for referral to a healthcare professional if indicated (Balady et al. 1998).

In the medical evaluation of an apparently healthy individual, the medical history should focus on risk of cardiovascular disease and the chance of injury if unsupervised. The latter may include severe obesity or neuromuscular disorders. Prior MI, bypass surgery, angioplasty, valvular heart disease, congestive heart failure, or congenital heart disease should be referred for further evaluation and possible testing prior to initiation of exercise. Symptoms of chest discomfort, shortness of breath with daily activities, and leg pain consistent with peripheral arterial disease should be considered cardiovascular disease equivalents and require referral for subsequent evaluation. All murmurs on exam should be regarded as indicating cardiovascular disease and triaged accordingly.

Absent any concerns generated in the history and physical examination, age is the predominant factor determining further evaluation (Fletcher et al. 2001):

- For men <45 years and women <55 years of age with no signs or symptoms of cardiovascular disease no further workup is required.
- Men ≥ 45 years and women ≥ 55 years with diabetes or 2 other risk factors for coronary artery disease should perform an exercise stress test if *vigorous* exercise is planned. An abnormal test should be followed up accordingly and the patient medically managed as if cardiovascular disease is present (Gibbons et al. 1997).

If a higher-risk individual chooses not to perform stress testing, modified exercise targets should be employed, and the patient referred for medical supervision by trained professionals (to include ACLS certification) during the initial phases of exercise. Supervised training for 6–12 sessions is recommended, and the individual should be trained in how to monitor his or her own activity.

Individuals with active/uncontrolled disease should be discouraged from participation in exercise. The AHA statement on exercise lists conditions that are contraindications to exercise (Fletcher et al. 2001), as well as specific recommendations for the amount of exercise that can be tolerated in patients with active cardiovascular disease.

EXERCISE PRESCRIPTION FOR CARDIOVASCULAR PREVENTION

A threshold of exercise intensity and frequency is likely required to achieve cardiovascular protection, and appears to be subject to individual variability. When assessing exercise intensity it is sometimes useful to differentiate between absolute intensity and relative intensity. *Absolute intensity* refers to the metabolic cost of each exercise, and is typically defined by METs (see above). *Relative intensity* refers to the percentage of maximum heart rate (or VO2 max) achieved. For practical purposes, defining activity based on METs is often the most useful when counseling middle-aged individuals for activity that confers cardiovascular protection. However, age must be taken into consideration. Due to the age-associated decline in heart rate and max VO2, an activity of moderate intensity for a middle-aged individual may represent exercise that is too light for an at-risk patient in his or her 30s, or too vigorous for an 80-year-old. At the extremes of age, relative intensity defined by heart rate may be a more appropriate metric to follow.

Higher intensity exercise is required to attain gains cardiovascular fitness, but not to provide cardiovascular protection (Hagberg et al. 1989; King et al. 1995). It is true, however, that increasing energy expenditure is related to incremental decrease in cardiovascular risk (Paffenberger, 1986). There is significant evidence to suggest that the threshold at which cardiovascular benefit occurs is at moderately intense exercise between 4 and 6 METs in trials involving middle-aged subjects (Fletcher et al. 2001). This would equate to exercise that burns 4–7kcal/min, and lies between 50–70 percent of maximum predicted heart rate. Examples of activities in this range can include brisk walking (3–4 miles per hour), yard work, leisurely cycling, and golf. This level of exertion should be achieved after a warm-up period lasting several minutes. Exercise can be increased to upwards of 85 percent (high intensity) of maximal heart rate if well tolerated. Older individuals will accrue cardiovascular benefit from activity as low as 2.0 METs (age 80–89). From a logistical standpoint, a moderate level of activity has the advantage of greater compliance the exercise program, while reducing the risk of complications or injury. If exercise is well tolerated, however, a more rigorous program has the advantages of achieving the same (if not more) cardiovascular protection in less time, as well as the opportunity to improve cardiovascular fitness.

To confer benefit, exercise does not need to be continuous but can be performed throughout the day in short intervals, allowing for integration into one's daily life. Emphasis should be placed on aerobic activity, with resistance training as a supplement. The American Heart Association and the American College of Sports Medicine recommend 30–60 minutes of moderate intensity five days a week, or 20 minutes of high intensity exercise three times per week (Haskell et al. 2007). This equates to a *minimum* of 150 minutes spent per week in moderate aerobic activity. Other societies have recommended similar targets, with slightly longer duration of intensive exercise at 75 minutes per week (U.S. Department of Health & Human Services 2008). Not surprisingly, the total amount of exercise performed does highly correlate with weight loss in addition to cardioprotection.

Significant health benefits can be derived from occupational and leisure-time activities. Leisure activity should target between 700–1000 kcal/week to confer benefit. As previously mentioned, prior studies have demonstrated reduced cardiac event rates in individuals with physically active jobs. However, unless one hour of brisk walking per day is reliably performed (i.e. postal route), supplemental activity off-hours should be incorporated into daily life. Heavy-lifting occupations that meet requirements are increasingly rare in today's society. To meet criteria, greater than 20lbs of lifting at least once an hour, or constant moving of loads without mechanical help, would be necessary to achieve cardiovascular benefit.

Flexibility and stretching exercises should be encouraged, but not take the place of, aerobic exercise. Emphasis should be given to the hamstring and lower back areas in an effort to reduce chronic lower back injury. In addition, individuals over 40 years of age should avoid repetitive high-impact aerobic activity, and vary the exercises performed accordingly.

Although resistance training affects cardiovascular risk factors less than aerobic exercise, it is an accepted and encouraged part of a comprehensive exercise regimen. In addition to its previously described benefits, increased muscle mass can reduce the chance of subsequent injury and increase the basal metabolic rate. Performance of 8–10 exercises targeting the large muscle groups (chest, arms, back, abdominals, and legs) is recommended. The exercises need only consist of a single set of 8–12 repetitions (10–15 repetitions at less weight for older persons to prevent injury) and be performed 2–3 times per week. This appears to be the minimum required for muscle group adaptation and maintenance. Any cardiovascular benefit from additional sets and frequency appears to be small (Feignenbaum and Pollock 1997).

Physical inactivity is the cardiac risk factor that affects the largest number of individuals in the population, and its reduction through exercise confers benefits on par with other well-established cardiovascular therapies. In addition to improving cardiovascular health, adherence to an exercise program has a broad range of benefits for the individual and the society. Greater emphasis on adherence to formal exercise programs involving research, health care policy, and pubic service announcements would reap considerable benefits for the population as a whole. In addition, a health care provider's act of encouraging, educating, and supporting regular daily exercise may provide the greatest opportunity to improve the long term health and quality of life of the individual.

REFERENCES

Ades, P. A., F. J Pashkow, and J. R. Nestor. 1997. Cost-effectiveness of cardiac rehabilitation after myocardial infarction. *J Cardiopulm Rehabil* 17: 222.

Albert, C. M, M. A. Mittleman, C. U. Chae, et al. 2000. Triggering of sudden death from cardiac causes by vigorous exertion. *NEJM* 343: 1355.

American Heart Association. 2002. *Heart disease and stroke statistics 2003 update.* Dallas, TX: American Heart Association.

Arroll, B., and R. Beaglehole. 1992. Does physical activity lower blood pressure: A critical review of the clinical trials. *Journal of Clinical Epidemiology* 45: 439–447.

Balady, G. J., B. Chaitman, D. Driscoll, et al. 1998. Recommendations for cardiovascular screening, staffing, and emergency policies at health/fitness facilities. *Circulation* 97: 2283–2293.

Balady, G. J., M. G. Larson, R. S. Vasan, et al. 2004. Usefulness of exercise testing in the prediction of coronary disease risk among asymptomatic persons as a function of the Framingham risk score. *Circulation* 110: 1920.

Blair, S. N., N. N. Goodyear, L. W. Gibbons, and K. H. Cooper. 1984. Physical fitness and incidence of hypertension in healthy normotensive men and women. *JAMA* 252: 487.

Blair, S. N., H. W. Kohl II, C. E. Barlow, et al. 1995. Changes in fitness and all-cause mortality. A prospective study of healthy and unhealthy men. *JAMA* 273: 1093–1098.

Blair, S. N., H. W. Kohl II, R. S. Paffenbarger, et al. 1989. Physical fitness and all-cause mortality. A prospective study of healthy men and women. *JAMA* 262: 2395–2401.

Blomqvist, C. G., and B. Saltin. 1983. Cardiovascular adaptations to physical training. *Annu Rev Physiol* 45: 169.

Braith, R. W., and K. J. Stewart. 2006. Resistance exercise training: Its role in the prevention of cardiovascular disease. *Circulation* 113: 2642–2650.

Cannistra, L. B., G. J. Balady, C. J. O'Malley, D. A. Weiner, and T. J. Ryan. 1992. Comparison of the clinical profile and outcome of women and men in cardiac rehabilitation. *Am J of Cardiology* 69: 1274–1279.

Capersen, C. J., M. A. Pereira, and K. M. Curran. 2000. Changes in physical activity patterns in the United States, by sex and cross-sectional age. *Med. Sci. Sports Exerc* 32(9): 1601–1609.

Cornelissen, V. A., R. H. Fagard. 2005. Effect of resistance training on resting blood pressure: a meta-analysis of randomized controlled trials. *J Hypertension* 23: 251–259.

Cuff, D. J., G. S. Meneilly, A. Martin, et al. 2003. Effective exercise modality to reduce insulin resistance in women with type 2 diabetes. *Diabetes Care* 26: 2977.

Currens, J. H., and P. D. White. 1961. Half century of running: Clinical, physiologic, and autopsy finding in the case of Clarence De Mar, "Mr. Marathoner." *NEJM* 265: 988–993.

Dietz, W. H., and S. L. Gortmaker. 1985. Do we fatten our children at the television set? Obesity and television viewing in children and adolescents. *Pediatrics* 75: 807–812.

Duncan, G. E., M. G. Perri, D. W. Theriaque, et al. 2003. Exercise training, without weight loss, increases insulin sensitivity and postheparin plasma lipase activity in previously sedentary adults. *Diabetes Care* 26: 557.

Ehsani, A. A., T. Ogawa, T. R. Miller, R. J. Spina, and S. M. Jilka. 1991. Exercise training improves left ventricular systolic function in older men. *Circulation* 83: 96–103.

Ekelund, L. G., W. L. Haskell, J. L. Johnson, et al. 1988. Physical fitness as a predictor of cardiovascular mortality in asymptomatic North American men. The Lipid Research Clinics Mortality Follow-up Study. *NEJM* 319: 1379–1384.

Fagard, R. H. 2001. Exercise characteristics and the blood pressure response to dynamic physical training. *Med Sci Sports Exerc* 33(6 suppl): S484–S492.

Feigenbaum, M. S., and M. L. Pollock. 1997. Strength training: rationale for current guidelines for adult fitness programs. *Physician Spports Med* 25: 44–64.

Fletcher, G., G. Balady, E. Amsterdam, et al. 2001. Exercise standards for testing and training: A statement for healthcare professionals from the American Heart Association. *Circulation* 104: 1694–1740.

Fletcher, G. F., G. Balady, S. N. Blair, et al. 1996. Statement on exercise. Benefits and recommendations for physical activity programs for all Americans. A statement for health professionals by the Committee on Exercise and Cardiac Rehabilitation of the Council on Clinical Cardiology. American Heart Association. *Circulation* 94: 857–862.

Forman, D. E., W. J. Manning, R. Hauser, et al. 1992. Enhanced left ventricular diastolic filling associated with long-term endurance training. *Journals of Gerontology* 47: M56–58.

Franco, O., C. de Laet, A. Peeters, et al. 2005. Effects of physical activity on life expectancy with cardiovascular disease. *Archives of Internal Medicine* 165: 2355.

Gerstenblith, G., E. G. Lakatta, M. L. Weisfeldt. 1976. Age changes in myocardial function and exercise response. *Prog Cardiovasc Dis* 19: 1.

Gibbons, R. J., G. J. Balady, J. W. Beasley, et al. 1997. ACC/AHA guidelines for exercise testing. A report of the American College of Cardiology/American Heart Association Task Force on Practive Guidelines (Committee on Exercise Testing). *JACC* 30: 260–311.

Green, H. J., L. L. Jones, and D. C. Painter. 1990. Effects of short-term training on cardiac function during prolonged exercise. *Med Sci Sports Exerc* 22: 488.

Gregg, E. W., R. B. Gerzoff, C. J. Caspersen, and D. F. Williamson. 2003. Relationship of walking to mortality among US adults with diabetes. *Arch Intern Med* 163: 1440.

Graham, T. E., and B. Saltin. 1989. Estimation of the mitochondrial redox state in human skeletal muscle during exercise. *J Appl Physiol* 66: 561.

Hagberg, J., S. Montain, W. Marrin, et al. 1989. Effect of exercise training in 60-69 year old persons with essential hypertension. *Am J Cardiol* 64: 348.

Hakim, A. A., H. Petrovitch, C. M. Burchfiel, et al. 1998. Effects of walking on mortality among nonsmoking retired men. *NEJM* 338: 94.

Haskell, W. L., I. M. Lee, R. R. Pate, et al. 2007. Physical activity and public health: updated recommendation for adults from the American College of Sports Medicine and the American Heart Association. *Circulation* 116: 1081.

Haskell, W. L., C. Sims, J. Myll, et al. 1993. Coronary artery size and dilating capacity in ultra-distance runners. *Circulation* 87: 1076–1082.

Helmrich, S. P., D. R. Ragland, R. W. Leung, and R. S. Paffenbarger Jr. 1991. Physical activity and reduced occurrence of non-insulin-dependent diabetes mellitus. *NEJM* 325: 147–152.

Hootman, J. M., C. A. Macera, B. E. Ainsworth, et al. 2002. Epidemiology of musculoskeletal injuries among sedentary and physically active adults. *Med Sci Sports Exerc* 34: 838–844.

Houmard, J. A., N. J. Bruno, R. K. Bruner, et al. 1994. Effects of exercise training on the chemical composition of plasma LDL. *Arterioscler Thromb* 14: 325.

Ishikawa-Takata K., T. Ohta, and H. Tanaka. 2003. How much exercise is required to reduce blood pressure in essential hypertensives: A dose-response study. *Am J Hypertens* 16: 629.

Jones, D., B. Ainsworth, J. Croft, C. Macera, E. Lloyd, and H. Yusuf. 1998. Moderate leisure-time physical activity: Who is meeting the Public Health Recommendation? A national cross-sectional study. *Arch Fam Med* 7: 285–289.

Jones, N. L. 1984. Normal values for pulmonary gas exchange during exercise. *Am Rev Respir Dis* 29(suppl): s44.

Kelder, S. H., C. L. Perry, and K. I. Klepp. 1993. Community-wide youth exercise promotion: Long-term outcomes of the Minnesota Heart Health Program and the Class of 1989 Study. *Journal of School Health* 63(5): 218–223.

Kelly, G. A., and K. S. Kelly. 2000. Progressive resistance exercise and resting blood pressure: a meta-analysis of randomized controlled trials. *Hypertension* 35: 838–843.

King, A. C., W. L. Haskell, D. R. Young, et al. 1995. Long-term effects of varying intensities and formats of physical activity on participation rates, fitness, and lipoproteins in men and women aged 50 to 65 years. *Circulation* 91: 2596.

Kodama, S., K. Saito, S. Tanaka, et al. 2009. Cardiorespiratory fitness as a quantitative predictor of all-cause mortality and cardiovascular events in healthy men and women: a meta-analysis. *JAMA* 301: 2024.

Kokkinos, P. F., J. C. Holland, P. Narayan, et al. 1995. Miles run per week and high-density lipoprotein cholesterol levels in healthy, middle-aged men. *Arch Intern Med* 155: 415.

Koller, A., A. Huang, D. Sun, et al. 1995. Exercise training augments flow-dependent dilation in rat skeletal muscle arterioles. Role of endothelial nitric oxide and prostaglandins. *Circ Res* 76: 544.

Kramsch, D. M., A. J. Aspen, B. M. Abramowitz, T. Kreimendahl, and W. B. Hood Jr. 1981. Reduction of coronary atherosclerosis by moderate conditioning exercise in monkeys on an atherogenic diet. *NEJM* 305: 1483–1489.

Kraus, W. E., J. A. Houmard, B. D. Duscha, et al. 2002. Effects of the amount and intensity of exercise on plasma lipoproteins. *NEJM* 347: 1483.

Kuh, D. J. L, and C. Cooper. 1992. Physical activity at 36 years: Patterns and childhood predictors in a longitudinal study. *Journal of Epidemiology and Community Health* 46: 114–119.

Kujala, U. M., J. Kaprio, S. Sarna, et al. 1998. Relationship of leisure-time physical activity and mortality: The Finnish Twin Cohort. *JAMA* 279: 440.

Lee, I. M., K. N. Rexrode, N. R. Cook, et al. 2001. Physical activity and coronary heart disease in women. Is "no pain, no gain" passé. *JAMA* 285: 1447.

Lee, I. M., H. D. Sesso, Y. Oguma, and R. S. Paffenbarger. 2003. Relative intensity of physical activity and risk of coronary heart disease. *Circulation* 107: 1110.

Leitzmann, M. F., Y. Park, A. Blair, et al. 2007. Physical activity recommendation and decreased risk of mortality. *Arch Intern Med* 167: 2453.

Leon, A. S., J. Connett, D. R. Jacobs, and R. Rauraman. 1987. Leisure-time physical activity levels and risk of coronary heart disease and death. The Multiple Risk Factor Intervention Trial. *JAMA* 258: 2388–2395.

Leon, A. S., and O. A. Sanchez. 2001a. Response of blood lipids to exercise training alone or combined with dietary intervention. *Med Sci Sports Exerc* 33 (6 supple): S502–S515.

Leon, A. S., and O. A. Sanchez. 2001b. Meta-analysis of the effects of aerobic exercise training on blood lipids. Abstract. *Circulation* 104 (suppl II): II–414–II415.

Lynch, J., S. P. Helmirch, T. A. Lakka, et al. 1996. Moderately intense physical activities and high levels of cardiorespiratory fitness reduce the risk of non-insulin-dependent diabetes mellitus in middle-aged men. *Archives of Internal Medicine* 156: 1307–1314.

Manini, T. M., J. E. Everhart, K. V. Patel, et al. 2006. Daily activity energy expenditure and mortality among older adults. *JAMA* 296: 171.

Manson, J. E., P. Greenland, A. LaCroix, et al. 2002. Walking compared with vigorous exercise for the prevention of cardiovascular events in women. *NEJM* 347 (10): 716–725.

Manson, J. E., F. B. Hu, J. W. Rich-Edwards, et al. 1999. A prospective study of walking as compared with vigorous exercise in the prevention of coronary heart disease in women. *NEJM* 341: 650.

Marcus, B. H., A. E. Albrecht, T. K. King, et al. 1999. The efficacy of exercise as an aid for smoking cessation in women. A randomized controlled trial. *Arch Intern Med* 159: 1229.

Martin, C. K., T. S. Church, A. M. Thompson, et al. 2009. Exercise dose and quality of life: a randominzed controlled trial. *Arch Intern Med* 169: 269.

Martinensen, E. W., A. Medhus, and L. Sandvik. 1985. Effects of aerobic exercise on depression: A controlled study. *British Medical Journal (Clinical Research Edition)* 291: 109.

Maron, B. J. 2003. Sudden death in young athletes. *NEJM* 349: 1064–1075.

Maron, B. J., et al. 2007. Recommendations and considerations related to preparticipation screening for cardiovascular abnormalities in competitive athletes: 2007 Update. *Circulation* 115: 1643–1655.

Maron, B. J., T. E. Gohman, and D. Aeppli. 1998. Prevalence of sudden cardiac death during competitive sports activities in Minnesota high school athletes. *JACC* 32: 1881–1884.

McHam, S. A., T. H. Marwick, F. J. Pashkow, et al. 1999. Delayed systolic blood pressure recovery after graded exercise: an independent correlate of angiographic coronary disease. *JACC* 34: 754–759.

Miller, T., G. Balady, and G. Fletcher. 1997. Exercise and its role in the prevention and rehabilitation of cardiovascular disease. *Ann Behav Med* 19 (3): 220–229.

Miller, J. P., R. E. Pratley, A. P. Goldberg, P. Gordon, M. Rubin, M. S. Treuth, A. S. Ryan, and B. F. Hurley. 1994. Strength training increases insulin action in healthy 50- to 65-year-old men. *J Appl Physiol* 77: 1122–1127.

Mittleman, M. A., M. Maclure, G. H. Tofler, et al. 1993. Triggering of acute myocardial infarction by heavy physical exertion: protection against triggering by regular exertion: Determinants of Myocardial Infarction Onset Investigators. *NEJM* 329: 1677–1683.

Mora, S., R. F. Redberg, Y. Cui, et al. 2003. Ability of exercise testing to predict cardiovascular and all-cause death in asymptomatic women: A 20-year follow-up of the Lipid Research Clinics prevalence study. *JAMA* 290: 1600.

Morales, M. C., N. L. Coplan, P. Zabetakis, and G. W. Gleim. 1991. Hypertension: The acute and chronic response to exercise (editorial). *Am Heart H* 122: 264.

Morbidity and Mortality Weekly Report. 2007. Prevalence of self-reported physically active adults United States, 2007. *MMWR* 57: 1297.

Morris, J. N., J. A. Heady, P. A. B. Raffle, C. G. Roberts, and J. W. Parks. 1953. Coronary heart disease and physical activity of work. *The Lancet* 2: 1053–1057, 1111–1120.

Mosca, L., L. Appel, E. Benjamin, et al. 2004. Evidence-based guidelines for cardiovascular disease prevention in women. *JACC* 43 (5): 900–921.

Mundal, R., S. E. Kjeldsen, L. Sandvik, et al. 1996. Exercise blood pressure predicts mortality from myocardial infarction. *Hypertension* 27: 324–329.

Myers, J., M. Prakach, V. Froelicher, et al. 2002. Exercise capacity and mortality among men referred for exercise testing. *NEJM* 346: 793.

Nelson, K. M., G. Reiber, E. J. Boyko. 2002. Diet and exercise amoung adults with type 2 diabetes: findings from the third National Health and Nutrition Examination Survey (NHANES III). *Diabetes Care* 25: 1722.

Niebauer, J., and J. P. Cooke. 1996. Cardiovascular effects of exercise: Role of endothelial shear stress. *JACC* 28: 1652–1660.

Paffenbarger Jr., R. S., R. T. Hyde, A. L. Wing, C. C. Hsieh. 1986. Physical activity, all-cause mortality, and longevity of college alumni. *NEJM* 314: 605–613.

Paffenbarger, R. S., R. T. Hyde, A. L. Wing, et al. 1993. The association of changes in physical-activity level and other lifestyle characteristics with mortality among men. *NEJM* 328: 538.

Pate, R. R., Pratt, M., Blair, S. N., Haskell, W. L., Macera, C. A., Bouchard, C., Buchner, D., Ettinger, W., Heath, G. W., King, A. C. & et al. 1995. Physical activity and public health. A recommendation from the Centers for Disease Control and Prevention and the American College of Sports Medicine. *JAMA, 273*: 402–7.

Patrick, K., K. J. Calfas, J. F. Sallis, and B. Long. 1996. Basic principles of physical activity counseling: Project PACE. In *The heart and exercise*, ed. R. Thomas and Igaku-shoin, 33–50. New York: Igaku-Shoin.

Patterson, J., C. Charabogos, and A. P. Goldberg. 1993. Aerobic versus strength training for risk factor intervention in middle-aged men at high risk for coronary heart disease. *Metabolism* 42: 177–184.

Pelliccia, A., F. Culasso, F. M. Di Paolo, et al. 1999. Physiologic left ventricular cavity dilation in elite athletes. *Ann Intern Med* 130: 23.

Pescatello, L. S., A. E. Fargo, C. N. Leach Jr., and H. H. Scherzer. 1991. Short term effect of dynamic exercise on arterial blood pressure. *Circulation* 83:1557–1561.

Pluim, B. M., A. H. Zwinderman, A. van der Laarse, and E. E. van der Wall. 2000.The athlete's heart: a meta-analysis of cardiac structure and function. *Circulation* 101: 336.

Poirier, P., A. Tremblay, C. Catellier, et al. 2000. Impact of time interval from the last meal on glucose response to exercise in subjects with type 2 diabetes. *J Clin Endocrinol Metab* 85: 2860.

Powell, K. E., and Blair, S. N. 1994. The public health burden of sedentary living habits: Theoretical but realistic estimates. *Med Sci Sports Exerc* 26: 851.

Powell, K. E., P. D. Thompson, C. J. Caspersen, and J. S. Kendrick. 1987. Physical activity and the incidence of coronary artery disease. *Annual Review of Public Health* 8: 253–287.

Pratt, M., C. A. Macera, and G. Wang. 2000. Higher direct medical costs associated with physical inactivity. *Physician Sports Med* 28: 63.

Putman, C. T., N. L. Jones, L. C. Lands, et al. 1995. Skeletal muscle pyruvate dehydrogenase activity during maximal exercise in humans. *Am J Physiol* 269: E458.

Rerych, S. K., P. M. Scholz, D. C. Sabiston Jr., and R. H. Jones. 1980. Effects of exercise training on left ventricular function in normal subjects: A longitudinal study by radionucleotide angiography. *American Journal of Cardiology* 45: 244–252.

Riddoch, C. J., and C. A. G. Boreham. 1995. The health-related physical activity of children. *Sports Medicine* 19: 86–102.

Rodnick, K. J., J. O. Holloszy, C. E. Mondon, and D. E. James. 1990. Effects of exercise training on insulin-regulatable glucose-transporter protein levels in rat skeletal muscle. *Diabetes* 39: 1425.

Ross, J. G., and G. G. Gilbert. 1985. The national children and youth fitness study. A summary of findings. *Journal of Physical Education and Recreational Dance* 56: 45–50.

Ross, J. G., and R. R. Pate. 1987. The national children and youth fitness study II. A summary of findings. *Journal of Physical Education and Recreational Dance* 58: 51–56.

Schneider, S. H., A. K. Khachadurian, L. F. Amorosa, et al. 1992. Ten-year experience with exercise-based outpatient life-style modification program in the treatment of diabetes mellitus. *Diabetes Care* 15: 1800.

Seals, D. R., and J. M. Hagberg. 1984. The effect of exercise training on human hypertension: A review. *Medicine and Science in Sports and Exercise* 16: 207–215.

Seals, D. R., J. M. Hagberg, R. J. Spina, et al. 1994. Enhanced left ventricular performance in endurance trained older men. *Circulation* 89: 198.

Seip, R. L., P. Moulin, T. Cocke, et al. 1993. Exercise training decreases plasma cholesteryl estertransfer protein. *Arterioscler Thromb* 13: 1359.

Sesso, H. D., R. S. Paffenbarger, I. M. Lee. 2000. Physical activity and coronary heart disease in men: the Harvard Alumni Health Study. *Circulation* 102: 975.

Shepard, R. J., and P. N. Shek. 1999. Exercise, immunity, and susceptibility to infection: A J-shaped relationship? *Physician and Sports Med* 27: 47.

Sigal, R. J., G. P. Kenny, N. G. Boule, et al. 2007. Effects of aerobic training, resistance training, or both on glycemic control in type 2 diabetes: A randomized trial. *Ann Intern Med* 147: 357.

Sigal, R., G. Kenny, D. Wasserman, C. Castaneda-Sceppa. 2004. Physical activity/exercise and type 2 diabetes. *Diabetes Care* 27 (10): 2518–2539.

Simons-Morton, D. G., K. J. Calfas, B. Oldenburg, et al. 1998. Effects of interventions in health care settings on physical activity or cardiorespiratory fitness. *Am J Prev Med* 15: 413–430.

Smutok, M. A., C. Reece, P. F. Kokkinos, C. Farmer, P. Dawson, R. Shulman, J. DeVane-Bell, N. J. Snowling, and W. G. Hopkins. 2006. Effects of different modes of exercise training on glucose control and risk factors for complications in type 2 diabetic patients: A meta-analysis. *Diabetes Care* 29: 2518.

Somers, V. K., J. Conway, J. Johnston, P. Sleight. 1991. Effects of endurance training on baroreceptor sensitivity and blood pressure in borderline hypertension. *Lancet* 337: 1363.

Spina, R. J., T. Ogawa, T. R. Miller, W. M. Kohrt, and A. A. Ehsani. 1993. Effect of exercise training on left ventricular performance in older women free of cardiopulmonary disease. *Am J of Cardiol* 71: 99–104.

Stainsby, W. N., W. E. Brechue, D. M. O'Drobinak, et al. 1989. Oxidative/reduction state of cytochrome oxidase during repetitive contractions. *J appl Physiol* 67: 2158.

Stefanick, M. L., S. Mackey, M. Sheehan, et al. 1998. Effects of diet and exercise in men and postmenopausal women with low levels of HDL cholesterol and high levels of LDL cholesterol. *NEJM* 339: 12.

Sue, D. Y., and J. E. Hansen. 1984. Normal values in adults during exercise testing. *Clin Chest Med* 5: 89.

Tanaka, H., K. D. Monahan, and D. R. Deals. 2001. Age-predicted maximal heart rate revisited. *J Am Coll Cardiol* 37: 153.

Tanasescu, M., M. F. Leitzmann, E. B. Rimm, and F. B. Hu. 2003. Physical activity in relation to cardiovascular disease and total mortality among men with type 2 diabetes. *Circulation* 107: 2435.

Taylor, H. L., E. Kelpetar, A. Keys, et al. 1962. Death rates among physically active and sedentary employees of the railroad industry. *American Journal of Public Health* 52: 1697–1707.

Terjung, R. L. 1995. Muscle adaptations to aerobic training. *Sports Sci Exchange* 8: 1.

Thompson, P., D. Buchner, I. Pina, G. Balady, et al. 2003. Exercise and physical activity in the prevention and treatment of atherosclerotic cardiovascular disease. A statement from the Council on Clinical Cardiology (subcommittee on Exercise, Rehabilitation, and Prevention) and the Council on Nutrition, Physical Activity, and Metabolism (subcommittee on Physical Activity). *Arterioscler Thromb Vasc Biol* 23: e42–e49.

Thompson, P. D., S. F. Crouse, B. Goodpaster, et al. 2001. The acute versus the chronic response to exercise. *Med Sci Sports Exerc* 33(6 suppl): S438–S445.

U.S. Department of Health & Human Services. 2008. Physical Activity Guidelines for Americans. http://www.health.gov/paguidelines/

Vaitkevicius, P. V., J. L. Fleg, J. H. Engel, et al. 1993. Effects of age and aerobic capacity on arterial stiffness in healthy adults. *Circulation* 88 (Part 1): 1456–1462.

Vander, L., B. Franklin, and M. Rubenfire. 1982. Cardiovascular complications of recreational physical activity. *Phys Sports Med* 10: 89.

Wade, O. L., and J. M. Bishop. 1962. *Cardiac output and regional blood flow*. Philadelphia: FA Davis.

Wang, J., C. J. Jen, and H. Chen. 1995. Effects of exercise training and deconditioning on platelet function in men. *Arterioscler Thromb Vasc Biol* 15: 1668.

Warburton, D. E., N. Gledhill, and A. Quinney. 2001. Musculoskeletal fitness and health. *Can J Appl Physiol* 26: 217.

Wasserman, K., and M. B. McIlroy. 1964. Detecting the threshold of anaerobic metabolism in cardiac patients during exercise. *Am J Cardiol* 14: 844.

Wei, M., L. W. Gibbons, J. B. Kampert, et al. 2003. Low cardiorespiratory fitness and physical inactivity as predictors of mortality in men with type 2 diabetes. *Circulation* 107: 2435.

Wenger, N.K., E. S. Froelicher, L. K. Smith, et al. 1995. Cardiac Rehabilitation. *Clinical Practice Guideline No. 17, ACHCPR Publication No 96-0672*. Rockville, MD: U.S. Department of Health and Human Services, Public Health Service, Agency for Health Care Policy and Research and the National Heart, Lung, and Blood Institute.

Whang, W., J. E. Manson, F. B. Hu, et al. 2006. Physical exertion, exercise, and sudden cardiac death in women. *JAMA* 295: 1399.

Williams, P. T., R. M. Krauss, P. D. Wood, et al. 1986. Lipoprotein subfractions of runners and sedentary men. *Metabolism* 35: 45.

Willich, S. N., M. Lewis, H. Lowel, et al. 1993. Physical exertion as a trigger of acute myocardial infarction: Triggers and mechanisms of myocardial infarction study group. *NEJM* 329: 1684–1690.

Wood, P. D., W. Haskell, H. Klein, et al. 1976. The distribution of plasma lipoproteins in middle-aged male runners. *Metabolism* 25: 1249.

Wood, P. D., M. L. Stefanick, D. M. Dreon, et al. 1988. Changes in plasma lipids and lipoproteins in overweight men during weight loss through dieting as compared with exercise. *New England Journal of Medicine* 319: 1173–1179.

Wood, P. D., M. L. Stefanick, P. T. Williams, et al. 1991. The effects on plasma lipoproteins of a prudent weight-reducing diet, with or without exercise, in overweight men and women. *NEJM* 325: 461–466.

Yusuf, S., S. Reddy, S. Ounpuu, et al. 2001. Global burden of cardiovascular diseases: Part I: General considerations, the epidemiologic transition, risk factors, and impact of urbanization. *Circulation* 104: 2746–53.

3

Botanical Medicine and Cardiovascular Disease

TIERAONA LOW DOG

KEY CONCEPTS

- A number of botanicals show promise in the field of cardiology, particularly when used within the context of an integrative approach.
- Hawthorn improves symptoms of congestive heart failure; hibiscus and garlic can lower blood pressure; red yeast rice and plant sterols effectively improve lipids; parsley seed has diuretic and naturietic activity; and pycnogenol and horse chestnut extract may be used to manage chronic venous insufficiency.
- Clinicians should inquire about patient use of all dietary supplements, including botanicals, and document that usage in the medical chart.
- Report adverse events from dietary supplements to FDA Medwatch and/or your local poison control center.

■

Introduction

Herbal medicine, also referred to as phytotherapy or botanical medicine, utilizes plants, plant parts, and preparations made from plants for therapeutic and/or preventive purposes. Herbal medicine gave rise to the modern sciences of botany, pharmacy, perfumery, and chemistry. The role of herbal medicine in the management of cardiovascular disease has been a long and distinguished one. Ancient physicians and healers noted that remedies such as squill and foxglove could ease the suffering from dropsy, an outdated term for congestive heart failure (CHF). Hawthorn was noted to benefit the aging heart centuries ago. As the science of pharmacy evolved, the first effective treatment for hypertension, reserpine, and for CHF, digoxin, were derived from plants (*Rauwolfia serpentina* and foxglove, respectively). Through isolating the potent actives in these plants, pharmaceutical products can be produced with a consistent and uniform composition. Indeed, one primary drug discovery model has been the identification, isolation, and production of single active compounds. These active compounds can then be researched, patented, and sold as drugs.

While some drugs are made directly from plant material, these isolated compounds are not considered herbal medicines in the classic sense, because in traditional practice, the plants themselves are considered medicinally functioning wholes. They are chemically complex mixtures and thus the entire plant, or the part being used (the root, leaf, or seed, for example), is considered the "active." Unfortunately, there has been little financial incentive to study herbal medicines that can be easily grown in the garden or harvested in the wild. And for herbal manufacturers that do spend the money to do clinical trials on their herbal product, there is no "patent protection" as there is for drugs. Furthermore, there is no way for consumers or clinicians to readily distinguish the clinically tested product from the myriad of "me-too" products in the marketplace which piggyback off the research of others.

All too often the research that is undertaken is focused on the use of one particular herb for one specific condition, though most experienced herbal practitioners individualize their prescriptions based upon the unique characteristics of the patient. Herbal mixtures are often preferred over single herbs as they are thought to offer greater efficacy, and to some degree, greater safety. Multi-herb formulations may have additive, or synergistic, effects, and secondary herbs can be included to modify potential side effects from the primary herb. For example, hawthorn may be combined with hibiscus or dandelion for a patient who has some early CHF. Hawthorn is a positive inotrope and has been shown to improve CHF symptoms, while hibiscus and dandelion have noted diuretic activity. Given the number of traditional medical systems that utilize herbal formulations, the focus on single-herb preparations may be a critical shortcoming in botanical research. Nevertheless, monotherapy is probably the best approach for the clinician who is just starting to use herbs in his or her practice. Getting to know each herb in this way allows the practitioner to gain greater familiarity and expertise with its use.

Knowledge and tradition are not stagnant, and the field continues to evolve alongside modern scientific research. Today, we know that plant sterols can effectively reduce cholesterol and are added to food products as part of a "heart-healthy" dietary approach. Flavonoids, responsible for the colors of flowers, fruit, and sometimes the leaves of plants, are thought to reduce the risk of coronary artery disease through the inhibition of platelet aggregation, reducing injury from ischemia and reperfusion (Aviram 1998). The monounsaturated fat in olive oil and multiple constituents within garlic have proven to be beneficial to the cardiovascular system when consumed as part of a healthy diet. Red yeast rice, which contains naturally occurring statins, has been shown to lower cholesterol. Parsley seed has significant diuretic and naturietic activity. Hibiscus lowers blood pressure. From the broadly useful to the very specific, from crude plant to highly refined extract, the field of herbal medicine continues to grow and flourish.

Quality of Botanical Products

Given the dizzying array of herbal medicines, it is understandable that both consumers and health care professionals have difficulty navigating the aisles of natural food stores and pharmacies. In addition to questions of efficacy and safety inherent to the individual plant, there are also concerns about the quality of dietary supplements in general, and botanical products in particular. Some long-established medical systems, such as Ayurveda and Traditional Chinese Medicine, occasionally include heavy metals and toxic herbs as part of their therapeutic approach. Indeed, a number of herbal products from India and China have been found to contain significant levels of heavy metals, toxic herbs, and undeclared pharmaceutical medications (Gardiner et al. 2008). In many cases where herbal products have been found to have had significant adverse effects, these effects were not due to the herbs listed on the label, but rather were the result of substitution or contamination of the declared ingredient, intentionally or accidentally, with a more toxic botanical, a poisonous metal, or a potent non-herbal drug substance (De Smet 1996).

With the passage of the new good manufacturing guidelines (GMP) by the Food and Drug Administration (FDA), the problems of contamination, adulteration, and poor quality will hopefully become less of an issue in the future (Food and Drug Administration 2007). The inspection of dietary supplement manufacturers by the FDA increased in 2009, when companies were required to come into compliance with the new guidelines. This burden on manufacturers, however, should actually help the industry in the long run, as consumers will become more confident in the products they purchase, and health care providers will be more comfortable making supplement recommendations.

Safety

With widespread consumer use, but a general lack of knowledge about the safe and effective use of dietary supplements, particularly herbal medicines, among the majority of health care providers, it is important to address concerns of safety. Overall, the majority of the herbs and herbal supplements generally available in the United States and Europe have a relatively good safety profile when used appropriately, if they are manufactured to high quality standards. As more concentrated herbal products are introduced into the marketplace, many of which will be taken for extended periods of time, new questions of safety will undoubtedly arise. The chronic use of certain herbs (e.g., comfrey, licorice) can cause hepatic, renal, or electrolyte abnormalities. Like any chemically active substance, whether an herb is safe or toxic depends upon the dose, type of product, and underlying constitution and health of the patient.

Perhaps more worrying to clinicians is the concern that concomitant use of botanical remedies with prescription or over-the-counter medications may lead to adverse interactions, especially in the elderly and those with diminished renal or hepatic function. A national survey noted that 16 percent of prescription drug users also reported taking one or more herbal supplements within the prior week (Kaufman, 2002). It is imperative that clinicians talk with patients about their use of botanical medicines and other dietary supplements, to help prevent potentially dangerous herb–drug interactions. There are wide variety of herbal practices and products available, which makes generalizations difficult; however, by asking a few open-ended questions, clinicians should be able to assess the patient's beliefs, cultural practices, and use of botanical remedies. Some questions clinicians might find useful follow.

- When you were growing up did you, or your family, ever use any medicinal plants or herbal remedies to improve your health or treat an illness?
- How do you use herbs or herbal remedies in your home?
- Are you taking any herbs or herbal medicines now? If so, what are you trying to treat and do you think the herbs are working?

Document all patient responses in their medical chart and be alert for potential adverse effects and herb–drug interactions, as well as any therapeutic benefit.

If you suspect a possible adverse effect, report it to FDA Medwatch at www.fda.gov/medwAtch. Another excellent resource is to contact your local poison control center. The new nationwide toll-free number for poison control is 800-222-1222.

Herbal Medicine in Cardiology

Since specific cardiovascular disorders are covered in depth throughout this text, this section will explore in broad terms the physiological action of plants that are utilized in the treatment of cardiovascular disease. When examining botanicals, it is useful to start with a basic understanding of how they work. In some cases, scientific research has identified key compounds within the plant that account for its physiological effects; in other cases, there are multiple compounds working in harmony that account for the overall therapeutic effect, making the hunt for an "active compound" futile at best. More than 2000 years ago, practitioners observed the physiologic action of plants and were able to use them effectively even in the absence of isolating specific compounds or having a detailed understanding of cellular physiology. Plants were effectively used to treat congestive heart failure, or dropsy as it was once known, though it would be centuries before the cardioactive glycosides were identified and isolated.

Thus, this chapter is a blending of traditional wisdom and modern science, observation and reductionism. It is beyond the scope of this chapter to address all herbal actions, thus, it will focus only on those commonly considered when addressing cardiovascular disease.

While this chapter focuses on the use of botanical medicines, it should be implicitly understood that the use of these remedies must exist within a framework that includes appropriate diagnosis and other integrative treatment approaches dietary recommendations, mind–body therapies, manual medicine, or other methods that may promote wellness and healing in the patient. For the specific integrative management of hypertension, dyslipidemia, congestive heart failure, or another specific condition, please see the appropriate chapters in this book.

ANTI-HYPERTENSIVE HERBS

There are a number of herbs that may be used to address mild cases of hypertension. Without question, *Rauwolfia serpentina* is the best known and understood. The roots of Rauwolfia have been used in India for centuries to relieve anxiety and treat psychiatric disorders. The isolated alkaloid, reserpine, revolutionized the management of hypertension in the 1950s. Reserpine depletes adrenergic neurons of norepinephrine, resulting in decreased sympathetic tone and vasodilation and also likely explaining its traditional use for certain psychiatric illnesses. Studies show that reserpine plus a thiazide diuretic has similar efficacy to nifedipine or enalapril (Griebenow et al. 1997; Manyemba 1997). There are concerns for side effects from reserpine (e.g., sedation, depression) one study noted adverse effects in eleven patients (17.2%) in the reserpine/diuretic group and nine patients (14.3%) in the enalapril group (Griebenow et al. 1997). Low dose reserpine is used in a number of poorer countries when diuretics are not sufficient to control blood pressure. Rauwolfia is still used by some naturopathic practitioners in non-standardized preparations. Given the variability of alkaloid levels in the root, this practice should not be encouraged.

More commonly, herbalists will use diuretics to lower blood pressure (discussed later in this chapter). A recent metaanalysis concluded that garlic (*Allium sativum*) preparations modestly reduce blood pressure in patients with hypertension. One study showed that grape seed extract reduces systolic and diastolic blood pressure by twelve and eight points, respectively (Sivaprakasapillai et al. 2009). Other plants such as linden flower (*Tilia platyphllos*) and mistletoe (*Viscum album*) are also used. But it is hibiscus (*Hibiscus sabdariffa*) that is gaining the most attention. The calyces (the outer parts of the flower) are used in the traditional medicines of India, Africa, Mexico, and South America. Commonly sold in the American southwest and Mexico as *Flor de Jamaica*, studies show that hibiscus is an effective hypotensive agent. It is a reliable diuretic and inhibits calcium influx into vascular smooth muscle cells (Ajay et al. 2007; Wright et al. 2007, Ajay 2007). Two studies have shown the standardized extract (9.6 mg anthocyanins) to be as effective as captopril and lisinopril in lowering blood pressure (Herrera-Arellano et al. 2004; Herrera-Arellano et al. 2007). A study of type 2 diabetics found significant reduction in systolic blood pressure after one month (Mozaffari-Khosravi et al. 2009).

CARDIOACTIVE HERBS

A number of plants contain potent cardioactive glycosides, or substances that increase the contractility and efficiency of the heart without increasing the need for oxygen. Cardioactive herbs traditionally found prominence in the treatment of heart failure. The most widely known in this class include foxglove *(Digitalis purpurea),* white squill *(Urginea maritima)* and lily-of-the-valley *(Convallaria majalis).* Of these, foxglove has been most broadly used and its glycosides the most researched. In 1785 William Withering, an English physician, published a treatise on his treatment of heart patients with foxglove extract, also known as *digitalis,* though the medicinal use of the plant stretches originated centuries earlier. A Cochrane review of 13 studies (7896 participants) of the use of digitalis in the treatment of CHF concluded that "The literature indicates that digitalis may have a useful role in the treatment of patients with CHF who are in normal sinus rhythm. New trials are needed to elucidate the importance of digitalis dosage, and its usefulness in the era of beta-blockers" (Hood et al. 2004).

While less known than foxglove, the dried sliced bulbs from white squill have been used to treat heart failure for more than 3,500 years. The remedy appears in the Egyptian Ebers papyrus (1500 BCE) and Hippocrates described its use in 5 BCE. The cardioactive glycosides in squill are poorly absorbed across the GI tract, thus it carries less risk of cumulative toxicity.

Lily-of-the-valley has a long and proven reputation in herbal medicine for the treatment of cardiac complaints. It is similar to digitalis but less cumulative, associated with fewer adverse effects, and as it has less effect on the conduction system, it is preferred for CHF with bradycardia. The German Commission E monograph approves the use of the herb for "mild cardiac insufficiency, heart insufficiency due to old age, and chronic *cor pulmonale* (Blumenthal 1998)."

Cardiac glycosides have a low therapeutic index and care must be taken when prescribing them. Given the variability of glycoside levels in the herbs, standardized products are highly recommended. Only qualified health care professionals who are well-versed in the management of cardiac patients should administer these cardioactive botanicals.

CARDIAC TONICS

In general, herbalists focus on cardiac tonics when addressing the aging heart and treating mild hypertension and early heart failure. While there are a number of cardiac tonics, those that dominate the field come from great herbal traditions. From Euro-American tradition we have hawthorn (*Crataegus spp*), from Ayurveda there is arjuna (*Terminalia arjuna*), and from the Mediterranean and Middle East comes Bishop's weed (*Ammi visnaga*). Papyrus writings from ancient Egypt describe the use of *Ammi visnaga* for the treatment of asthma, painful kidney stones, and angina. Arjuna tree bark has been used to treat angina for more than 3,000 years (Narayana and Kumaraswamy 1996). Experimental studies show that it exerts significant positive inotropic and hypotensive effects, increasing coronary artery flow and protecting the myocardium against ischemic damage. It also has mild diuretic, antithrombotic, prostaglandin- enhancing, and hypolipidaemic activity (Dwivedi 2007).

Hawthorn, a flowering shrub in the rose family, has been used by physicians and herbalists for roughly 2,000 years, and its efficacy and uses have been particularly widely researched. Hawthorn is widely accepted in Europe as a treatment for mild cases of CHF and minor arrhythmias. While there have been many clinical studies, the largest was the Survival and Prognosis: Investigation of Crataegus Extract WS 1442 in Congestive Heart Failure (SPICE) trial. Conducted in 13 European countries, researchers randomized 2681 patients with NYHA class II-III heart failure and a left-ventricular ejection fraction (LVEF) <35% to receive either WS-1442 or placebo for two years, in addition to their standardized CHF therapy (Holubarsch et al. 2007). Overall, no beneficial effect was noted. However, in a prospectively planned subgroup analysis, patients who received hawthorn and had an LVEF of 25 to 35 percent showed a significantly reduced risk of sudden cardiac death from month 12 to month 24; no such signal emerged for patients with the poorest ventricular function. This is consistent with the notion that hawthorn is a tonic and that it is most beneficial in cases of modest dysfunction. It also speaks to its anti-arrhythmic action. Herbalists generally combine hawthorn with omega-3

Tea is good for the heart. A metaanalysis (Peters, Poole, and Arab 2001) of tea consumption in relation to stroke, myocardial infarction, and all coronary heart disease concluded that the incidence rate of myocardial infarction was estimated to decrease by 11% with an increase in tea consumption of 3 cups per day (95% CI: 0.79, 1.01) (1 cup = 237 ml) fatty acids, likely resulting in an additive effect. Importantly, the SPICE trial found no evidence of herb–drug interactions with any of the drugs taken by the participants. Cochrane reviewers concluded that when taken in totality, the evidence "suggests that there is a significant benefit in symptom control and physiologic outcomes from hawthorn extract as an adjunctive treatment for chronic heart failure" (Pittler, Guo, and Ernst 2008).

DIURETICS

Diuretics, both in conventional and herbal medicine, are used in the management of hypertension and heart failure. Many plants have diuretic effects, but those that have shown the most promise using modern scientific methods include parsley (*Petroselinum sativum*), horsetail (*Equisetium spp*), fennel (*Foeniculum vulgare*), hibiscus (*Hibiscus sabdariffa*), and the African traditional medicine *Spergularia purpurea*, with all showing diuretic and naturietic effects (Wright et al. 2007).

Parsley is both a culinary herb and an herbal medicine. While the herb can be used as a diuretic, the seeds are stronger. Parsley seed reduces the activity of Na+–K+ ATPase in both the renal cortex and medulla, leading to a reduction in sodium and potassium and resulting in osmotic water flow into the lumen and diuresis (Kreydiyyeh and Usta 2002). The German Commission E recognizes both the root and leaf of dandelion for the stimulation of diuresis (Blumenthal 1998), though studies indicate that the leaf is superior (Wright et al. 2007).

> *Diuretics are often used in conjunction with hawthorn for those with mild hypertension. Serum electrolytes should be periodically monitored.*

HYPOLIPIDEMIC PLANT PRODUCTS

Several plant and natural products that are well known for lipid management include plant sterols, psyllium (*Plantago ovata*), red yeast rice (*Monascus purpureus*), garlic (*Allium sativum*), guggul (*Commiphora mukul*), artichoke (*Cynara scolymus*), and policosanol. The most beneficial in clinical trials are phytosterols, psyllium, and red yeast rice. Phytosterols impair intestinal absorption of cholesterol, resulting in a 10–15 percent reduction in LDL-C with daily intakes of 2 to 3 grams (Plat and Mensink 2001). Plant sterols can be safely combined with statins, niacin, or red yeast rice, and both the American Heart Association and the National Cholesterol Education Program Expert Panel endorse their use. Psyllium and other soluble fibers should be encouraged for cardiovascular and overall health.

Red yeast rice products are prepared from cooked, non-glutinous white rice fermented by the yeast *Monascus purpureus*. Red yeast rice contains naturally occurring statins referred to as monocolins, as well as isoflavones and plant sterols (McCarthy 1998), all of which contribute to its lipid-lowering effects. A metaanalysis of randomized controlled trials reported that LDL-C is lowered by 27–32 percent, triglycerides are lowered by 27–38 percent, and HDL-C is raised by 15–22 percent (Liu et al. 2006). Quality control is a concern, however, as laboratory testing has found that red yeast products vary widely in their monocolin content and some contain the mycotoxin citrinin, which is nephrotoxic in animals (Consumerlabs 2009; Heber et al. 2001). Strict regulations and guidelines are needed to limit the total daily amount of monocolin and guarantee the absence of mycotoxins.

Red yeast rice can be a suitable choice in patients who do not tolerate statins. Given the variability in monocolin content, it is advisable to draw labs 8 to 10 weeks after initiation of therapy to determine effectiveness and possible impact on liver function. Coenzyme Q-10 is often recommended in conjunction with red yeast rice, as it is with prescription statin drugs.

NERVINE RELAXANTS

Nervine relaxants are those herbs that have a mild tranquilizing or calmative effect. As chronic stress and depression have both been associated with increased risk of cardiovascular disease, herbalists generally consider the addition of a nervine relaxant in their treatment protocol. Those that are typically used specifically for the cardiovascular system include motherwort (*Leonurus cardiaca*) and valerian (*Valeriana officinalis*). Motherwort is often included in formulae for hypertensive individuals with a nervous/stress component. The alkaloids in motherwort, stachydrine, and leonurine are mildly sedating and hypotensive. Research suggests that leonurine is an inhibitor of vascular smooth muscle tone, probably acting by inhibiting Ca2+ influx and the release of intracellular Ca2+ (Chen and Kwan 2001). Lavandulifolioside, another constituent, is responsible for the negative chronotropic and hypotensive effects reported with motherwort administration (Milkowska-Leyck, Filipek, and

Strzelecka 2002). Those with a "nervous heart" often find relief from palpitations and anxiety-provoked simple tachycardia.

Valerian is often considered in cases where hypertension is accompanied by stress and insomnia. It is unclear if the hypotensive activity reported by clinicians is due to the general calming effect of the herb or a direct vasodilatory effect. One study found that when valerian was given for seven days to individuals performing psychological stress tests, there was a significant decrease in systolic blood pressure and heart rate compared to controls (Cropley et al. 2002). Valerian has been used for at least 1000 years as a calming agent and sedative. It was officially categorized as a tranquilizer in the United States Pharmacopoeia from 1820 to 1942. Unlike conventional benzodiazepines, valerian is not addictive and has been shown to reduce anxiety (Andreatini et al. 2002) and total stress severity and to induce sleep (Wheatley 2001).

VASCULAR TONICS

Relieving the discomfort of varicose veins or chronic venous insufficiency (CVI) has long been under the herbalist's purview. The seeds and bark of the horse chestnut tree have been used as vascular tonics in Europe for at least 400 years. The seed was primarily used for the treatment of varicose veins, hemorrhoids, phlebitis, neuralgia, and rheumatic complaints. A metaanalysis of six trials found that horse chestnut extract was superior to placebo for CVI, and one trial indicated it is as effective as treatment with compression stockings (Pittler and Ernst 2006). Pycnogenol (patented trade name for a water extracted French maritime pine bark [*Pinus pinaster* ssp. *Atlantica*]) has been shown in clinical trials to rapidly improve CVI, and when taken both internally and applied topically, it heals venous ulcerations (Belcaro et al. 2005; Cesarone et al. 2006). Other vascular tonics include bilberry (*Vaccinium myrtillis*) and ginkgo (*Ginkgo biloba*).

Summary

When reviewing the history and contemporary research, it is clear that herbal medicines have played, and continue to play, a significant role in treating disease and improving health. Given the vast number of botanicals that have yet to be explored for their medicinal effects, it is likely that plants will continue to contribute to our understanding and management of cardiovascular disease. However, there remains much work to be done from "bench to bedside" to determine which botanicals are most efficacious and how they are best used in clinical practice. Unlike many pharmaceutical drugs, there are few long-term outcome studies using medicinal plants. While this chapter cites the clinical trials that are being conducted on herbal medicines for cardiovascular health, the research literature reflects only a very small percentage of plants that have potential benefit. There is a definite need for more rigorous and creative research in this area.

The following is a list of resources that clinicians may use to obtain current, authoritative information regarding the safe and effective use of herbal therapies.

GOVERNMENT WEB SITES

The National Center for Complementary and Alternative Medicine (NCCAM)

www.nccam.nih.gov

NCCAM provides information on complementary and alternative medicine for consumers, health care providers, and researchers. The site include fact sheets, an online newsletter, clinical trial information, and general health information in both English and Spanish.

Office of Dietary Supplements (ODS)

www.ods.od.nih.gov/index.aspx

This is a very helpful site with a wealth of free material available. In the "Quick Links" section you can access dietary supplement fact sheets and a link to the International Bibliographic Information on Dietary Supplements (IBIDS).

Health Canada

www.hc-sc.gc.ca

The Canadian government regulates natural health products by licensing those with proof of safety and efficacy. This is a helpful Web site that provides a list of products licensed in Canada and also contains a number of monographs.

OTHER WEB SITES

American Botanical Council

www.herbalgram.org

The American Botanical Council is a nonprofit and international member-based organization providing education using science-based and traditional information on herbal medicine. The Web site offers an excellent online bookstore and an "Herb Clip" service summarizing current research articles, as well as an educational resource section offering continuing education credits for health care professionals.

Natural Medicines Comprehensive Database

www.naturaldatabase.com

Th herbal monographs available on this site include extensive information about common uses, evidence of efficacy, safety, mechanisms, interactions, and dosage. This site also provides continuing medical education courses, information organized by medical condition, a listserv, and a section on supplement–drug interactions. This Web site is available by subscription only.

Natural Standard

www.naturalstandard.com

This subscription-only site is an independent collaboration of international clinicians and researchers who have created a database that can be searched by CAM subject or by medical condition. The quality of evidence is ranked for each supplement.

Consumer Labs

www.consumerlabs.com

This site, available by subscription, evaluates commercially available dietary supplements for composition, purity, bioavailability, and consistency of products.

REFERENCES

Ajay, M., H. J. Chai, A. M. Mustafa, A. H. Gilani, and M. R. Mustafa. 2007. Mechanisms of the anti-hypertensive effect of Hibiscus sabdariffa L. calyces. *J Ethnopharmacol* 109(3): 388–93.

Andreatini, R., V. A. Sartori, M. L. Seabra, and J. R. Leite. 2002. Effect of valepotriates (valerian extract) in generalized anxiety disorder: A randomized placebo-controlled pilot study. *Phytother Re.* 16(7): 650–54.

Aviram, M., and B. Fuhrman. 1998. Polyphenolic flavonoids inhibit macrophage-mediated oxidation of LDL and attenuate atherogenesis. *Atherosclerosis* 137: S45–S50.

Belcaro, G., M. R. Cesarone, B. M. Errichi, A. Ledda, A. Di Renzo, S. Stuard, M. Dugall, L. Pellegrini, P. Rohdewald, E. Ippolito, A. Ricci, M. Cacchio, I. Ruffini, F. Fano, M. Hosoi. 2005. Venous ulcers: microcirculatory improvement and faster healing with local use of Pycnogenol. *Angiology* 56(6): 699–705.

Bharani A., A. Ganguli, L. K. Mathur, Y. Jamra, and P. G. Raman. 2002. Efficacy of Terminalia arjuna in chronic stable angina: A double-blind, placebo-controlled, crossover study comparing *Terminalia arjuna* with isosorbide mononitrate. *Indian Heart Journal* 54(2): 170–75.

Blumenthal M, W. R. Busse, A. Goldberg, J. Gruenwald, T. Hall, C.W. Riggins, R. S. Rister, S. Klein. The Complete German Commission E Mongraphs: Therapeutic Guide to Herbal Medicines. Thieme Medical Publishers, 1998.

Cesarone, M. R., G. Belcaro, P. Rohdewald, L. Pellegrini, A. Ledda, G. Vinciguerra, A. Ricci, G. Gizzi, E. Ippolito, F. Fano, M Dugall, G. Acerbi, M. Cacchio, A. Di Renzo, M. Hosoi, S. Stuard, M. Corsi. 2006. Comparison of Pycnogenol and Daflon in treating chronic venous insufficiency: A prospective, controlled study. *Clin Appl Thromb Hemost.* 12(2): 205–12.

Chen, C. X., and C. Y. Kwan. 2001. Endothelium-independent vasorelaxation by leonurine, a plant alkaloid purified from Chinese motherwort. *Life Sci* 68(8): 953–60.

Consumer Labs. Product review: Red yeast rice supplements. http://www.consumer-lab.com/reviews/Red_Yeast_Rice_Supplements-Lovastatin_Monacolin/Red_Yeast_Rice/

Cropley, M., Z. Cave, J. Ellis, and R. W. Middleton. 2002. Effect of kava and valerian on human physiological and psychological responses to mental stress assessed under laboratory conditions. *Phytother Res* 16(1): 23–27.

De Smet PAGM, P.F. D'Arcy. Drug interactions with herbal and other non- orthodox remedies. In: D'Arcy PF, McElnay JC, Welling PG, Eds. Mechanisms of Drug Interactions. New York, NY: Springer-Verlag; 1996:327–352.

Dwivedi, S. 2007. *Terminalia arjuna* Wight & Arn. A useful drug for cardiovascular disorders. *J Ethnopharmacol* 114(2): 114–29.

Food and Drug Administration. Dietary supplement current good manufacturing practices and interim final rule facts. Federal Register 72(121): June 25 2007. Washington DC.

Gardiner, P., D. N. Sarma, T. Low Dog, M.L. Barrett, M.L. Chavez, R. Ko, G.B. Mahady, R. J. Marles, L.S. Pellicore, G.I. Giancaspro GI. 2008. The state of dietary supplement adverse event reporting in the United States. *Pharmacoepidemiol Drug Saf* 17(10): 962–70.

Griebenow, R., D. B. Pittrow, G. Weidinger, E. Mueller, E. Mutschler, and D. Welzel. 1997. Low-dose reserpine/thiazide combination in first-line treatment of hypertension: Efficacy and safety compared to an ACE inhibitor. *Blood Press* 6(5): 299–306.

Heber, D., A. Lembertas, Q.Y. Lu, S. Bowerman, V. L. Go. 2001. An analysis of nine proprietary Chinese red yeast rice dietary supplements: Implications of variability in chemical profile and contents. *J Altern Complement Med* 7(2): 133–39.

Herrera-Arellano, A., S. Flores-Romero, M. A. Chávez-Soto, and J. Tortoriello. 2004. Effectiveness and tolerability of a standardized extract from Hibiscus sabdariffa in patients with mild to moderate hypertension: a controlled and randomized clinical trial. *Phytomedicine* 11(5): 375–82.

Herrera-Arellano, A., J. Miranda-Sánchez, P. Avila-Castro, et al. 2007. Clinical effects produced by a standardized herbal medicinal product of Hibiscus sabdariffa on patients with hypertension. A randomized, double-blind, lisinopril-controlled clinical trial. *Planta Med* 73(1): 6–12.

Holubarsch, C. J. F., W. S. Colucci, T. Meinertz, et al. 2007. Crataegus extract WS 1442 postpones cardiac death in patients with congestive heart failure class NYHA II-III: A randomized, placebo-controlled, double-blind trial in 2681 patients. Paper presented at the American College of Cardiology 2007 Scientific Sessions, March 27, in New Orleans, Louisiana.

Hood, W. B., A. Dans, G. H. Guyatt, R. Jaeschke, and J. V. McMurray. 2004. Digitalis for treatment of congestive heart failure in patients in sinus rhythm (Cochrane Review). *CochraneDatabase Syst Rev* 2: CD002901.

Kaufman DW, J.P. Kelly, L. Rosenberg, T. E. Anderson, A. A. Mitchell. 2002. Recent patterns of medication use in the ambulatory adult population of the United States the Slone survey. *JAMA*. 287(3): 337–344.

Kreydiyyeh, S. I., and J. Usta. 2002. Diuretic effect and mechanism of action of parsley. *J Ethnopharmacol* 79(3): 353–57.

Liu J, J. Zhang, Y. Shi, S. Grimsgaard, T. Alraek, V. F nneb . 2006. Chinese red yeast rice (Monascus purpureus) for primary hyperlipidemia: a meta-analysis of randomized controlled trials. *Chin Med*. Nov 23; 1: 4.

Manyemba, J. 1997. A randomised crossover comparison of reserpine and sustained-release nifedipine in hypertension. *Cent Afr J Med* 43(12): 344–49.

McCarthy, M. 1998. FDA bans red yeast rice product. *Lancet* 351: 1637.

Milkowska-Leyck, K., B. Filipek, and H. Strzelecka. 2002. Pharmacological effects of lavandulifolioside from *Leonurus cardiaca*. *J Ethnopharmacol* 80(1): 85–90.

Mozaffari-Khosravi, H., B. A. Jalali-Khanabadi, M. Afkhami-Ardekani, F. Fatehi, and M. Noori-Shadkam. 2009. The effects of sour tea (*Hibiscus sabdariffa*) on hypertension in patients with type II diabetes. *J Hum Hypertens* 23(1): 48–54.

Narayana, A., and R. Kumaraswamy. 1996. A medico-historical review of Arjuna. *Bull Indian Inst Hist Med Hyderabad* 26(1–2): 1–10.

Peters, U., C. Poole, and L. Arab. 2001. Does tea affect cardiovascular disease? A meta-analysis. *American Journal of Epidemiology* 154(6): 495–503.

Pittler, M. H., and E. Ernst. 2006. Horse chestnut seed extract for chronic venous insufficiency. *Cochrane Database Syst Rev*. Jan. 25(1): CD003230.

Pittler, M. H., R. Guo, and E. Ernst. 2008. Hawthorn extract for treating chronic heart failure. *Cochrane Database Syst Rev* Jan 23(1): CD005312.

Plat, J., and R. P. Mensink. 2001. Effects of plant sterols and stanols on lipid metabolism and cardiovascular risk. *Nutr Metab Cardiovasc Dis* 11(1): 31–40.

Sivaprakasapillai, B., I. Edirisinghe, J. Randolph, F. Steinberg, and T. Kappagoda. 2009. Effect of grape seed extract on blood pressure in subjects with the metabolic syndrome. *Metabolism* [Epub ahead of print].

Wheatley, D. 2001. Stress-induced insomnia treated with kava and valerian: singly and in combination. *Hum Psychopharmacol* 16(4): 353–56.

Wright, C. I., et al. 2007. Herbal medicines as diuretics: A review of the scientific evidence. *J Ethnopharmacol* 114(1): 1–31.

4

An Aspirin a Day Is Even Better than an Apple a Day!

JAMES E. DALEN

KEY CONCEPTS

- Aspirin is effective in the primary and secondary prevention of myocardial infarction and ischemic stroke.
- The primary side effect of aspirin is bleeding. As compared to placebo, aspirin, at doses from 81 to 325 mg/day, is associated with an excess of one to three cases of major bleeding per 1,000 patients per year.
- The incidence of major bleeding is not dose related at doses from 81 to 325 mg/day.
- Doses less than 162 mg/day have been ineffective in preventing stroke and myocardial infarction in 6 primary prevention trials.
- The author recommends a dose of 162 mg (two baby aspirin per day) for the primary and secondary prevention of stroke and myocardial infarction.

■

Daily aspirin consumption for the prevention of myocardial infarction and stroke is a classic example of an unconventional therapy that has become conventional therapy.

Aspirin was first synthesized in 1853 by Bayer. It began to be used for the treatment of rheumatism in 1899 (Dalen 1991). The first report suggesting that aspirin may have a cardiovascular indication was a paper by Craven published in 1950. He reported that aspirin prevented heart attacks. Six years later, Craven reported that aspirin also prevented strokes (1956). Craven based his reports on clinical observations and a clinical trial without controls. As a busy general practitioner, he noted an increased incidence of bleeding in patients in whom he had performed a tonsillectomy. He noted that the increase in bleeding occurred about the same time that he began to use aspergum (aspirin) as a post-operation pain reliever. He concluded that aspirin was a mild anticoagulant. At that time, patients with myocardial infarction were treated with dicumarol, an oral anticoagulant. He reasoned that dicumarol might prevent heart attacks in those at increased risk. He worried that dicumarol would cause excess bleeding; but his newly discovered mild anticoagulant, aspirin, might just do the trick. In 1948 he advised all his male patients aged 45 to 65 to take 10 to 30 grains (650 mg to 2 grams) of aspirin a day. After 2 years, he noted that none of his 400 patients had suffered a myocardial infarction (Craven, 1950). He continued his trial, and in 1953 he reported that not a single member of his study group of 1465 healthy overweight and sedentary men had suffered a myocardial infarction (Craven, 1953). He did not have a control group, and there was limited statistical analysis. He stated that "in such a large group of subjects of this type most likely to experience coronary episodes it is—to say the least—remarkable that all remained healthy and active" (Craven, 1953).

In 1953, Craven decreased the aspirin dose to 325 mg per day. In 1956 he reported that none of his now 8000 patients taking aspirin had suffered a myocardial infarction and that none had suffered a stroke or transient ischemic attack (TIA)—so he reported that aspirin also prevents strokes (Craven, 1956).

After I published an article in 1991 (Dalen 1991) about Craven's reports I received a call from a *New York Times* reporter asking for me for more information about Dr. Craven. I suggested that he call the local medical society in Glendale, California to determine if any physicians remembered Craven. He located two physicians who knew Craven. One said that Craven was a genius, the other said that he was crazy! I do not know if he was a genius, but he certainly was right about aspirin.

After hundreds of randomized clinical trials it has become clear that aspirin is effective in the primary and secondary prevention of stroke and myocardial infarction. (Dalen, 1991) A metaanalysis of more than 100 randomized trials found that aspirin prevents vascular death by 15 percent, and non-fatal vascular events (myocardial infarction and stroke) by 30 percent (Antithrombotic Trialists Collaboration 2002). Not bad for an over-the-counter drug costing pennies!

Aspirin inhibits platelet activation by inactivating platelet COX-I activity. The inhibition of platelet activation decreases the incidence of thrombosis in atherosclerotic coronary and cerebral arteries. Aspirin does not decrease the incidence of atherosclerosis; it decreases the incidence of myocardial infarction and stroke in patients who have atherosclerosis involving the coronary or cerebral arteries. Aspirin is not effective in preventing venous thrombosis.

At present more than 30 million Americans, including 49 percent of all Americans ages 65 and older, take aspirin for prevention of stroke and myocardial infarction. Aspirin therapy for prevention has evolved into conventional, mainstream therapy.

Complications of Aspirin

The primary complication of aspirin therapy is bleeding, especially gastrointestinal bleeding. The incidence of minor bleeding increases with the dose of aspirin. However, in doses ranging from 50 mg/day to 325 mg/day, the incidence of major bleeding is not related to the dose of aspirin. The excess of major bleeding compared to placebo is one to three cases per 1000 patients per year (Berger et al. 2009; Patrono et al. 2008). In five placebo-controlled trials involving 368,000 patient years of aspirin therapy, there was no difference in the risk of fatal bleeding between aspirin (50–500 mg/day) and placebo, as shown in Table 4.1 (Collaborative Group of the Primary Prevention Project 2001; Hansson et al. 1998; Peto et al. 1988; Ridker et al. 2005; Steering Committee of the Physicians' Health Study Group 1989).

Contraindications to Aspirin

The only absolute contraindications to aspirin are a documented allergy to aspirin or non-steroidal antiinflammatory drugs, or the presence of active

Table 4.1. Fatal Bleeding During Aspirin Therapy

			Fatal Bleeds	
Study	Dose/Day	Pt/years	ASA	Placebo
WHS, 2005	50 mg	199,380	2	3
HOT, 1998	75 mg	17,850	7	8
PPP, 2001	100 mg	80,928	1	3
PHS, 1989	160 mg	55,175	1	0
UK, 1988	500 mg	15,41	3	3
TOTAL			14	17

WHS = Women's Health Study HOT = Hypertension Optimal Treatment Study PPP = Primary Prevention Project PHS = Physician's Health Study UK = British Physician Study bleeding. The relative contraindications are a history of peptic ulcer or GI bleeding.

What is the Right Dose?

The appropriate dose for primary and secondary prevention of stroke remains controversial. All agree that it is 325 mg/day or less. However, some suggest 81mg (one baby aspirin), some say 162 mg (two baby aspirin), and some suggest 325 mg (one adult aspirin). Others suggest any dose from 81 to 325 mg. Determining the recommended dose should not be so difficult. The price of aspirin is minimal and there is no difference in the incidence of major bleeding in doses ranging from 81 to 325 mg.

There is some evidence that the dose for secondary prevention in patients with a history of coronary artery disease or stroke is less than the dose required for primary prevention The European Stroke Prevention Study found that 50 mg of aspirin per day decreased the risk of recurrent stroke by 18% in patients with a history of stroke or TIA. (Diener, 1996).

In patients with stable angina pectoris Juul-Moller reported a 34% reduction in myocardial infarction (MI) or death as compared to placebo in patients treated with 75 mg of aspirin daily. (Juul-Moller, 1992.) In a study of 796 men with unstable angina there was a 31% reduction in myocardial infarction or sudden death with 75 mg of aspirin per day. (RISC Group,1990). Other studies of secondary prevention in patients with a history of stroke or myocardial, infarction have found doses of 160 mg or 300 mg per day to be effective.(Lewis, 1983; ISIS-2, 1988; CAST,1997).

The most commonly recommended dose for primary prevention of myocardial infarction and stroke is 81 mg/day (Bhatt et al. 2008). I believe that this dose is too low. Doses less than 162 mg/day failed to prevent stroke and myocardial infarction in six primary prevention trials (Collaborative Group of the Primary Prevention Project 2001; Hansson et al. 1998; Ogawa et al. 2008; Ridker et al. 2005; Belch et al. 2008; Fowkes. 2009.

Strong evidence that an aspirin dose of 162 mg/day is effective in the primary prevention of myocardial infarction was reported by the US Physicians' Health study. (Physicians' Health Study Group, 1989). More than 20,000 US physicians were randomized to 325 mg of aspirin every other day or placebo. After five years of follow-up there was a 44% reduction in MIs in those taking aspirin.

I am convinced that the optimal dose for primary and secondary prevention of myocardial infarction and stroke in men and women is 162 mg/day (Dalen 2010) . This can be given as 2 baby aspirin a day, one-half adult aspirin a day, or one adult aspirin every other day; whichever is most convenient for the patient. There is no clear evidence that buffered aspirin or enteric-coated aspirin are less effective or have fewer side effects than regular aspirin.

What about Aspirin Resistance?

Some patients who have been prescribed long-term aspirin therapy develop myocardial infarction or stroke. When this occurs does it mean treatment failure, or does it indicate that the patient is resistant to aspirin? Or, is there another explanation?

Treatment failure is certainly a reasonable explanation. No therapy, conventional or unconventional, is 100 percent effective. Patients have myocardial infarction and/or stroke despite effective therapy of hypertension or hyperlipidemia, so why should aspirin therapy be any different?

Some suggest that the explanation for the occurrence of vascular event in patients prescribed aspirin is aspirin resistance, that is, the failure of aspirin to suppress thromboxane generation and thus not prevent platelet aggregation. Some have suggested that all 30 million patients taking aspirin therapy should be tested for aspirin resistance.

The gold standard for determining aspirin's effect on platelets is optical aggregometry, also called light transmission aggregometry. Several other platelet function tests that can be performed at the bedside are also available (Dalen 2007).

Unfortunately, these tests are not concordant. The incidence of aspirin resistance utilizing optical aggregometry is less than 1 percent in most reports. The incidence with the two bedside tests is much higher; in the range of 20 to 30 percent (Dalen 2007).

Reports that patients with laboratory evidence of aspirin resistance are at increased risk of myocardial infarction or stroke are inconclusive. The clinical relevance of aspirin resistance is uncertain. I agree with the recent recommendation from the American College of Chest Physicians that routine testing for aspirin resistance is not indicated (Patrono et al. 2008).

There is a third explanation for the occurrence of stroke or myocardial infarction in patients prescribed aspirin: noncompliance (Dalen 2007). A very significant study reported on 190 patients with myocardial infarction who had been prescribed 81 to 325 mg aspirin/day. Seventeen (9 percent) were aspirin resistant by light aggregometry. When the 17 were questioned, 10 admitted that they were not taking the aspirin. When the test was repeated after the 17 were observed ingesting 325 mg aspirin, only one patient was found to be aspirin resistant (Schwartz, 2005).

Several other studies have confirmed the findings of Schwartz: aspirin resistance is very rare in patients who actually take aspirin. Noncompliance is the most common explanation for aspirin resistance as measured by laboratory tests. The most common cause of stroke or myocardial infarction in patients who are compliant with aspirin therapy is treatment failure. There is no evidence that myocardial infarction or stroke occurring in patients prescribed aspirin is due to aspirin resistance.

Who should take Aspirin?

In the absence of contraindications, all patients with evidence of coronary artery disease— including patients with a history of myocardial infarction, coronary artery bypass surgery, angioplasty, or angina, and patients in whom coronary disease has been diagnosed by angiography—should take 162 mg aspirin/day for their entire lives. Lifelong aspirin therapy is also indicated in patients with a history of ischemic stroke, and patients with peripheral arterial disease. Aspirin is also recommended in patients who are at increased risk of having asymptomatic coronary artery disease. Patients with multiple risk factors—including diabetes, hypertension, hypercholesterolemia, and smoking—should take aspirin unless there are contraindications.

In addition, age is a risk factor for coronary artery disease in the United States. One should consider aspirin therapy in men age 50 and older, and postmenopausal women.

In patients with atrial fibrillation, aspirin (325 mg/day) is indicated when there are contraindications to long-term warfarin therapy. Aspirin decreases the incidence of stroke and arterial embolism in patients with atrial fibrillation by 21 percent, compared to 68 percent with warfarin therapy (Singer et al. 2008).

REFERENCES

Antithrombotic Trialists Collaboration. 2002. Collaborative meta-analysis of randomized trof antiplatelet therapy for prevention of death, myocardial infarction and stroke in high-risk patients. *BMJ* 324: 71–86.

Berger, J. S., Krantz, M. J., Kittelson, J. M. & Hiatt, W. R. 2009. Aspirin for the prevention of cardiovascular events in patients with peripheral artery disease: a meta-analysis of randomized trials. *JAMA*, 301: 1909–19.

Bhatt, D. L., Scheiman, J., Abraham, N. S., Antman, E. M., Chan, F. K., Furberg,C. D., Johnson, D. A., Mahaffey, K. W., Quigley, E. M., Harrington, R. A., Bates, E. R.,

Bridges, C. R., Eisenberg, M. J., Ferrari, V. A., Hlatky, M. A., Kaul, S., Lindner, J. R., Moliterno, D. J., Mukherjee, D., Schofield, R. S., Rosenson, R. S., Stein, J. H., Weitz, H. H. & Wesley, D. J. 2008. ACCF/ACG/AHA 2008 expert consensus document on reducing the gastrointestinal risks of antiplatelet therapy and NSAID use: a report of the American College of Cardiology Foundation Task Force on Clinical Expert Consensus Documents. *J Am Coll Cardiol,* 52: 1502–17.

CAST (Chinese Acute Stroke Trial) Collaborative Group. 1997. CAST: randomised placebo-controlled trial of early aspirin use in 20,000 patients with acute ischaemic stroke. *Lancet* 349: 1641–1649.

Collaborative Group of the Primary Prevention Project (PPP). 2001. Low-dose aspirin and vitamin E in people at cardiovascular risk: A randomised trial in general practice. *Lancet* 357: 89–95.

Craven, L. L. 1950. Acetylsalicylic acid, possible preventive of coronary thrombosis. *Ann West Med Surg* 4: 95.

Craven, L. L. 1953. Experiences with aspirin (acetylsalicylic acid) in the nonspecific prophylaxis of coronary thrombosis. *Miss Valley Med J* 75: 38.

Craven, L. L. 1956. Prevention of coronary and cerebral thrombosis. *Miss Valley Med J* 78: 213.

Dalen, J. E. 1991. An apple a day or an aspirin a day? *Arch Intern Med* 151: 1066–69.

Dalen, J. E. (2006). Aspirin to prevent heart attack and stroke: what's the right dose? *Am J Med* 119: 198–202.

Dalen, J. E. (2007). Aspirin resistance: Is it real? Is it clinically significant? *Am J Med* 120: 1–4.

Dalen J. E. 2010. Aspirin for the primary prevention of stroke and myocardial infarction: ineffective or wrong dose? *Am J Med* 123: 101–102.

Diener, H. C., Cunha, L., Forbes, C., Sivenius, J., Smets, P. & Lowenthal, A. 1996. European Stroke Prevention Study. 2. Dipyridamole and acetylsalicylic acid in the secondary prevention of stroke. *J Neurol Sci,* 143: 1–13.

Fowkes G. 2009. Aspirin for asymptomatic atherosclerosis trial. Presented at European Society of Cardiology 2009 Congress, August 30, 2009, Barcelona, Spain.

Hansson, L., Zanchetti, A., Carruthers, S. G., Dahlof, B., Elmfeldt, D., Julius, S., Menard, J., Rahn, K. H., Wedel, H. & Westerling, S. 1998. Effects of intensive blood-pressure lowering and low-dose aspirin in patients with hypertension: principal results of the Hypertension Optimal Treatment (HOT) randomised trial. HOT Study Group. *Lancet,* 351: 1755–62.

ISIS-2 (Second International Study of Infarct Survival) Collaborative Group. 1988. Randomised trial of intravenous streptokinase, oral aspirin, both, or neither among 17,87 cases of suspercted acute myocardial infarction: ISIS-2. *Lancet* 332: 349–360.

Juul-Moller, S., Edvardsson, N., Jahnmatz, B., Rosen, A., Sorensen, S. & Omblus, R. 1992. Double-blind trial of aspirin in primary prevention of myocardial infarction in patients with stable chronic angina pectoris. The Swedish Angina Pectoris Aspirin Trial (SAPAT) Group. *Lancet,* 340: 1421–5.

Lewis, H. D., JR., Davis, J. W., Archibald, D. G., Steinke, W. E., Smitherman, T. C., Doherty, J. E., 3rd, Schnaper, H. W., Lewinter, M. M., Linares, E., Pouget, J. M., Sabharwal, S. C., Chesler, E. & DEMOTS, H. 1983. Protective effects of aspirin against acute myocardial infarction and death in men with unstable angina. Results of a Veterans Administration Cooperative Study. *N Engl J Med*, 309: 396–403.

Ogawa, H., Nakayama, M., Morimoto, T., Uemura, S., Kanauchi, M., Doi, N., Jinnouchi, H., Sugiyama, S. & Saito, Y. 2008. Low-dose aspirin for primary prevention of atherosclerotic events in patients with type 2 diabetes: a randomized controlled trial. *JAMA*, 300: 2134–41.

Patrono, C., C. Baigent, J. Hirsh, and G. Roth. 2008. Antiplatelet drugs. American College of Chest Physicians Evidence-based Clinical Practice Guidelines. (8th Edition). *Chest*, 1336: 199S–233S.

Peto, R., Gray, R., Collins, R., Wheatley, K., Hennekens, C., Jamrozik, K., Warlow, C., Hafner, B., Thompson, E., Norton, S. & et al. 1988. Randomised trial of prophylactic daily aspirin in British male doctors. *Br Med J (Clin Res Ed)*, 296: 313–6.

Ridker, P. M., Cook, N. R., Lee, I. M., Gordon, D., Gaziano, J. M., Manson, J. E., Hennekens, C. H. & Buring, J. E. 2005. A randomized trial of low-dose aspirin in the primary prevention of cardiovascular disease in women. *N Engl J Med*, 352: 1293–304.

RISC Group. 1990. Risk of myocardial infarction and death during treatment with low dose aspirin and intravenous heparin in men with unstable coronary artery disease. *Lancet* 336: 827–830.

Schwartz, K. A., Schwartz, D. E., Ghosheh, K., Reeves, M. J., BarbeR, K. & Defranco, A. 2005. Compliance as a critical consideration in patients who appear to be resistant to aspirin after healing of myocardial infarction. *Am J Cardiol*, 95: 973–5.

Singer, D. E., Albers, G. W., Dalen, J. E., Fang, M. C., Go, A. S., Halperin, J. L., Lip, G. Y. & Manning, W. J. 2008. Antithrombotic therapy in atrial fibrillation: American College of Chest Physicians Evidence-Based Clinical Practice Guidelines (8th Edition). *Chest*, 133: 546S–592S.

Steering Committee of the Physicians' Health Study Group. 1989. Final report of the aspirin component of the ongoing physicians' health study. *N Engl J Med* 321: 129–35.

5

Metabolic Cardiology

STEPHEN T. SINATRA

KEY CONCEPTS

- Attention to the energy demands of diseased hearts is often missing in conventional cardiology practice.
- Disease states and the use of certain medications are associated with depletion of key factors needed for cardiac energy production.
- Metabolic support with D-ribose, Coenzyme Q10, L-carnitine, and magnesium can be important for the maintenance of myocardial energy reserves.

■

Optimal cardiovascular function is dependent on maintaining adequate energy reserves. Metabolic cardiology highlights the importance of sustaining key enzymatic and biochemical reactions that revitalize the energy charge in oxidative ischemic or hypoxic hearts (Sinatra 2005; 2009).

Efforts to support the metabolic needs of the heart have well documented benefits, yet are not known to most cardiologists. The therapies to be outlined carry the added advantage of an excellent safety profile a key factor in light of the finding that the fourth leading cause of death in the United States is properly prescribed medications (Lazaron, Pomeranz, and Corey 1989). The importance of supporting energy production in myocytes and the preservation of the mitochondria in these cells will be the focus of this discussion.

Cardiac Energy Metabolism: Bench to Bedside

Bioenergetics is the study of energy transformation in living organisms. Understanding the distinction between the concentration of ATP in the cell and the efficiency of ATP turnover and recycling is central to our appreciation of cellular bioenergetics. It is now widely accepted that one characteristic of the failing heart is the persistent and progressive loss of energy. The requirement for energy to support the systolic and diastolic work of the heart is absolute. Therefore, a disruption in cardiac energy metabolism, and the energy supply/demand mismatch that results, can be identified as the pivotal factor contributing to the inability of failing hearts to meet the hemodynamic requirements of the body. In her landmark book, *ATP and the Heart*, Joanne Ingwall, PhD, describes the metabolic process associated with the progression of CHF, and identifies the mechanisms that lead to a persistent loss of cardiac energy reserves as the disease process unfolds (2002).

The heart consumes more energy per gram than any other organ, and the chemical energy that fuels the heart comes primarily from adenosine triphosphate, or ATP (Figure 5.1). The chemical energy held in ATP is resident in the phosphoryl bonds, with the greatest amount of energy residing in the outermost bond holding the ultimate phosphoryl group to the penultimate group. When energy is required to provide the chemical driving force to a cell, this ultimate phosphoryl bond is broken and chemical energy is released. The cell then converts this chemical energy to mechanical energy to do work.

The consumption of ATP in the enzymatic reactions that release cellular energy yields the metabolic byproducts adenosine diphosphate (ADP) and inorganic phosphate (Pi) (Figure 5.2). A variety of metabolic mechanisms have evolved within the cell to provide rapid re-phosphorylation of ADP to restore ATP levels and maintain the cellular energy pool. But, these metabolic mechanisms can easily become disrupted, tipping the balance in a manner that creates a chronic energy supply/demand mismatch that results in an energy deficit.

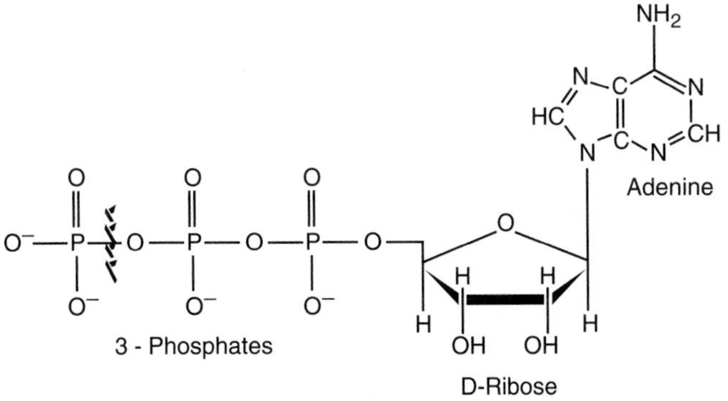

FIGURE 5.1. ATP is composed of D-ribose, adenine, and three phosphate groups. Breaking the chemical bond attaching the last phosphate group to ATP releases chemical energy that is converted to mechanical energy to perform cellular work.

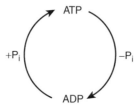

FIGURE 5.2. When ATP is used the remaining byproducts are adenosine diphosphate (ADP) and inorganic phosphate (Pi). ADP and Pi can then recombine to form ATP in the cellular processes of energy recycling. When oxygen and food (fuel) is available, energy recycling occurs unimpeded millions of times per second in every cell in the body. Lack of oxygen or mitochondrial dysfunction severely limits the cell's ability to recycle its energy supply.

The normal non-ischemic heart is capable of maintaining a stable ATP concentration despite large fluctuations in workload and energy demand. In a normal heart, the rate of cellular ATP synthesis via re-phosphorylation of ADP closely matches ATP utilization. The primary site of cellular ATP re-phosphorylation is the mitochondria, where fatty acid and carbohydrate metabolic products flux down the oxidative phosphorylation pathways. ATP recycling can also occur in the cytosol via the glycolytic pathway of glucose metabolism, but in normal hearts this pathway accounts for only about 10 percent of ATP turnover.

ATP levels are also maintained through the action of creatine kinase in a reaction that transfers a high-energy phosphate creatine phosphate (PCr) to ADP to yield ATP and free creatine. Because the creatine kinase reaction is approximately 10 times faster than ATP synthesis via oxidative phosphorylation, creatine phosphate acts as a buffer to assure a consistent availability of ATP in times of acute high metabolic demand. Although there is approximately twice as much creatine phosphate in the cell as ATP, there is still only enough to supply energy to drive about 10 heartbeats, making the maintenance of high levels of ATP availability critical to cardiac function. The content of ATP in heart cells progressively falls in CHF, frequently reaching and then stabilizing at levels that are 25 percent to 30 percent lower than normal (Ingwall 2004; 2006). The fact that ATP falls in the failing heart means that the metabolic network responsible for maintaining the balance between energy supply and demand is no longer functioning normally. It is well established that oxygen deprivation in ischemic hearts contributes to the depletion of myocardial energy pools, but the loss of energy substrates in the failing heart is a unique example of chronic metabolic failure in the myocardium.

One of the mechanisms responsible for energy depletion in heart failure is the loss of energy substrates and the delay in their resynthesis. In conditions where energy demand outstrips supply, ATP is consumed at a rate that is faster than it can be restored via oxidative phosphorylation or the alternative pathways of ADP re-phosphorylation. The cell has a continuing need for energy, so it will use all its ATP stores and then break down the by-product, adenosine diphosphate (ADP), to pull the remaining energy out of this compound as well, resulting in the production of adenosine monophosphate (AMP).

Since a growing concentration of AMP is incompatible with sustained cellular function, it is quickly broken apart and the by-products are washed out of the cell. The net result of this process is a depletion of the cellular pool of energy substrates. When the by-products of AMP catabolism are washed out of the cell, they are lost forever (Figure 5.3). It takes a long time to replace these lost energy substrates, even if the cell is fully perfused with oxygen again. This reduction in energy is like a depleted car battery struggling to start the engine. In diseased hearts the energy pool depletion via this mechanism can

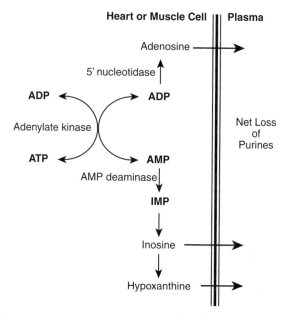

FIGURE 5.3. When the cellular concentration of ATP falls and ADP levels increase, two molecules of ADP can combine. This reaction provides one ATP, giving the cell additional energy, and one AMP. The enzyme adenylate kinase (also called myokinase) catalyzes this reaction. The AMP formed in this reaction is then degraded and the byproducts are washed out of the cell. The loss of these purines decreases the cellular energy pool and is a metabolic disaster to the cell.

be significant, reaching levels that exceed 40 percent in ischemic heart disease and 30 percent in heart failure.

Under high workload conditions, even normal hearts display a minimal loss of energy substrates. These substrates must be restored via the de novo pathway of ATP synthesis. This pathway is slow and costly in terms of energy, requiring consumption of six high-energy phosphates to yield one newly synthesized ATP molecule. The slow speed and high energy cost of de novo synthesis highlights the importance of cellular mechanisms designed to preserve energy pools. In normal hearts the salvage pathways are the predominant means by which the ATP pool is maintained.

While de novo synthesis of ATP proceeds at a rate of approximately 0.02 nM/min/g in the heart, the salvage pathways operate at a rate that is 10 times higher (Manfredi and Holmes 1985). The function of both the de novo and salvage pathways of ATP synthesis is limited by the cellular availability of 5-phosphoribosyl-1-pyrophosphate, or PRPP (Figure 5.4). PRPP initiates these synthetic reactions, and is the sole compound capable of donating the D-ribose-5-phosphate moiety required to re-form ATP and preserve the energy pool. In muscle tissue, including that of the heart, formation of PRPP is slow and rate limited, impacting the rate of ATP restoration via the de novo and salvage pathways.

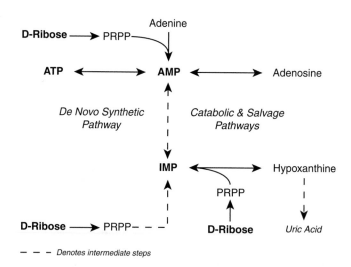

FIGURE 5.4. Replacing lost energy substrates through the de novo pathway of energy synthesis begins with D-ribose. D-ribose can also "salvage" AMP degradation products capturing them before they can be washed out of the cell. Both the de novo and salvage pathways of energy synthesis are rate limited by the availability of D-ribose in the cell.

Energy Starvation in the Failing Heart

The chronic mechanism explaining the loss of ATP in CHF is decreased ATP synthesis relative to ATP demand. In part, the disparity between energy supply and demand in hypertrophied and failing hearts is associated with a shift in relative contribution of fatty acid versus glucose oxidation to ATP synthesis. The major consequence of the complex readjustment toward carbohydrate metabolism is that the total capacity for ATP synthesis decreases. At the same time, the demand for ATP continually increases as hearts work harder to circulate blood in the face of the increased filling pressures that are associated with congestive heart failure and cardiac dilation.

The net result of this energy supply/demand mismatch is a decrease in the absolute concentration of ATP in the failing heart, and this decrease in absolute ATP level is reflected in a lower energy reserve in the failing and/or hypertrophied heart. A declining energy reserve is directly related to heart function, with diastolic function being the first to be affected, followed by systolic function, and finally global performance (Figure 5.5). In ischemic or hypoxic hearts, the cell's ability to match ATP supply and demand is disrupted leading

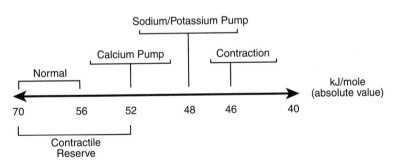

FIGURE 5.5. Cellular energy levels can be measured as the free energy of hydrolysis of ATP, or the amount of chemical energy available to fuel cellular function. Healthy, normal hearts contain enough energy to fuel all the cellular functions, with a contractile reserve for use in emergency. Cellular mechanisms used in calcium management and cardiac relaxation (Diastole) require the highest level of available energy. Sodium/potassium pumps needed to maintain ion balance are also significant energy consumers. The cellular mechanisms associated with contraction require the least amount of cellular energy. Thus, when ATP levels drop, and since more energy is required to break calcium bonds, diastolic dysfunction deteriorates. Therefore, filling the heart with blood requires more ATP than emptying the heart.

to both depletion of the cardiac energy pool and dysfunction in mitochondrial ATP turnover mechanisms. When ATP levels drop, diastolic heart function deteriorates.

Diastolic dysfunction is an early sign of myocardial failure, despite the presence of normal systolic function and preserved ejection fraction. High concentrations of ATP are required to activate calcium pumps necessary to facilitate cardiac relaxation and promote diastolic filling. This observation leads to the conclusion that, in absolute terms, more ATP is needed to fill the heart than to empty it, consistent with Starling's Law, which requires more energy in diastole than in systole. This absolute requirement for ATP in the context of cardiac conditions in which energy is depleted makes a metabolic therapeutic approach such a reasonable intervention.LaPlace's law confirms that pressure overload increases energy consumption in the face of abnormalities in energy supply. In failing hearts these energetic changes become more profound as left ventricle remodeling proceeds (Gourine et al. 2004; Hu et al. 2006; Ye et al. 2001),[8] but they are also evident in the early development of the disease (Maslov et al. 2007). It has additionally been found that similar adaptations occur in the atrium, with energetic abnormalities constituting a component of the substrate for atrial fibrillation in CHF (Cha et al. 2003).

Left ventricular hypertrophy is initially an adaptive response to chronic pressure overload, but it is ultimately associated with a 10-fold greater likelihood of subsequent chronic CHF. While metabolic abnormalities are persistent in CHF and left ventricular hypertrophy, at least half of all patients with left ventricular hypertrophy-associated heart failure have preserved systolic function, a condition referred to as a diastolic heart failure.

Oxidative phosphorylation is directly related to oxygen consumption, which is not decreased in patients with pressure-overload left ventricular hypertrophy (Bache et al. 1999). Metabolic energy defects, instead, relate to the absolute size of the energy pool and the kinetics of ATP turnover through oxidative phosphorylation and creatine kinase. Dysfunctional ATP kinetics is similar in both systolic and diastolic heart failure, and may be both an initiating event and a consequence.Inadequate ATP availability would be expected to initiate and accentuate the adverse consequences of abnormalities in energy-dependent pathways. Factors that increase energy demand, such as adrenergic stimulation and systolic overload, exaggerate the energetic deficit. Consequently, the hypertrophied heart is more metabolically susceptible to stressors such as increased chronotropic and inotropic demand, and ischemia. In humans, this metabolic deficit is shown to be greater in compensated left ventricular hypertrophy (with or without concomitant CHF) than in dilated cardiomyopathy (Smith et al. 2006; Weiss, Gerstenblith, and Bottomley 2005).

Hypertensive heart disease alone was not shown to contribute to alterations in high energy phosphate metabolism, but it can contribute to left ventricular hypertrophy and diastolic dysfunction, which can later alter cardiac energetics (Beer et al. 2002; Lamb et al. 1999). Further, for a similar clinical degree of heart failure, volume overload hypertrophy does not, but pressure overload does, induce significant high-energy phosphate impairment (Neubauer et al. 1997).

Type 2 diabetes has also been shown to contribute to altering myocardial energy metabolism early in the onset of diabetes, and these alterations in cardiac energetics may contribute to left ventricular functional changes (Diamant et al. 2003). The effect of age on progression of energetic altering has also been reviewed, with results of both human (Schocke et al. 2003) and animal (Perings et al. 2000) studies, suggesting that increasing age plays a moderate role in the progressive changes in cardiac energy metabolism that correlates to diastolic dysfunction, left ventricular mass, and ejection fraction.

Cardiac energetics also provide important prognostic information in patients with heart failure, and determining the myocardial contractile reserve has been suggested as a method of differentiating which patients would most likely respond to cardiac resynchronization therapy (CRT) seeking to reverse LV remodeling (Ypenburg et al. 2007). Patients with a positive contractile reserve are more likely to respond to CRT and reverse remodeling of the left ventricle. Non-responders show a negative contractile reserve, suggesting increased abnormality in cardiac energetics.

Taken together, results of clinical and laboratory studies confirm that energy metabolism in CHF and left ventricular hypertrophy is of vital clinical importance. Impaired diastolic filling and stroke volume limit the delivery of oxygen-rich blood to the periphery. This chronic oxygen deprivation forces peripheral muscles to adjust and down-regulate energy turnover mechanisms, a contributing cause of symptoms of fatigue, dyspnea and muscle discomfort associated with CHF.

The following discussion will review metabolic interventions intended to preserve myocardial energy substrates. Therapies to be discussed include: D-ribose, Coenzyme Q10, L-carnitine, and magnesium.

ENERGY NUTRIENTS FOR CONGESTIVE HEART FAILURE

D-ribose (Ribose)

The effect of the pentose monosaccharide, D-ribose, in cardiac energy metabolism has been studied since the 1970s, with clinical studies describing its value as an adjunctive therapy in ischemic heart disease first appearing in 1991. Ribose is a naturally occurring simple carbohydrate that is found in every living tissue, and natural synthesis occurs via the oxidative pentose phosphate pathway of glucose metabolism. But the poor expression of gate-keeper enzymes glucose-6-phosphate dehydrogenase and 6-phosphogluconate dehydrogenase limit its natural production in heart and muscle tissue. The primary metabolic fate of ribose is the formation of 5-phosphoribosyl-1-pyro-phosphate (PRPP) required for purine synthesis and salvage via the purine nucleotide pathway. PRPP is rate limiting in purine synthesis and salvage, and concentration in tissue defines the rate of flux down this pathway. In this way, ribose is rate limiting for preservation of the cellular adenine nucleotide pool.

As a pentose, ribose is not used by cells as a primary energy fuel. Instead, ribose is preserved for the important metabolic task of stimulating purine nucleotide synthesis and salvage. Approximately 98 percent of consumed ribose is quickly absorbed into the bloodstream and is circulated to remote tissue with no first pass effect by the liver. As ribose passes through the cell membrane it is phosphorylated by membrane bound ribokinase before entering the pentose phosphate pathway downstream of the gatekeeper enzymes. In this way, administered ribose is able to increase intracellular PRPP concentration and initiate purine nucleotide synthesis and salvage.

The use of ribose in congestive heart failure was first reported in the *European Journal of Heart Failure* in 2003 in a double-blind, placebo controlled, crossover study which included patients with chronic coronary artery disease and NYHA Class II/III CHF (Omran et al. 2003). Patients underwent two treatment periods of three weeks each, during which either oral ribose (5 g t.i.d.) or placebo (glucose; 5 g t.i.d.) was administered. Following a one-week washout period, the alternate test supplement was administered for three weeks. Before and after each three-week trial period, assessment of myocardial function was made by echocardiography, and the patient's exercise capacity was determined using a stationary exercise cycle. Participants also completed a quality of life questionnaire. Ribose administration resulted in significantly enhanced indices of diastolic heart function and exercise tolerance, and was also associated with improved quality of life score. By comparison, none of these parameters were changed with glucose (placebo) treatment.

In addition to impaired pump function, CHF patients exhibit compromised ventilation and oxygen uptake efficiency that presents as dyspnea. Ventilation efficiency slope and oxygen uptake efficiency slope are highly sensitive predictors of CHF patient survival that can be measured using sub-maximal exercise protocols that included pulmonary assessment of oxygen and carbon dioxide levels. In one study, ribose administration (5 g, t.i.d.) to NYHA Class III/IV

CHF patients significantly improved ventilation efficiency, oxygen uptake efficiency, and stroke volume (Vijay et al. 2005).

A second study (Carter et al. 2005) showed that in NYHA Class II/III CHF patients ribose administration significantly maintained VO2max when compared to placebo and improved ventilatory efficiency to the respiratory compensation point. A third (Sharma et al. 2005), similar, study involving patients with NYHA Class III CHF patients investigated the effect of ribose on Doppler derived Myocardial Performance Index (MPI), VO2max, and ventilatory efficiency—all powerful predictors of heart failure survival in a Class III heart failure population. Results showed that ribose improved MPI and ventilatory efficiency while preserving VO2max. Results of these studies show that ribose stimulates energy metabolism along the cardiopulmonary axis, thereby improving gas exchange.

Increased cardiac load produces unfavorable energetics that deplete myocardial energy reserves. Because ribose is the rate limiting precursor for adenine nucleotide metabolism, its role in preserving energy substrates in remote myocardium following infarction was studied in a rat model (Befera et al. 2007). In this study, male Lewis rats received continuous venous infusion of ribose or placebo via an osmotic mini-pump for 14 days. One to two days after pump placement, animals underwent ligation of the left anterior descending coronary artery to produce an anterior wall myocardial infarction. Echocardiographic analysis performed preoperatively and at two and four weeks following infarction was used to assess functional changes as evidenced by ejection indices, chamber dimensions, and wall thickness.

By all three measured indices, ribose administration better maintained the myocardium. Contractility and wall thickness were increased, while less ventricular dilation occurred. This study showed that the remote myocardium exhibits a significant decrease in function within four weeks following myocardial infarction, and that, to a significant degree, ribose administration attenuates this dysfunction.

A note about D-Ribose dosage: the data presented suggests that D-Ribose may have significant value as an adjunct to traditional therapy for congestive heart failure. A dose range of 10 to 15 g/day is recommended. If patients respond favorably after two to three weeks, a lower dose of 5 g/dose two times per day could be tried. Individual doses of greater than 10 grams are not recommended, because high single doses of hygroscopic carbohydrate may cause mild gastrointestinal discomfort or transient lightheadedness. It is suggested that ribose be administered with meals or mixed in beverages containing a secondary carbohydrate source. D-Ribose may actually lower glucose levels so, in diabetic patients prone to hypoglycemia, ribose should be administered in fruit juices.

Coenzyme Q10

Coenzyme Q10 or ubiquinone, so named for its ubiquitous nature in cells, is a fat-soluble compound that functions as an antioxidant and coenzyme in the energy-producing pathways. As an antioxidant, the reduced form of CoQ10 inhibits lipid peroxidation in both cell membranes and serum-low density lipoprotein, and also protects proteins and DNA from oxidative damage. Coenzyme Q10 also has membrane stabilizing activity. However, its bioenergetic activity and electron transport function for its role in oxidative phosphorylation is probably its most important function.

In CHF, oxidative phosphorylation slows due to a loss of mitochondrial protein and lack of expression of key enzymes involved in the cycle. Disruption of mitochondrial activity may lead to a loss of Coenzyme Q10 that can further depress oxidative phosphorylation. In patients taking statin drugs, the mitochondrial loss of Coenzyme Q10 may be exacerbated by restricted Coenzyme Q10 synthesis resulting from HMG-CoA reductase inhibition (Figure 5.6). It has been reported that long term treatment with atorvastatin may increase plasma levels of brain natriuretic peptide (BNP) in coronary artery disease when associated with a greater reduction in plasma Coenzyme Q10 (Suzuki et al. 2008).

Although Coenzyme Q10 is found in relatively high concentrations in the liver, kidney, and lungs, the heart requires the highest levels of ATP activity

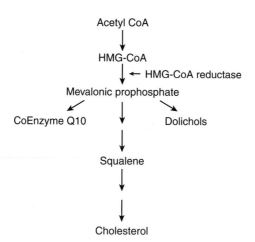

FIGURE 5.6. Statin drugs (HMG-CoA reductase inhibitors) can reduce natural coenzyme Q10-synthesis in the body.

because it is continually aerobic and contains more mitochondria per gram than any other tissue in the body. Cardiomyocytes, for example, contain more than 3,500 mitochondria per cell, compared to a bicep muscle cell that houses approximately 200 mitochondria per cell. Tissue deficiencies and low serum blood levels of Coenzyme Q10 have been reported across a wide range of cardiovascular diseases, including diastolic dysfunction, CHF, hypertension, aortic valvular disease and coronary artery disease and research suggests that Coenzyme Q10 support may be indicated in these disease conditions (Langsjoen and Langsjoen 1999; Langsjoen, Littarru, and Silver 2005).

While the medical literature generally supports the use of Coenzyme Q10 in CHF, the evaluated dose-response relationships for this nutrient have been confined to a narrow dose range, with the majority of clinical studies having been conducted on subjects who were taking only 90 to 200 mg daily. At such doses, some patients have responded, while others have not. In 22 controlled trials of supplemental CoQ10 in congestive heart failure, 19 have shown benefit while 3 failed to demonstrate improvement in any significant cardiovascular function (Langsjoen and Langsjoen 1999; Langsjoen, Littarru, and Silver 2005). The three that concluded no benefit had limitations that will be discussed.

In the study conducted by Permanetter et al, (1992), a 100-mg dose of Coenzyme Q10 failed to show benefit. However, actual blood levels of CoQ10 were not obtained in this investigation; thus it is impossible to know if a therapeutic blood level was ever achieved. In the second trial by Watson et al. (2001), a mean treatment plasma CoQ10 level of only 1.7 g/ml was obtained with only two of the 30 patients having a plasma level greater than 2.0g/ml. The third study, performed by Khatta and colleagues (2000), demonstrated a mean treatment plasma CoQ10 level of 2.2 +/− 1.1 g/ml, and indicated that approximately 50 percent of the patients had plasma levels as low as 1.0 g/ml. Unfortunately, these last two clinical trials are frequently quoted as CoQ10 failures, despite the fact that adequate blood levels were not achieved.

In patients with CHF or dilated cardiomyopathy, higher doses of Coenzyme Q10 in ranges of at least 300 mg or more daily is required to obtain therapeutic blood levels, defined as greater than 2.5 g/ml and preferably 3.5 g/ml (Sinatra 2000). In a previous analysis in three patients with refractory congestive heart failure, such higher doses of CoQ10 were required in order to get such a therapeutic result (Sinatra 1997).

In a later investigation at the Lancisi Heart Institute in Italy, researchers studied 23 patients with a mean age of 59, using a double-blind, placebo-controlled, cross-over design. Patients were assigned to receive 100 mg of oral CoQ10 three times per day plus supervised exercise training. The study concluded that CoQ10 supplementation improved functional capacity, endothelial function and left ventricular contractility in CHF without any side effects (Belardinelli et al. 2006).

In a long-term study of 424 patients with systolic and/or diastolic dysfunction in the presence of CHF, dilated cardiomyopathy, or hypertensive heart disease, a dose of 240 mg/day maintained blood levels of Coenzyme Q10 above 2.0 g/ml, and allowed 43 percent of the participants to discontinue one to three conventional drugs over the course of the study (Langsjoen et al. 1994). Patients were followed for an average of 17.8 months, and during that time, a mild case of nausea was the only reported side effect. This long-term study clearly shows Coenzyme Q10 to be a safe and effective adjunctive treatment for patients with systolic and/or diastolic left ventricular dysfunction with or without CHF, dilated cardiomyopathy, or hypertensive heart disease.

These results are further confirmed by an investigation involving 109 patients with hypertensive heart disease and isolated diastolic dysfunction showing that Coenzyme Q10 supplementation resulted in clinical improvement, lowered elevated blood pressure, enhanced diastolic cardiac function and decreased myocardial thickness in 53%of study patients (Langsjoen, Willis, and Folkers 1994).

Plasma CoQ(10) concentration has been shown to be an independent predictor of mortality in patients with congestive heart failure (Molyneux et al. 2008). New Zealand researchers studied the relationship of plasma CoQ10 levels and survival in patients with chronic heart failure. In their cohort of 236 patients (mean age 77 years), they concluded that plasma CoQ10 concentration was an independent predictor of mortality. A blood level of 0.73 Mol/l* or more was the best predictor for survival. Researchers suggested that lower concentrations of plasma CoQ10 might be detrimental in the long-term prognosis of CHF.

The effect of Coenzyme Q10 administration on 32 heart transplant candidates with end-stage CHF and cardiomyopathy was reported in 2004 (Berman et al. 2004). The study was designed to determine if Coenzyme Q10 could improve the pharmacological bridge to transplantation and the results showed three significant findings. Following six weeks of Coenzyme Q10 therapy, the study group showed elevated blood levels from an average of 0.22 mg/l to 0.83 mg/l*, an increase of 277 percent (note that different labs in other countries have different standardizations of CoQ10). By contrast, the placebo group measured 0.18 mg/l at the onset of the study and 0.178 mg/l at six weeks. Second, the study group showed significant improvement in 6-minute walk test distance, shortness of breath, NYHA functional classification, fatigue, and episodes of waking for nocturnal urination. No such changes were found in the placebo group. These results strongly show that Coenzyme Q10 therapy may augment pharmaceutical treatment of patients with end-stage CHF and cardiomyopathy.

I have suggested that a new emerging field in "Metabolic Cardiology" will most likely be realized by those who treat the energy-starved heart at the mitochondrial level (Sinatra 2004).

Levocarnitine (L-Carnitine or Carnitine)

Carnitine is derived naturally in the body from the amino acids lysine and methionine. Biosynthesis occurs in a series of metabolic reactions involving these amino acids, complemented with niacin, vitamin B_6, vitamin C, and iron. Although carnitine deficiency is rare in a healthy, well-nourished population consuming adequate protein, CHF, left ventricular hypertrophy, and other cardiac conditions causing renal insufficiency can lead to cellular depletion and conditions of carnitine deficiency.

The principal role of carnitine is to facilitate the transport of fatty acids across the inner mitochondrial membrane to initiate beta-oxidation. The inner mitochondrial membrane is normally impermeable to activated coenzyme A (Co A) esters. To affect transfer of the extracellular metabolic byproduct acyl-Co A across the cellular membrane, the mitochondria delivers its acyl unit to the carnitine residing in the inner mitochondrial membrane. Carnitine (as acetyl-carnitine) then transports the metabolic fragment across the membrane and delivers it to coenzyme A residing inside the mitochondria. This process of acetyl transfer is known as the carnitine shuttle, and the shuttle also works in reverse to remove excess acetyl units from the inner mitochondria for disposal. Excess acetyl units that accumulate inside the mitochondria disturb the metabolic burning of fatty acids. Other crucial functions of intracellular carnitine include the metabolism of branched-chain amino acids, ammonia detoxification, and lactic acid clearance from tissue. Carnitine also exhibits antioxidant and free radical scavenger properties.

Although the role of carnitine in the utilization of fatty acids and glucose in cardiac metabolism has been known for decades, the relationship between carnitine availability in heart tissue, carnitine metabolism in the heart, and carnitine's impact on left ventricular function has been elucidated only recently. Two independent studies have investigated the relationship between tissue carnitine levels and heart function and have evaluated the possibility that plasma or urinary carnitine levels might actually serve as markers for impaired left ventricular function in patients with CHF.

In the first study of carnitine tissue levels and CHF, the myocardial tissue from 25 cardiac transplant recipients with end-stage CHF and 21 control donor hearts was analyzed for concentrations of total carnitine, free carnitine, and carnitine derivatives. Compared to controls, the concentration of carnitines in the heart muscle of heart transplant recipients was significantly lower in patients, and the level of carnitine in the tissue was directly related to ejection fraction. This study concluded that carnitine deficiency in the heart tissue might be directly related to heart function (El-Aroussy 2000).The second study measured plasma and urinary levels of L-carnitine in 30 patients with CHF and cardiomyopathy and compared them to 10 control subjects with no heart disease (Narin 1997). Results showed that patients with CHF had higher plasma and urinary levels of carnitine, suggesting that carnitine was being released from the challenged heart muscle cells. Similarly, the study demonstrated that the level of plasma and urinary carnitine was related to the degree of left ventricular systolic dysfunction and ejection fraction. This finding suggests that elevated plasma and urinary carnitine levels, reflecting loss of carnitine from compromised cardiomyocytes, might represent measurable physiological markers for myocardial damage and impaired left ventricular function.

A previous investigation examined the effect of long-term carnitine administration on mortality in patients with CHF and dilated cardiomyopathy. This study followed 80 patients with moderate to severe heart failure (NYHA class III/IV) for three years. After a three-month period of stable cardiac function on standard medical therapy, patients were randomly assigned to receive either two grams of carnitine per day or a matched placebo. After an average of 33.7 months of follow up, 70 patients remained in the study (33 taking placebo and 37 supplementing with carnitine) and at the end of the study period 63 had survived (27 placebo and 36 carnitine). This study determined that carnitine provided a benefit to longer-term survival in late-stage heart failure in dilated cardiomyopathy (Rizos 2000).

A similar placebo-controlled study evaluated 160 myocardial infarction survivors for twelve months (Davini et al. 1992). Eighty subjects were included in each group; the study group received a daily dose of 4 grams of L-carnitine; the controls received a placebo. Both the carnitine and control groups continued their conventional therapeutic regimen while on the test substance. Subjects in both groups showed improvement in arterial blood pressure, cholesterol levels, rhythm disorders, and signs and symptoms of CHF over the study period, but all-cause mortality was significantly lower in the carnitine compared to the placebo group (1.2 percent and 12.5 percent, respectively). A further double-blind, placebo-controlled trial by Singh and coworkers studied 100 patients with suspected myocardial infarction. Patients taking carnitine (2 g/day for 28 days) showed improvement in arrhythmia, angina, onset of heart failure, and mean infarct size, as well as a reduction in total cardiac events. There was a significant reduction in cardiac death and non-fatal infarction in the carnitine group versus the placebo group (15.6 percent vs. 26 percent respectively) (Singh et al. 1996).

In a European study of 472 patients published in the *Journal of the American College of Cardiology*, nine grams per day of carnitine was administered intravenously for five days followed by six grams per day orally for the next twelve months (Iliceto et al. 1995). The study validated previous findings, demonstrating an improvement in ejection fraction and a reduction in left ventricular size in carnitine-treated patients. Although the European study was not designed to demonstrate outcome differences, the combined incidence of CHF death after discharge was lower in the carnitine group than placebo group (6.0 percent vs. 9.6 percent, respectively)—a reduction of more than 30 percent.

A newer form of carnitine, glycine propionyl L-carnitine (GPLC), demonstrated significant advantages in the production of nitric oxide and lower malondialdehyde (MDA)—a marker of lipid peroxidation and oxidative damage. This form of carnitine resulted in vasodilation via a nitric oxide mechanism inhibition. GPLC also blocked key steps in the process of platelet aggregation and adhesion, as well as reducing levels of lipid peroxidation and oxidative damage (Bloomer, Smith, and Fisher-Wellman 2007).

Magnesium: Switching on the Energy Enzymes

Magnesium is an essential mineral critical for a wide range of energy requiring processes including: protein synthesis, membrane integrity, nervous tissue conduction, neuromuscular excitation, muscle contraction, hormone secretion, maintenance of vascular tone, and intermediary metabolism. Deficiency may lead to changes in neuromuscular, cardiovascular, immune, and hormonal function. Magnesium deficiency is now considered to contribute to many diseases, and the role of magnesium as a therapeutic agent is expanding.

A German study of 16, 000 patients were assigned to subgroups based on gender, age, and state of health (Schimatschek and Rempis 2001). Hypomagnesemia was identified in 14.5 percent of all persons examined, and suboptimal levels were found in yet another 33.7 percent, for a total of 58.2 percent—more than half of those evaluated.

Magnesium deficiency reduces the activity of important enzymes used in energy metabolism. Hypomagnesemia can result in progressive vasoconstriction, coronary spasm, and even sudden death (Turlapaty and Altura 1980). In anginal episodes due to coronary artery spasm, treatment with magnesium has been shown to be efficacious (McLean 1994). Magnesium deficiency, which is better detected by mononuclear blood cell magnesium than the standard serum level performed at most hospitals, predisposes to excessive mortality and morbidity in patients with acute MI (Elin 1998).

While magnesium is found in most foods—particularly beans, figs, and vegetables—deficiencies are common. Softened water, depleted soils, and a trend toward lower vegetable consumption are the culprits contributing to these rising deficiencies. Major magnesium deficiencies exist especially in the insulin resistance/metabolic syndrome as well as in prolapse mitral valve.

Magnesium has shown considerable efficacy in relieving symptoms of mitral valve prolapse (MVP). In a double-blind study of 181 participants, serum magnesium levels were assessed in 141 patients with symptomatic MVP and compared to those of 40 healthy control subjects (Lichodziejewska et al. 1997). While decreased serum magnesium levels were found in 60 percent of patients with MVP, only 5 percent of the control subjects showed similar decreases. The second phase of the study investigated response to treatment. Participants with magnesium deficits were randomly assigned to receive magnesium supplement or placebo. The frequency of symptoms was significantly reduced with magnesium supplementation; significant reductions were noted in weakness, chest pain, shortness of breath, palpitations, and even anxiety.

The combination of magnesium and coenzyme Q10 has been extremely promising. I have seen this combination alleviate 80 to 90 percent of symptoms, including chest pain, shortness of breath, easy fatigability, and palpitations. The combination of magnesium and CoQ10 is more efficacious than beta blockers. The enhanced quality of life is probably due to some improvement in diastolic dysfunction, which often is present in women with MVP.

Summary

Attention to the energy demands of diseased hearts is often missing in conventional cardiology practice. Metabolic support with D-ribose, Coenzyme Q10, L-carnitine, and magnesium can be important for the maintenance of contractile reserve and energy charge in minimally oxidative ischemic or hypoxic hearts. Preservation of cellular energy charge provides the chemical driving force needed to maintain cell and tissue viability and function.

Summarized below is a metabolic cardiology approach to mild to moderate congestive heart failure, severe congestive heart failure, dilated cardiomyopathy, and mitral valve prolapse. The program that I have found to be most effective for the patients I treat in my practice includes the following:

Congestive heart failure

1. Multivitamin/mineral foundation program with 1 gram of fish oil
2. Coenzyme Q10: 300–360 mg

3. L-carnitine: 2,000–2,500 mg
4. D-ribose: 10–15 grams
5. Magnesium: 400–800 mg

Severe congestive heart failure, dilated cardiomyopathy, patients awaiting heart transplantation

1. Multivitamin/mineral foundation program with 1 gram of fish oil
2. Coenzyme Q10: 360–600 mg
3. L-carnitine: 2,500–3,500 mg
4. D-ribose: 15 grams
5. Magnesium: 400–800 mg

Note: If quality of life is still not satisfactory, add 1500 mg of hawthorn berry and 2–3 grams of taurine, as the addition of these two nutraceuticals has helped many of my patients with severe refractory congestive heart failure.
Mitral valve prolapse

1. Multivitamin/mineral foundation program with 1 gram of fish oil
2. Coenzyme Q10: 90–180 mg daily
3. L-carnitine: 500–1000 mg
4. D-ribose: 5 grams
5. Magnesium: 600–800 mg

Conclusion

Cardiovascular function depends on the operational capacity of myocardial cells to generate the energy to expand and contract. Insufficient myocardial energy contributes significantly to CHF. Literally, heart failure is an "energy-starved heart."

Although there may be several causes of myocardial dysfunction, the energy deficiency in cardiac myocytes plays a significant role. It is no longer enough that physicians focus on the fluid retention aspects of "pump failure." For instance, diuretic therapies target the kidneys indirectly to relieve the sequelae of CHF without addressing the root cause. Inotropic agents attempt to increase contractility directly, yet fail to offer the extra energy necessary to assist the weakened heart muscle. Metabolic solutions, on the other hand, treat the heart muscle cells directly. "Metabolic cardiology" supports the biochemical interventions that can be employed to directly improve energy substrates and therefore energy metabolism in heart cells.

D-Ribose, Coenzyme Q10, L-carnitine and magnesium all promote cardiac energy metabolism and help normalize myocardial adenine nucleotide concentrations. These naturally occurring compounds exert a physiological benefit that, by providing energy substrates, support the production of ATP. All of these interventions positively impact on cardiac systolic and diastolic function. Acknowledging this metabolic support for the heart provides a missing link that offers great potential for the future treatment of cardiovascular disease.

REFERENCES

Bache, R. J., J. Zhang, Y. Murakami, Y. Zhang, Y. K. Cho, H. Merkle, G. Gong, A. H. From, and K. Ugurbil. 1999. Myocardial oxygenation at high workstates in hearts with left ventricular hypertrophy. *Cardiovasc Res* 42(3): 567–570.

Beer, M., T. Seyfarth, J. Sandstede, W. Landschutz, C. Lipke, H. Kostler, M. von Kienlin, K. Harre, D. Hahn, and S. Neubauer. 2002. Absolute concentrations of high-energy phosphate metabolites in normal, hypertrophied, and failing human myocardium measured noninvasively with (31)P-SLOOP magnetic resonance spectroscopy. *JACC* 40(7): 1267–1274.

Befera, N., A. Rivard, G. Gatlin, S. Black, J. Zhang, and J. E. Foker. 2007. Ribose treatment helps preserve function of the remote myocardium after myocardial infarction. *J Surg Res* 137(2): 156.

Belardinelli, R., A. Mucaj, F. Lacalaprice, M. Solenghi, G. Seddaiu, F. Principi, L. Tiano, and G. P. Littarru. 2006. Coenzyme Q10 and exercise training in chronic heart failure. *Eur Heart J* 27(22): 2675–81.

Berman, M., A. Erman, T. Ben-Gal, et al. 2004. Coenzyme Q10 in patients with end-stage heart failure awaiting cardiac transplantation: A randomized, placebo-controlled study. *Clin Cardiol* 27: 295–99.

Bloomer, R. J., W. A. Smith, and K. H. Fisher-Wellman. 2007. Glycine Propionyl-L-Carnitine increases plasma nitrate/nitrite in resistance trained men. *J International Society of Sports Nutr* 4: 22.

Carter, O., D. MacCarter, S. Mannebach, J. Biskupiak, G. Stoddard, E. M. Gilbert, and M. A. Munger 2005. D-Ribose improves peak exercise capacity and ventilatory efficiency in heart failure patients. *JACC* 45(3 Suppl A): 185A.

Cha Y-M, P. P. Dzeja, W. K. Shen, A. Jahangir, C. Y. T. Hart, A. Terzic, and M. M. Redfield. 2003. Failing atrial myocardium: energetic deficits accompany structural remodeling and electrical instability. *Am J Physiol Heart Circ Physiol* 284: H1313–H1320.

Davini, P., A. Bigalli, F. Lamanna, and A. Boem. 1992. Controlled study on L-carnitine therapeutic efficacy in post-infarction. *Drugs under Experimental and Clinical Research* 18: 355–65.

Diamant, M., H. J. Lamb, Y. Groeneveld, E. L. Endert, J. W. Smith, J. J. Bax, J. A. Romijm, A. de Roos, J. K. Radder. 2003. Diastolic dysfunction is associated with altered myocardial metabolism in asymptomatic normotensive patients with well-controlled type 2 diabetes mellitus. *JACC* 41(2): 328–35.

El-Aroussy, W., A. Rizk, G. Mayhoub, et al. 2000. Plasma carnitine levels as a marker of impaired left ventricular functions. *Mol Cell Biochem* 213(1–2): 37–41.

Elin, R. J. 1998. Magnesium metabolism in health and disease. *Dis Mon* 34: 161.

Gourine, A. V., Q. Hu, P. R. Sander, A. I. Kuzmin, N. Hanafy, S. A. Davydova, D. V. Zaretsky, and J. Zhang. 2004. Interstitial purine metabolites in hearts with LV remodeling. *Am J Physiol Heart Circ Physiol* 286: H677–H684.

Hu, Q., Q. Wang, J. Lee, A. Mansoor, J. Liu, L. Zeng, C. Swingen, G. Zhang, J. Feygin, K. Ochiai, T. L. Bransford, A. H. From, R. J. Bache, and J. Zhang. 2006. Profound bioenergetic abnormalities in peri-infarct myocardial regions. *Am J Physiol Heart Circ Physiol* 291: H648–H657.

Iliceto, S., D. Scrutinio, P. Bruzzi, et al. 1995. Effects of L-carnitine administration on left ventricular remodeling after acute anterior myocardial infarction: The L-Carnitine Ecocardiografia Digitalizzata Infarto Miocardioco (CEDIM) Trial. *JACC* 26(2): 380–87.

Ingwall, J. S. 2002. *ATP and the heart.* Boston: Kluwer Academic Publishers.

Ingwall, J. S. 2006. On the hypothesis that the failing heart is energy starved: Lessons learned from the metabolism of ATP and creatine. *Cur Hypertens Rep* 8: 457–464.

Ingwall, J. S., R. G. Weiss. 2004. Is the failing heart energy starved? On using chemical energy to support cardiac function. *Circ Res* 95: 135–45.

Khatta, M., B. S. Alexander, C. M. Krichten, et al. 2000. The effect of coenzyme Q10 in patients with congestive heart failure. *Ann Intern Med* 132(8): 636–40.

Lamb, H. J., H. P. Beyerbacht, A. van der Laarse, B. C. Stoel, J. Doornbos, E. E. van der Wall, and A. de Roos. 1999. Diastolic dysfunction in hypertensive heart disease is associated with altered myocardial metabolism. *Circ* 99(17): 2261–2267.

Langsjoen, P. H., and A. M. Langsjoen. 1999. Overview of the use of CoQ10 in cardiovascular disease. *Biofactors* 9(2–4): 273–84.

Langsjoen, P. H., P. Langsjoen, R. Willis, et al. 1994. Usefulness of Coenzyme Q10 in clinical cardiology: A long-term study. *Mol Aspects Med* 15: S165–175.

Langsjoen, P. H., G. P. Littarru, and M. A. Silver. 2005. Role of concomitant coenzyme Q10 with statins for patients with hyperlipidemia. *Curr Topics Nutr Res* 3(3): 149–58.

Langsjoen, P. H., R. Willis, and K. Folkers. 1994. Treatment of essential hypertension with Coenzyme Q10. *Mol Aspects Med* 15(suppl): 265–72.

Lazaron, J., B. Pomeranz, and P. Corey. 1998. Incidence of adverse drug reaction in hospitalized patients. *JAMA* 279: 1200–05.

Lichodziejewska, B., J. Klos, J. Rezler, et al. 1997. Clinical symptoms of mitral valve prolapse are related to hypomagnesemia and attenuated by magnesium supplementation. *Am J Cardiol* 79(6): 768.

Manfredi, J. P., and E. W. Holmes. 1985. Purine salvage pathways in myocardium. *Ann Rev Physiol* 47: 691–705.

Maslov, M. Y., V. P. Chacko, M. Stuber, A. L. Moens, D. A. Kass, H. C. Champion, and R. G. Weiss. 2007. Altered high-energy phosphate metabolism predicts contractile dysfunction and subsequent ventricular remodeling in pressure-overload hypertrophy mice. *Am J Physiol Heart Circ Physiol* 292: H387–H391.

McLean, R. M. 1994. Magnesium and its therapeutic uses: A review. *Am J Med* 96: 63.

Molyneux, S., C. Florkowski, P. George, A. Pilbrow, C. Frampton, M. Lever, and A. M. Richards. 2008. Coenzyme Q10: An independent predictor of mortality in chronic heart failure. *JACC* 52(18): 1435–41.

Narin, F., N. Narin, H. Andac, et al. 1997. Carnitine levels in patients with chronic rheumatic heart disease. *Clin Biochem* 30(8): 643–45.

Neubauer, S., M. Horn, T. Pabst, K. Harre, H. Stromer, G. Bertsch, J. Sandstede, G. Ertl, D. Hahn, and K. Kochsiek. 1997. Cardiac high-energy phosphate metabolism in patients with aortic valve disease assessed by 31P-magnetic resonance spectroscopy. *J Investig Med* 45(8): 453–62.

Omran, H., S. Illien, D. MacCarter, J. A. Cyr, B. Luderitz. 2003. D-Ribose improves diastolic function and quality of life in congestive heart failure patients: A prospective feasibility study. *Eur J Heart Failure* 5: 615–19.

Perings, S. M., K. Schulze, U. Decking, M. Kelm, B. E. Strauer. 2000. Age-related decline of PCr/ATP-ratio in progressively hypertrophied hearts of spontaneously hypertensives rats. *Heart Vessels* 15(4): 197–202.

Permanetter, B., W. Rossy, G. Klein, F. Weingartner, K. F. Seidl, and H. Blomer. 1992. Ubiquinone (coenzyme Q10) in the long-term treatment of idiopathic dilated cardiomyopathy. *Eur Heart J* 13(11): 1528–33.

Rizos, I. 2000. Three-year survival of patients with heart failure caused by dilated cardiomyopathy. *Am Heart J* 139(2 Pt 3): S120–23.

Schimatschek, H. F., and R. Rempis. 2001. Prevalence of hypomagnesemia in an unselected German population of 16,000 individuals. *Magnes Res* 14(4): 283–90.

Schocke, M. F., B. Metzler, C. Wolf, P. Steinboeck, C. Kremser, O. Pachinger, W. Jaschike, and P. Lukas. 2003. Impact of aging on cardiac high-energy phosphate metabolism determined by phosphorous-31 2-dimensional chemical shift imaging (31P 2D CSI). *Magn Reson Imaging* 21(5): 553–59.

Sharma, R., M. Munger, S. Litwin, O. Vardeny, D. MacCarter, St., J. A. Cyr. 2005. D-Ribose improves Doppler TEI myocardial performance index and maximal exercise capacity in stage C heart failure. *J Mol Cell Cardiol* 38(5): 853.

Sinatra, S. T. 1997. Coenzyme Q10: a vital therapeutic nutrient for the heart with special application in congestive heart failure. *Conn Med* 61(11): 707–11.

Sinatra, S. T. 2000. Letter to Editor: Coenzyme Q10 and congestive heart failure. *Ann Intern Med* 133(9): 745–46.

Sinatra, S. T. 2004. Letter to Editor: Coenzyme Q10 in patients with end-stage heart failure awaiting cardiac transplantation: A randomized, placebo-controlled study. *Clin Cardiol* 27(10): A26.

Sinatra, S. T. 2005. *The Sinatra Solution*. Laguna Beach, CA: Basic Health Publications, Inc.

Sinatra, S. T. 2009. Metabolic cardiology: The missing link in cardiovascular disease. *Alternative Therapies in Health and Medicine*. 15: 48–50.

Singh, R. B., M. A. Niaz, P. Agarwal P et al. 1996. A randomized, double-blind, place-bo-controlled trial of L-carnitine in suspected acute myocardial infarction. *Postgrad Med* 72: 45–50.

Smith, C. S., P. A. Bottomley, S. P. Schulman, G. Gerstenblith, and R. G. Weiss. 2006. Altered creatine kinase adenosine triphosphate kinetics in failing hypertrophied human myocardium. *Circ* 114: 1151–58.

Suzuki, T., T. Nozawa, M. Sobajima, N. Igarashi, A. Matsuki, N. Fujii, and H. Inoue. 2008. Atorvastatin-induced changes in plasma coenzyme Q10 and brain natriuretic peptide in patients with coronary artery disease. *Int Heart J* 49(4): 423–33.

Turlapaty, P. D. M. V., and B. M. Altura. 1980. Magnesium deficiency produces spasms of coronary arteries: relationship to etiology of sudden death ischemic heart disease. *Science* 208: 198.

Vijay, N., D. MacCarter, M. Washam, St. J. Cyr. 2005. Ventilatory efficiency improves with d-ribose in congestive heart failure patients. *J Mol Cell Cardiol* 38(5): 820.

Watson, P. S., G. M. Scalia, A. J. Gaibraith, D. J. Burstow, C. N. Aroney, and J. H. Bett. 2001. Is coenzyme Q10 helpful for patients with idiopathic cardiomyopathy? *Med J Aust* 175(8): 447 and author reply 447–48.

Weiss, R. G., G. Gerstenblith, and P. A. Bottomley. 2005. ATP flux through creatine kinase in the normal, stressed, and failing human heart. *Proc Nat Acad Sci* 102(3): 808–13.

Ye, Y., G. Gong, K. Ochiai, J. Liu, and J. Zhang. 2001. High-energy phosphate metabolism and creatine kinase in failing hearts: a new porcine model. *Circ* 103: 1570–76.

Ypenburg, C., A. Sieders, G. B. Bleeker, E. R. Holman, E. E. van der Wall, M. J. Schalij, and J. J. Bax. 2007. Myocardial contractile reserve predicts improvement in left ventricular function after cardiac resynchronization therapy. *Am Heart J* 154(6): 1160–65.

6

Acupuncture in Cardiovascular Medicine

JOHN LONGHURST

KEY CONCEPTS

- Meridians and acupoints along the meridians in Traditional Chinese Medicine serve as a guide for therapists, directing them where to achieve the best clinical responses. Neither meridians nor acupoints are represented by an anatomical structure, but many are located over major neural pathways.
- Acupuncture works by stimulating somatic sensory neural pathways to activate regions of the brain that regulate autonomic neural outflow, and hence cardiovascular function.
- A number of excitatory and inhibitory neurotransmitters/neuromodulators in both long- and short-loop pathways in the hypothalamus, midbrain, and medulla underlie acupuncture's ability to lower elevated blood pressure.
- Manual and low frequency electroacupuncture are the most effective forms of stimulation used to lower elevated blood pressure.
- Key features of acupuncture differentiating it from simple somatosensory stimulation are its point-specific effects, slow onset (requiring minutes to days before a response is observed), and prolonged action (which can last for hours to weeks after therapy).
- Acupuncture's principal cardiovascular effect is to normalize blood pressure.
- Small trials suggest that acupuncture may be able to reduce angina in patients with demand-induced myocardial ischemia.

- Although theoretically acupuncture should be able to modify many cardiovascular risk factors, such as obesity, smoking, hypercholesterolemia and hypertension, only hypertension has been shown to be modified in well-constructed clinical trials. Better prospective randomized clinical trials are necessary to determine acupuncture's influence on other risk factors.

■

Traditional Chinese Medicine

Acupuncture originated over 2,000 years ago as a therapy in Traditional Chinese Medicine (TCM). The technique and practice of acupuncture was shaped empirically through trial, error, and success and, in fact, even today much teaching of this ancient technique is based on observations of masters and practitioners that were recorded in texts and passed down to students as dogma. Only in the last few decades has modern science begun to provide insight into the mechanisms and actions of acupuncture. Since the early 1970s there have been over 500 randomized controlled clinical trials investigating the clinical influence of acupuncture (Klein and Trachtenberg 1997; Vickers 1998), yet its influence has been proven rigorously for only a few diseases, most notably pain and nausea and vomiting.

Acupuncture is a form of energy-based medicine, and the energy is referred to as *Qi*. This energy flows through a system of twelve principal channels, or meridians, that lie along the skin's surface and are named after and connect to twelve Chinese organs. Although somewhat controversial, there is no proven anatomical basis for the meridians and they cannot be reliably detected with instruments that measure skin resistance. Furthermore, the Chinese organs, while sometimes named similarly to Western visceral organs, are not exactly equivalent. For example, the heart meridian connects to the Chinese heart, which actually represents the Western equivalent of the heart and the brain. Along these meridians are small nodes or acupuncture points (acupoints) through which therapists place sterile stainless steel needles during treatment. Although neither the meridians nor acupoints have a physical basis, they are useful because they direct the therapist where stimulation should occur to obtain the best clinical result. Thus, meridians and acupoints act as road maps for acupuncture therapy. A number of acupoints have been shown experimentally to exert strong cardiovascular responses (Figure 6.1).

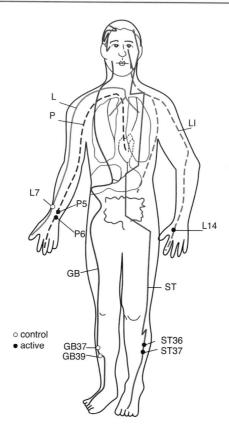

FIGURE 6.1. Diagram of acupoints along meridians that cause strong (active points, filled circles) or weak (control points, open circles) cardiovascular responses. See text for discussion of individual points. Meridians are identified according to Traditional Chinese Medicine theory as belonging to the principal Chinese organs to which they connect and influence, including the gallbladder (GB), large intestine (LI), lung (L), pericardial (P) and stomach (ST) meridians. The numbers for acupoints refer to standardized reference system to distinguish points along each meridian. Modified from Li, Ayannusi, Reed, & Longhurst 2004.

Acupuncture is an empirically developed ancient therapy. Modern science has found substantial truth in many of its concepts, particularly Qi, the energy that circulates through meridians. Western science translates Qi to acupuncture-triggered neural impulses in somatic sensory nerves that transmit information to the brain to alter cardiovascular function.

MECHANISM OF ACTION

Acupuncture is one of the few areas of integrative medicine for which the mechanism of cardiovascular action has been explored (Lin et al. 2001; Longhurst, J. 1998; Longhurst, J. C. 2002).

Over the last two decades, studies in both China and the United States have used a number of experimental preparations that lend themselves to acupuncture and careful measurement of its action to modify cardiovascular function. We now recognize that many meridians overlie neural pathways containing both motor and sensory nerves, which can be activated by needle stimulation. Motor nerve activation during electroacupuncture is useful because it provides a gauge to adjust the stimulation intensity, which generally is set at motor threshold. Sensory nerves, on the other hand, carry information resulting from acupuncture stimulation to the brain, which biologically transduces the input from different sources of acupoint stimulation to modify autonomic and humoral output to the heart and vascular system. Thus, from a physiological perspective, acupuncture needle stimulation activates sensory neural pathways, which provide input to regions of the central nervous system that regulate cardiovascular function (Longhurst J.C. 2007b). Acupuncture-related activation of thin fiber somatic sensory pathways (including both finely myelinated group III and unmyelinated group IV nerve fibers) provides input to the spinal cord dorsal horn and ultimately the intermediolateral columns (containing sympathetic motor nerves), arcuate nucleus in the ventral hypothalamus, midbrain ventrolateral periaqueductal gray (vlPAG), especially the caudal vlPAG and the rostral ventrolateral, and raphe pallidus nuclei in the medulla (rVLM and NRP)—regions that regulate sympathetic (and probably parasympathetic) outflow. Input derived from manual acupuncture and low frequency, low intensity electroacupuncture to these lower brain regions leads to the release of a number of modulatory (inhibitory) neuropeptide systems, including opioids (endorphins and enkephalins), γ-aminobutyric acid (GABA), nociceptin, serotonin, and endocannabinoids, as well as excitatory amino acids like glutamate and acetylcholine, which ultimately inhibit sympathetic (and likely parasympathetic) outflow to the heart and vascular system (Longhurst, J. C. 2002; 2007b). In the spinal cord, acupuncture appears to inhibit sensory inflow and sympathetic outflow through both opioid and nociceptin mechanisms of blockade (Zhou et al. 2006, Zhou et al. 2009).

When blood pressure is within the normal range, acupuncture causes only minimal changes (Li et al. 2004). Conversely, acupuncture inhibits sympathetic outflow and reduces blood pressure when it is elevated during excitatory reflex activation—for example, during stimulation of sensory nerves associated with visceral organs like the gallbladder with bradykinin (related to inflammatory pain), or gastric distension, or in spontaneously hypertensive rats or in humans during exercise (Li et al. 2002; Li et al. 2004; Longhurst, J. C. 1998; Tjen-A-Looi, Pan, and Longhurst 1998; Vickers 1998).

Acupuncture can be differentiated with respect to its cardiovascular actions from non-specific somatosensory stimulation with regard to both point specificity and the prolonged nature of its action. Relatively brief somatosensory reflex cardiovascular responses lasting for a few seconds or minutes that adapt quickly to maintained stimulation, and which return to baseline values shortly after termination of stimulation, can be elicited from stimulating almost any somatic or sensory nerve. Strong somatosensory stimulation generally increases blood pressure, while low-intensity stimulation typically does not alter or only briefly lowers blood pressure. The concept of point specificity refers to the differential physiological cardiovascular and clinical response to stimulation of individual acupoints (Longhurst, J.C. 2007b). In this respect, some acupoints (such as P5 and P6, which lie along the pericardial meridian overlying the median nerve in the wrist) exert a stronger influence on the cardiovascular system than other nearby acupoints (such as LI6 and LI7, located along the large intestine meridian on the forearm over the superficial radial nerve) (Tjen-A-Looi, Li, and Longhurst 2004). Studies also have shown that the extent of influence on sympathetic outflow from stimulation of each individual acupoint is highly correlated with the extent of input that they provide to regions of the brainstem that control autonomic and ultimately cardiovascular function. The existence of point specificity is controversial, but clearly evidence for its presence, shown in multiple studies, is valuable, because the ability to stimulate some acupoints that cause a strong physiological response (e.g., to reduce blood pressure) may be important clinically (Fu, Guo, and Longhurst 2008; Li et al. 2002; Li et al. 2004; Li, Tjen-A-Looi, and Longhurst 2006; Tjen-A-Looi, Li, and Longhurst 2004; Zhou et al. 2005; Zhou et al. 2006).

Acupuncture's prolonged action is determined by the mode of sensory nerve stimulation, duration of stimulation, and network processing in cardiovascular centers in the hypothalamus, midbrain, and brainstem that are activated by acupuncture-induced somatic sensory nerve stimulation. In addition, the extent of release of neurotransmitters in the CNS over time with repeated stimulation, which increases genetic expression of neuromodulatory neurotransmitter precursors, likely accounts for the long-term action of electroacupuncture on blood pressure (Li and Longhurst 2007; Li, Tjen-A-Looi, and Longhurst 2009). Low frequency (2–6 Hz) or manual acupuncture provided at acupoints known to have a strong cardiovascular effect for

30 to 45 minutes seems to be most effective, reducing sympathetic outflow after 10 to 15 minutes of stimulation, and lasting for many minutes to hours or even days after acupuncture, depending on the model of investigation and the extent of repeated stimulation (Li and Longhurst 2007; Lin et al. 2001; Zhou et al. 2005). The cardiovascular influence of electroacupuncture in anesthetized experimental studies can last for 1 to 2 hours, and for 10 to 12 hours in studies conducted in awake subjects (Lin et al. 2001), whereas repetitive acupuncture administered once weekly over a course of eight weeks in patients with mild to moderate hypertension can exert a cardiovascular influence for several weeks (Li and Longhurst 2007; Longhurst, J. C. 2007a). Studies are needed to determine how frequently these blood- pressure-lowering effects of acupuncture must be reinforced.

Acupuncture seems to have the ability to reduce activity of neurons in regions controlling cardiovascular function that have been stimulated. Without an increase in neuronal discharge, there is nothing for acupuncture to influence, and thus, in normotensive conditions, acupuncture does not alter blood pressure. But if sympathetic activity is elevated, it can be reduced by acupuncture to lower blood pressure. Conversely, preliminary studies suggest that if the parasympathetic system is activated, to lower heart rate and blood pressure, acupuncture may be able to reduce vagal outflow and hence restore low blood pressure. Hence, acupuncture appears to be able to normalize elevated or depressed blood pressure.

Clinical Actions of Acupuncture

A number of cardiovascular risk factors, including hypertension, obesity, and hypercholesterolemia potentially can be influenced by acupuncture. In addition it may be efficacious in stroke, coronary and peripheral vascular disease (Longhurst, J. C. 2007a), although clearly more studies are warranted.

HYPERTENSION

Because acupuncture can decrease elevated sympathetic outflow and sympathoexcitatory reflex responses associated with elevated blood pressure, there is a rationale for using it to treat hypertension particularly in patients who do not want to take antihypertensive medications or who want the possibility of reducing the dosage of these drugs (Longhurst, J.C. 2007a). However, the results of clinical trials are mixed. Experimental studies in quadriplegic rats suggest that transcutaneous electrical stimulation (TENS), which shares some features with electroacupuncture, decreases the exaggerated blood pressure responses associated with colon distension (Collins and DiCarlo 2002). Although acupuncture appears to be safe (Averill et al. 2000), no clinical trials are available on its effect in spinal patients experiencing autonomic dysreflexia. Blood pressure in spontaneously hypertensive rats is reduced by acupuncture of acupoints located over the deep peroneal nerve for periods lasting up to 12 hours (Yao, Andersson, and Thoren 1982). A small study of fifty patients suggested that thirty minutes of acupuncture lowers both systolic and diastolic pressure (Chiu, Chi, and Reid 1997). However, the SHARP trial (Stop Hypertension with Acupuncture Research Trial), which treated patients with moderate hypertension over a twelve-week period, demonstrated no influence on blood pressure over and above the response to an invasive sham control, when blood pressure was measured intermittently with mercury sphygmoma-nometers (Macklin et al. 2006). However, large and small trials incorporating ambulatory monitoring have demonstrated small, but consistent, decreases in blood pressure in patients with mild to moderate hypertension, especially if acupoints are used that have been shown to have a strong cardiovascular influence (P5, P6, St36, and St37, referring to points along the pericardial and stomach meridians overlying the median and deep peroneal nerves—see Fig. 6.1) (Flachskampf, Gallasch, and Gefeller 2007; Li and Longhurst 2007a). Acupuncture may influence systolic and mean arterial pressure more than dia-stolic blood pressure. The onset action is slow, frequently requiring several acupuncture treatments over a course of several weeks before a sustained decrease in blood pressure is observed. Blood pressure decreases by five to twenty mmHg and tends to remain low for up to four weeks following cessa-tion of a two-month period of treatment.

CHOLESTEROL

In addition to hypertension, experimental studies demonstrate that acupunc-ture can lower cholesterol. Daily acupuncture for a two-week period reduces the increase in cholesterol in experimental models fed high cholesterol diets (Li and Zhang 2007; Wu and Hsu 1979). There are no good randomized control clinical trials, but a small non-randomized, unblinded trial of electroa-cupuncture that did not incorporate a control acupoint group demonstrated similar or greater weight loss, LDL cholesterol and triglyceride reduction, and greater HDL reduction, compared to a control group that were fed a low caloric diet (Cabioglu and Ergene 2005). More adequately powered, prospec-tive clinical trials incorporating adequate controls need to be conducted to determine if acupuncture effectively lowers cholesterol in patients with coronary disease.

OBESITY

Stimulation of auricular acupoints used to treat overweight patients provides input to regions of the brain that regulate food ingestion, including the ventromedial and ventrolateral hypothalamus (Shiraishi et al. 2009). However, the efficacy of acupuncture to consistently assist with weight loss in obesity is less certain. Experimental studies (Asamoto and Takeshige 1992) in rats have shown that auricular acupuncture leads to a 5 percent loss in weight over a period of two to three weeks. The results of clinical trials are mixed, with uncontrolled studies showing small decreases (Dung 1986; Huang, Yang, and Hu 1996; Mazzoni et al. 1999; Mok et al. 1976; Sacks 1975; Shafshak 1995; Soong 1975; Sun and Xu 1993) and many showing either very modest or no weight loss that could be ascribed to acupuncture. Most trials lack suitable controls. Thus, weight loss trials using acupuncture represent another area of needed research.

SMOKING CESSATION

Because acupuncture leads to the release of endogenous opioids, it has been thought that it may be useful in treating addictive habits like smoking. With respect to addiction, acupuncture reduces symptoms in subjects addicted to opiates like morphine (Han and Zhang 1993; Wen and Cheung 1973). However, metanalyses of relevant clinical trial with respect to smoking cessation reveals that many are low quality and short term, lack suitable controls, and do not provide sufficient information to assess their quality (White, Resch, and Ernst 1999). Thus, at present, insufficient data are available to determine the efficacy of acupuncture in smoking cessation. More research needs to be conducted in this area.

Acupuncture appears to lower blood pressure or reduce ischemia in only 70 percent of patients. Although more research is required, experimental studies suggest that antagonistic neuropeptides, such as cholecystokinin, may prevent acupuncture's normal action to release opioid neurotransmitters that limit sympathetic outflow.

MYOCARDIAL ISCHEMIA

Through an opioid mechanism, acupuncture lowers myocardial oxygen demand, and hence reduces demand-supply imbalances and regional ventricular dysfunction in experimental myocardial ischemia (Chao et al. 1999; Li et al. 1998). Similarly, small studies demonstrate that both TENS and acupuncture reduce myocardial ischemia that occurs during exercise in patients with angina and ECG evidence of ischemia (Ballegaard et al. 1990; 1995; 1999; Ballegaard, Meyer, and Trojaborg 1991; Ballegaard, Norrelund, and Smith 1996; Emanuelsson et al. 1987; Mannheimer et al. 1982; 1985; 1989; Richter, Herlitz, and Hjalmarson 1991). TENS is not exactly equivalent to acupuncture, since much stronger intensities of stimulation and higher frequencies are used during the transcutaneous stimulation, which also is not directed at specific locations (acupoints) over neural pathways. Although there is some debate about whether acupuncture increases coronary blood flow, it does lower the increase in blood pressure and the double product (but not the elevated heart rate) associated with exercise, hence reducing myocardial oxygen demand (Li et al. 2004).

A few studies have examined the influence of acupuncture in situations that can provoke angina. For example, acupuncture also decreases the reflex excitatory responses to mental stress (Middlekauff, Yu, and Hui 2001). It is important to note that the influence of acupuncture is not universal, since it occurs in only 70 percent of individuals (Li et al. 2004; Middlekauff, Yu, and Hui 2001). This raises the question of which individuals are most likely to respond. In this regard, individuals demonstrating changes in pain threshold and finger skin temperature in response acupuncture appear to be most responsive to acupuncture (Ballegaard et al. 1990; Ballegaard, Meyer, and Trojaborg 1991).

Several small studies have evaluated the influence of acupuncture in patients with symptomatic coronary artery disease. A course of acupuncture therapy employed over a period of several weeks decreases nitroglycerin consumption and the rate of anginal attacks in patients with stable angina (Ballegaard et al. 1990; Ballegaard, Meyer, and Trojaborg 1991; Liu et al. 1986; Richter, Herlitz, and Hjalmarson 1991). A prospective non-randomized study of patients in which acupuncture was administered as part of a lifestyle program incorporating stress reduction and healthy eating documented decreases in medication usage, in-patient days and the accumulated mortality rate (Ballegaard et al. 1999; 2004; Ballegaard, Norrelund, & Smith 1996). The specific contribution of acupuncture to these beneficial effects has not been determined.

PERIPHERAL VASCULAR DISEASE

TENS increases the survival of skin flaps in experimental models as well as in patients undergoing reconstructive surgery (Cramp et al. 2002; Lundeberg, Kjartansson, and Samuelson 1998). Spinal cord stimulation, which may involve activation of many of the same central neural regions as acupuncture (Longhurst, J. 2001), increases skin temperature, reduces pain and ulcer formation, and leads to tissue salvage in patients with peripheral vascular insufficiency (Augustinsson et al. 1985; Jivegard et al. 1987; 1995). No trials of acupuncture's influence in patients with peripheral vascular disease have been published. Thus, symptomatic peripheral arterial disease represents yet another area of needed future study.

Summary and Conclusions

Acupuncture through stimulation of sensory nerve pathways that project to cardiovascular regulatory regions in the brain and spinal cord has the ability to markedly reduce sympathetic outflow, and hence lower elevated blood pressure and myocardial oxygen demand. Interestingly, acupuncture does not alter blood pressure when it is in the normal range. In addition to lowering blood pressure, acupuncture may be able to reduce demand-induced myocardial ischemia mainly by lessening demand, rather than increasing the blood supply. The efficacy of acupuncture in reducing cardiovascular risk is much less apparent. It may assist in weight loss, although the changes typically are quite small. It also may reduce elevated cholesterol, but does not appear to consistently help smokers quit. Studies showing the cardiovascular effects are reasonably strong in experimental animals. Clinical trials of acupuncture, however, are not as numerous and tend to be small and frequently are not prospective or adequately controlled. It is clear that much more research on the role of acupuncture in cardiovascular disease is needed. Both mechanistic studies defining acupuncture's action and prospective, and adequately powered and carefully controlled randomized clinical trials should be conducted. Mechanistic studies can help guide the clinical studies by identifying points that can exert the strongest cardiovascular influence, the best modalities of stimulation, and the best combinations of acupoints stimulated to achieve optimal responses.

However, in designing trials for acupuncture, a number of issues that often have not been addressed in past studies need to be taken into account. One of the most important considerations in constructing clinical trials of acupuncture is the sham control. The literature suggests that simply placing (but not manipulating or electrically stimulating) a needle in an active acupoint or stimulation of an "inactive" acupoint may serve as an adequate strong control (Mayer 2000; Zhou et al. 2005), since in the absence of neural stimulation (i.e., stimulation outside a classical meridian) *deqi*, the neurological sensation associated with good responses during acupuncture, may not occur. It is clear that acupuncture trials cannot be reliably double-blinded, since it is not possible to prevent the acupuncturist from knowing exactly where to place the needle.

Another issue to consider in constructing acupuncture trials is the method for choosing acupoints. On one hand, TCM theory dictates that acupoints should be selected after obtaining a history followed by tongue and pulse physical diagnosis. This method leads to selection of variable combinations of points that are stimulated, depending on the individual acupuncturist's assessment. The different locations of stimulation increase the number of patients that have to be studied to adequately power studies, and thus determine statistically significant responses to acupuncture. This approach has led to more failures than successes in studies addressing clinically significant cardiovascular responses to acupuncture. A more standardized approach, commonly adapted in Western medical trails, is to select a fixed number of points that are always stimulated. Although the desire to simulate the actual practice of TCM is understandable, we have been able to use observations in experimental studies to help guide in the selection of the best points to stimulate to evoke reproducible acupuncture responses in approximately 70 percent of our preparations and in a preliminary clinical trial for hypertension (Li and Longhurst 2007). This more standardized approach, guided by modern biology, clearly is repugnant to many TCM practitioners, but it does allow critical testing of acupuncture's clinical responses—a necessary condition if this therapy is ever to be fully accepted by Western medicine. Without such critical testing, acupuncture will likely remain relegated largely to street corner clinics unassociated with mainstream medicine.

Clinical Application of Acupuncture in Cardiovascular Disease

At present, acupuncture probably can be used safely to treat patients with mild to moderate hypertension, i.e., blood pressures below 170/105 mmHg. Approximately 70 percent of patients likely will respond to the intervention, but unfortunately at the present time, we cannot determine which patients are more likely to be responsive. It should be kept in mind that acupuncture, especially electroacupuncture, is most effective in reducing systolic and mean blood pressure and is less effective in reducing diastolic pressure. Hence, it may be useful in subjects with reduced vascular compliance, including older patients. It can be used in patients off pharmacological therapy or in combination with antihypertensive drugs. Practitioners should be aware that the onset of action of the blood-pressure-lowering effects of acupuncture may take several weeks to develop, if it is employed once weekly for 30 minutes, using low frequency (2 Hz), low intensity (2–6 mA) electroacupuncture at acupoints that display cardiovascular activity, e.g., P5-P6 and St36-St37. Initial trials have determined that short courses (2 months) of electroacupuncture are effective, but few data are available to guide its use more chronically. Reinforcement of the initial therapy most likely will be required, either once each week or once every other week. If a patient is on drugs when the acupuncture is begun, there is a possibility that the drug therapy over time can be reduced, or possibly even stopped. However, drug therapy manipulation should be done in active collaboration with a physician. Thus, interaction between acupuncturists and Western physicians is recommended as the safest course for therapy at this time.

Future Research

A number of important clinical issues still need to be addressed in studies of acupuncture's role in cardiovascular medicine.

First, we need properly constructed trials on smoking, weight loss, and cholesterol reduction.

Second, the potential for acupuncture to raise blood pressure in subjects who have symptomatic hypotension needs to be evaluated, since early experimental results suggest that acupuncture can increase blood pressure when it has been lowered. The concept in these studies is that acupuncture does not just lower blood pressure if it is elevated, but rather it normalizes pressure, by raising it if it is too low, lowering it when it is high, and not altering it within the normal range. The idea of achieving homeostasis with acupuncture is entirely consistent with TCM theory, which states that stimulation of acupoints along meridians normalizes the imbalance of energy flow (*Qi*, see above), which occurs in disease states.

Third, although we are beginning to accept the possibility that acupuncture may be able to lower blood pressure in patients with hypertension, perhaps for prolonged periods of time, we do not know how often we need to reinforce this beneficial effect after the initial course of therapy.

Fourth, the importance of stimulating multiple points, although commonly used by most acupuncturists, has not been evaluated prospectively in sufficiently large sample sizes to provide a definitive answer. In fact, current experimental data suggest that stronger effects may not always be achieved by simultaneously stimulating two strong sets of cardiovascular acupoints (Zhou et al. 2005). However, there is evidence that acupuncture can have an influence at multiple levels in the brain and spinal cord (Longhurst, J.C. 2007b). Thus, the regional cardiovascular influence of acupuncture in the spinal cord (Zhou et al. 2006) likely can be supplemented by its more global actions in higher centers in the hypothalamus, midbrain, and medulla (Longhurst, J.C. 2007b).

Fifth, another concern that must be addressed in future acupuncture research is why only 70 percent of individuals respond to acupuncture, even when needles are carefully placed in acupoints known to have strong cardio-vascular effects (Li et al. 2004). It is likely that counter-regulatory neurotrans-mitter systems like cholecystokinin can antagonize the action of opioid neuromodulators that are released by acupuncture during its action on cardio-vascular centers in the brain (Huang 2007; Tang 1997). A reasonable, testable hypothesis, therefore, is that administration of an inhibitor of the CCK_A or CCK_B receptor system may convert some non-responders into responders or may enhance the effect of acupuncture in responsive individuals.

Sixth, the method of acupuncture application needs further consideration. As noted above, TENS causes many of the same cardiovascular responses that occur with acupuncture. In addition, it is well known that TENS can help con-trol pain much like acupuncture (Longhurst, J. 1998). Although there are fun-damental differences between acupuncture and TENS (see above), it may be possible to construct a noninvasive skin electrode system that could be used with stimulation parameters that are more like electroacupuncture (i.e., low intensity and low frequency) and that can be directed to stimulate specific acu-points known to have a strong cardiovascular influence. Such an electrode system then could be used in patients who cannot regularly visit an acupunc-turist or in military personnel who need a means to help them deal with the emotional and cardiovascular stress that they regularly encounter. A noninva-sive system would make acupuncture much more available for individuals who want to take responsibility for their own health care.

REFERENCES

Asamoto, S., and C. Takeshige. 1992. Activation of the satiety center by auricular acu-puncture point stimulation. *Brain Res Bulletin* 29(2): 157–64.

Augustinsson, L. E., C. A Carlson, J.,Holm, and L. Jivegard. 1985. Epidural electrical stimulation in severe limb ischemia: Pain relief, increased blood flow and possible limb saving effect. *Ann Surg* 202: 104–10.

Averill, A., A. C. Cotter, S. Nayak, R. J. Matheis, and S. C. Shiflett. 2000. Blood pressure response to acupuncture in a polulation at risk for autonomic dyreflexia. *Arch. Phys. Med. Rehabil* 81(11): 1494–97.

Ballegaard, S., E. Borg, B. Karpatschof, J. Nyboe, and A. Johannessen. 2004. Long-Term effects of integrated rehabilitation in patients with advanced angina pectoris: a nonrandomized compartive study. *J. Altern. Complement. Med* 10: 777–83.

Ballegaard, S., A. Johannessen, B. Karpatschof, and J. Nyeboe 1999. Addition of acupuncture and self-care education in the treatment of patients with severe angina pectoris may be cost beneficial: an open, prospective study. *J. Altern. Complement. Med* 5: 405–13.

Ballegaard, S., B. Karpatschof, J. A. Holck, C. N. Meyer, and W. Trojaborg. 1995. Acupuncture in angina pectoris. Do psycho-social and neurophysiological factors relate to the effect? *Acupunct. Electrother. Res* 20: 101–16.

Ballegaard, S., C. N. Meyer, and W. Trojaborg. 1991. Acupuncture in angina pectoris: does acupuncture have a specific effect? *J. Intern. Med* 229: 357–62.

Ballegaard, S., S. Norrelund, and D. F. Smith. 1996. Cost benefit of combines use of acupuncture, shiatsu and lifestyle adjustment for treatment of patients with severe angina pectoris. *Acupunct. Electrother. Res* 21: 187–97.

Ballegaard, S., F. Pedersen, A. Pietersen, V. H. Nissen, and N. V. Olsen. 1990. Effects of acupuncture in moderate stable angina pectoris. *J Intern Med* 227: 25–30.

Cabioglu, M. T. and N. Ergene. 2005. Electroacupuncture therapy for weight loss reduces serum total cholesterol, triglycerides, and LDL cholesterol levels in obese women. *American Journal of Chinese Medicine* 33(4): 525–33.

Chao, D. M., L. L. Shen, S. Tjen-A-Looi, K. F. Pitsillides, P. Li, and J. C. Longhurst. 1999. Naloxone reverses inhibitory effect of electroacupuncture on sympathetic cardiovascular reflex responses. *American Journal of Physiology* 276: H2127–H2134.

Chiu, Y. J., A. Chi, and I. A. Reid. 1997. Cardiovascular and endocrine effects of acupuncture in hypertensive patients. *Clinical and Experimental Hypertension* 19(7): 1047–63.

Collins, H. and S. DiCarlo. 2002. TENS attenuates response to colon distension in paraplegic and quadriplegic rats. *Am J Physiol Heart Circ Physiol* 283: H1734–H1739.

Cramp, F. L., G. R. McCullough, A. S. Lowe, and D. M. Walsh. 2002. Trancutaneous electric nerve stimulation: The effect of intensity on local and distal cutaneous blood flow and skin temperature in healthy subjects. *Arch. Phys. Med. Rehabil* 83: 5–9.

Dung, H. 1986. Role of the vagus nerve in weight reduction through auricular acupuncture. *Am J Acupuncture* 14: 249–54.

Emanuelsson, H., C. Mannheimer, F. Waagstein, and C. Wilhelmsson. 1987. Catecholamine metabolism during pacing-induced angina pectoris and the effect of transcutaneous electrical nerve stimulation. *Am Heart J* 114: 1360–66.

Flachskampf F. A., J. Gallasch, and O. Gefeller. 2007. Randomized trial of acupuncture to lower bldood pressure. *Circulation* 115: 3121–29.

Fu, L. W., Z. L. Guo, and J. C. Longhurst. 2008. Undiscovered role of endogenous TxA_2 in activation of cardiac sympathetic afferents during ischemia. *J Physiol* 586: 3287–300.

Han, J. S. and R. L. Zhang. 1993. Suppression of morphine abstinence syndrome by body electroacupuncture of different frequencies in rats. *Drug Alcohol Depend* 31(2): 169–75.

Huang C., Z. P. Hu, S. Z. Jiang, H. T. Li, J. S. Han, Y. Wang. 2007. CCKB receptor antagonist L365,260 potentiates the efficacy to and reverses chronic tolerance to electroacupuncture-induced analgesia in mice. *Brain Res Bulletin* 71: 447–51.

Huang, M. H., R. C.Yang, and S. H. Hu. 1996. Preliminary results of triple therapy for obesity. *Int J Obes Relat Metab Disord* 20(9): 830–36.

Jivegard, L. D., L. E. Augustinsson, C. A. Carlsson, and J. Holm. 1987. Long-term results by epidural spinal electrical stimulation (ESES) in patents with inoperable severe lower limb ischaemia. *Eur J Vasc Surg* 1(5): 345–49.

Jivegard, L. D., L. E. Augustinsson, J. Holm, B. Risberg, and P. Ortenwall. 1995. Effects of spinal cord stimulation (SCS) in patients with inoperable sever lower limb ischemia: A prospective randomised controlled study. *Eur J Vasc Endovasc Surg* 9(4): 421–25.

Klein L., A. I. Trachtenberg. 1997. National Library of Medicine. Reference Section. Acupuncture: January 1970 through October 1997. (Series: Current Bibliographies in Medicine.) Bethesda, MD: U.S. Dept. of Health and Human Services, Public Health Service, National Institutes of Health, National Library of Medicine.

Li, M., S. Tjen-A-Looi, and J. Longhurst, J. 2009. Electroacupuncture enhances preproenkephalin mrna expression in rostral ventrolateral medulla of rats. *FASEB* 23: 958.

Li, M., and Y. Zhang. 2007. Modulation of gene expression in cholesterol-lowering effect of electroacupuncture at Fenglong acupoint (ST40): A cDNA microarray study. *Int J Mol Med* 19(4): 617–29.

Li, P., O. Ayannusi, C. Reed, and J. Longhurst. 2004. Inhibitory effect of electroacupuncture (EA) on the pressor response induced by exercise stress. *Clinical Autonomic Research* 14: 182–88.

Li, P., and J. Longhurst. 2007. Long-lasting inhibitory effect of EA on blood pressure in patients with mild to moderate hypertension. *Society for Neuroscience* 35: 417.

Li, P., K. Pitsillides, S. Rendig, H. L. Pan, and J. Longhurst. 1998. Reversal of reflex-induced myocardial ischemia by median nerve stimulation: A feline model of electroacupuncture. *Circulation* 97: 1186–94.

Li, P., K. Rowshan, M. Crisostomo, S. Tjen-A-Looi, and J. Longhurst. 2002. Effect of electroacupuncture on pressor reflex during gastric distention. *American Journal of Physiology* 283: R1335–R1345.

Li, P., S. Tjen-A-Looi, and J. Longhurst. 2006. Excitatory projections from arcuate nucleus to ventrolateral periaqueductal gray in electroacupuncture inhibition of cardiovascular reflexes. *American Journal of Physiology* 209: H2535–H2542.

Lin, M. C., R. Nahin, M. E. Gershwin, J. C. Longhurst, and K. K. Wu. 2001. State of complementary & alternative medicine in cardiovascular, lung and blood. *Circulation* 103: 2038–41.

Liu, F., J. Li, G. Liu, Y. Wang, H. Chi, B. Gao, J. Meng, R. Liu, and H. Xu. 1986. Clinical observation of effect of acupuncture on angina pectoris. In *Research on acupuncture, moxibustion and acupuncture anesthesia*, ed. H. T. Chang, 861–75. Beijing: Science Press and Springer Verlag.

Longhurst, J. 1998. Acupuncture's beneficial effects on the cardiovascular system. *Preventive Cardiology* 1(4): 21–33.

Longhurst, J. 2001. Alternative approaches to the medical management of cardiovascular disease: acupuncture, electrical nerve and spinal cord stimuation. *Heart Dis* 3: 236–41.

Longhurst, J. C. 2002. Central and peripheral neural mechanisms of acupuncture in myocardial ischemia. In *Acupuncture: Is there a physiological basis?*, ed. A. Sato, P. Li, and J. L. Campbell, 79–87. New York: Elsevier Science.

Longhurst, J. C. 2007a. Acupuncture. In *Integrative cardiology: Complementary and alternative medicine for the heart*, ed. J. Vogel and M. Krucoff, 113–31. New York: McGraw Hill.

Longhurst, J.C. 2007b. Integrative cardiology: Mechanisms of cardiovascular action of acupuncture. In *Integrative cardiology: Complementary and alternative medicine for the heart*, ed. J. Vogel and M. Krucoff, 382–98. New York: McGraw Hill.

Lundeberg, T., J. Kjartansson, and U. E. Samuelson. 1998. Effect of electrical nerve stimulation on healing of ischaemic skin flaps. *Lancet* 24: 712–14.

Macklin, E.A., P. M. Wayne, L. Kalish, P. Valaskatgis, J. Thompson, M. Pian-Smith, Q. Zhang, S. Stevens, C. Goertz, R. J. Prineas, B. Buczynski, and R. Zusman. 2006. Stop hypertension with the acupuncture research program (SHARP): Results of a randomized, controlled clinical trial. *Hypertension* 48(5): 838–45.

Mannheimer, C., C. A. Carlsson, H. Emanuelsson, A. Vedin, F. Waagstein, and C. Wilhelmsson. 1985. The effects of transcutaneous electrical nerve stimulation in patients with severe angina pectoris. *Circulation* 71(2): 308–16.

Mannheimer, C., C.A. Carlsson, K. Eriksson, A. Vedin, and C. Wilhelmsson. 1982. Transcutaneous electrical nerve stimulation in severe angina pectoris. *European Heart Journal* 3: 297–302.

Mannheimer, C., H. Emanuelsson, F. Waagstein, and C. Wilhelmsson. 1989. Influence of naloxone on the effects of high frequency transcutaneous electrical nerve stimulation in angina pectoris induced by atrial pacing. *Br.Heart J* 62(1): 36–42.

Mayer, D. J. 2000. Acupuncture: An evidence-based review of the clinical literature. *Ann Rev Med* 51(49): 63.

Mazzoni, R., E. Mannucci, S. Rizzello, V. Ricca, and C. Rotella. 1999. Failure of acupuncture in the treatment of obesity: A pilot study. *Eat Weight Disord* 4(4): 198–202.

Middlekauff, H. R., J. L.Yu, and K. Hui. 2001. Acupuncture effects on reflex responses to mental stress in humans. *Am J Physiol Regul Integr Comp Physiol* 280(5): R1462–R1468.

Mok, M., L. Parker, S. Voina, and G. Bray. Treatment of obesity by acupuncture. *Am J Clin Nutr* 29(8): 832–35.

Richter, A., J. Herlitz, and A. Hjalmarson. 1991. Effect of acupuncture in patients with angina pectoris. *European Heart Journal* 12: 175–78.

Sacks, L. L. 1975. Drug addiction, alcoholism, smoking, obesity, treated by auricular staplepuncture. *Am J Acupuncture* 3: 147.

Shafshak, T. 1995. Electroacupuncture and exercise in body weight reduction and their application in rehabilitating patients with knee osteoarthritis. *American Journal of Chinese Medicine* 23(1): 15–25.

Shiraishi, T., M. Onoe, T. Kojima, Y. Sameshima, and T. Kageyama. 2009. Effects of auricular stimulation on feeding-related hypothalamic neuronal activity in normal and obese rats. *Brain Res Bulletin* 36(2): 141–48.

Soong, Y. 1975. The treatment of exogenous obesity employing auricular acupuncture. *American Journal of Chinese Medicine* 3(3): 285–87.

Sun, Q., and Y. Xu. 1993. Simple obesity and obesity hyperlipemia treated with otoacupoint pellet pressure and body acupuncture. *J Tradit Chin Med* 13(1): 22–26.

Tang N. M., H. W. Dong, X. M. Wang, Z. C. Tsui, and J. S. Han. 1997. Cholecystokinin antisense RNA increases the analgesic effect induced by electroacupuncture or low dose morphine: conversion of low responder rats into high responders. *Pain.* 71: 71–80.

Tjen-A-Looi, S., H. L. Pan, and J. C. Longhurst. 1998. Endogenous bradykinin activates ischaemically sensitive cardiac visceral afferents through kinin B_2 receptors in cats. *Journal of Physiology* 510(2): 633–41.

Tjen-A-Looi, S. C., P. Li, and J. C. Longhurst. 2004. Medullary substrate and differential cardiovascular response during stimulation of specific acupoints. *American Journal of Physiology* 287: R852–R862.

Vickers, A. J. 1998. Bibliometric analysis of randomized trials in complementary medicine. *Complement Ther Med* 6: 185–89.

Wen, H. L., and S. Y. C. Cheung. 1973. Treatment of drug addiction by acupuncture and 14 electrical stimulation. *Asian J Med* 9: 138–41.

White, A. R., K. Resch, and E. Ernst. 1999. A meta-analysis of acupuncture techniques for smoking cessation. *Tob Control* 8(4): 393–97.

Wu, C. C., and C. Hsu. 1979. Neurogenic regulation of lipid metabolism in the rabbit. A mechanism for the cholesterol-lowering effect of acupuncture. *Atherosclerosis* 33(2): 153–64.

Yao, T., S. Andersson, and P. Thoren. 1982. Long-lasting cardiovascular depression induced by acupuncture-like stimulation of the sciatic nerve in unanaesthetized spontaneously hypertensive rats. *Brain Research* 240: 77–85.

Zhou, W., L. W. Fu, S. C. Tjen-A-Looi, P. Li, and J. C. Longhurst. 2005. Afferent mechanisms underlying stimulation modality-related modulation of acupuncture-related cardiovascular responses. *Journal of Applied Physiology* 98(3): 872–80.

Zhou, W., I. Hsiao, V. Lin, and J. Longhurst. 2006. Modulation of cardiovascular excitatory responses in rats by transcutaneous magnetic stimulation: Role of the spinal cord. *Journal of Applied Physiology* 100(3): 926–32.

Zhou W., A. Mahajan, and J. C. Longhurst. 2009. Spinal nociceptin mediates electroacupuncture-related modulation of visceral sympathoexcitatory reflex responses in rats. *American Journal of Physiology.* 297: H859–H865.

7

Spirituality and Heart Health

MARY JO KREITZER AND KEN RIFF

KEY CONCEPTS

- Spirituality has been defined in a multitude of ways and is generally understood to be related to, but distinct from, religiosity. In the broadest sense, spirituality is focused on purpose, meaning, and connectedness with self, others, and a higher power. Spirituality is recognized as an integral part of being human that is very interconnected with health and well-being.
- A *spiritual assessment or screening* can be conducted by a physician, nurse, spiritual care provider, or other health professional as a routine part of providing care. It is common for screening questions to be incorporated into standard health history interviews and forms.
- Emotional and spiritual pain, loneliness, despair, and isolation are examples of spiritual issues that are known to be related to heart disease.
- Commonly used spiritual practices include prayer, meditation, journaling, labyrinth walking, and interacting with nature.

■

In a compelling book titled *Love and Survival: The Scientific Basis for the Healing Power of Intimacy,* Dean Ornish, most well-known for demonstrating that comprehensive lifestyle changes can reverse even severe coronary heart disease, writes about the emotional, psychological, and spiritual dimensions of "opening your heart." He notes that in his experience, when the emotional heart and the spiritual heart begin to open, the physical heart often follows. The core message conveyed is that "anything that promotes a sense of isolation often leads to illness and suffering. Anything that promotes a sense of love and intimacy, connection and community, is healing" (Ornish 1998, 14).

The approach to care that Ornish is describing reflects the growing sense that we need to move beyond the biopsychosocial model of care proposed by Engel (1977) to one that encompasses what is often called whole-person care, a biopsychosocial-spiritual model. A growing number of medical schools teach content or even entire courses in spirituality (Puchalski and Larson 1998), and the Joint Commissions on Healthcare Organization (2008) requires that spiritual care be available to patients in hospital settings. This chapter will explore the implications of spirituality for heart health by examining definitions of spirituality, the relationship between spirituality and clinical outcomes, the role of the health professional in meeting the spiritual needs of patients and families, and ways to support and nurture the spirituality of professional caregivers.

Throughout history, and across all cultures, spiritual beliefs and practices have been expressed in a myriad of ways. The word "spirit" comes from the Hebrew work *ruah*, which means wind, breath, or air that which gives life (Golberg,1998). Greeks viewed the spirit in opposition to the body and any material reality. In Chinese, spirit means *chi* or vital energy (Chiu, 2000). The Latin word, *spiritus*, means breath. Spirituality, in its broadest sense, is recognized as an integral part of being human that is deeply interconnected with health and well-being.

The healing professions of nursing and medicine, were grounded in spirituality from their earliest beginnings. In ancient societies, the connection between spirituality and healing was so close that the roles of priest, shaman, and healer were one and the same. Hildegard of Bingen, a twelfth-century Christian mystic was well known for her use of herbs, art, music and prayer. The first hospitals were founded by religious orders and missionary movements across centuries and continents; from the beginning, they have recognized the need for spiritual healing along side physical healing.

It has only been since the time of the scientific revolution and the advent of dualism, in the seventeeth century, that a wall of separation has divided the physical and spiritual care of people into mutually exclusive, and often antagonistic, camps. Medicine was charged with caring for the body, and later the mind, while religion was left with the care and feeding of the soul. As a result, contemporary Western science, including the disciplines of medicine and nursing, has often dealt with the spiritual side of human nature by ignoring it and viewing it as beyond the scope of their professional practice.

Over the past 20 years, there has been a growing interest in both the lay press and the professional literature on the topic of spirituality and its impact on health and well-being. Increasingly, consumers are demanding care that is holistic and attentive to the whole person—mind, body, and spirit. Clinicians are beginning to recognize the importance of both assessing and addressing spiritual needs of patients, and researchers are establishing a link between spirituality and spiritual interventions and health outcomes.

The role of the health professional in addressing the spiritual issues of patients is not without some controversy. As noted by Post, Puchalski, and Larson (2000), there are physicians who may still think that it is inappropriate to discuss spiritual matters with patients, either because they see themselves as lacking the expertise to do so, or feel that it may be an intrusion. Post, Puchalski, and Larson note, however, that there is a preponderance of evidence that confirms that many patients welcome such discussion. Davidson (2008) asserts that good medicine should include sensitivity to the spiritual dimension of patients' lives, and Magyar-Russell et al. (2008) argue that the physician who knows little about a patient's family status, occupation, and spiritual and religious beliefs may provide inadequate therapeutic guidance despite being technically competent. The goal of the clinician, suggests Hart (2008), should be "to figure out what the patient finds supportive or important and then to encourage such healthy practices in each patient's life rather than injecting practitioners' own thoughts or belief systems into the patient's life". Hart goes on to emphasize that a clear, ethical plan for how to address the issue of spirituality with patients is important.

Defining Spirituality

Spirituality is a multidimensional construct that has been defined in a multitude of ways, and is generally understood to be related to but distinct from religiosity (Albaugh 2003; Ameling and Povilonis 2001; Chiu et al. 2004; Fry 1998; Narayanasamy 1999; Tanyi 2002). Religious beliefs are associated with a particular faith tradition. Participation in or commitment to a religion may involve adherence to certain beliefs (ideology), religious practices (prayer, sacraments, and rituals), religious proscriptions (dietary modifications or avoidance of tobacco, alcohol, or drugs), and participation in a religious community. Spirituality is understood to be a broader concept that includes many dimensions. Murray and Zentner (1989) define spirituality as a quality that goes beyond religious affiliation and that strives for inspiration, reverence, awe, meaning, and purpose, even in those who do not believe in God. The spiritual dimension, they suggest, is in harmony with the universe, strives for answers about the infinite, and comes into focus when the person faces

Table 7.1. Characteristics of Spirituality

Connectedness/relationships with self, others, Higher Power, nature
Meaning and purpose in life
Transcendence
Love/compassion
Wholeness
Energy

emotional stress, physical illness, or death. Spirituality has also been described as a process and sacred journey (Mische 1982), the essence or life principle of a person (Colliton 1981), an experience of the radical truth of things (Legere,1984), and the propensity to make meaning (Reed 1992). Waldfogel (1997) notes that the experiences of joy, love, forgiveness, and acceptance all depend on, and are manifestations of, optimal spiritual well-being. Cohen (1993) adds that spirituality involves finding deep meaning in everything, including illness and death, and living life according to a set of values. Chiu et al. describe spirituality as a power, force, or energy that stimulates creativity, motivation, or a striving for inspiration (2004). The simplest and most straightforward definition is from Pargament (1997), who defined spirituality as the "search for the sacred." Table 7.1 lists characteristics commonly associated with spirituality.

RELATIONSHIP BETWEEN SPIRITUALITY AND HEALTH OUTCOMES

A number of studies report findings suggesting that spiritual and religious beliefs overall contribute to positive health benefits, including stress reduction and an increased sense of well-being (Larson et al. 1992). A metaanalysis of 42 studies revealed that attendance at church, synagogue, mosque, or Buddhist monastery is related to longer life (McCullough et al. 2000). The odds of survival were significantly greater for people who scored higher on measures of religious involvement than for people who scored lower, even after controlling for a variety of social and health-related variables.

These findings mirror a number of earlier studies that focused on the relationship between social support, isolation, and heart disease. Ruberman et al. (1984) studied over 2,300 men who had survived a heart attack. Men who identified themselves as being socially isolated and having a high degree of life stress had more than four times the risk of death as men who reported low levels of isolation and stress, even when controlling for factors such as smoking, diet, weight, and exercise. Interestingly, these psychosocial effects had a much more powerful effect on premature deaths than did the beta-blocker drugs that were the primary focus of the study. Williams et al. (1992) studied over 1,300 men and women who had undergone coronary angioplasty and were found to have at least one severely occluded coronary artery. In following these patients five years post-procedure, it was found that men and women who were not married and who did not have a close confidant were three times more likely to have died than those who were married, had a confidant, or both.

In addition to the extensive body of literature on the health-related benefits of social support and community, many studies have been conducted that have focused more specifically on the relationship between spiritual health and heart health. Haskell (2003) reported that patients who score higher on spirituality or religious scales have lower mortality due to coronary artery disease or cardiac surgery-related complications. Similarly, Morris (2001), in reporting on Ornish's Lifestyle Heart Trial, reported that the degree of spiritual well-being may be an important factor in the progression or regression of coronary artery disease. Patients with the lowest scores on spiritual well-being had the most progression of coronary obstruction, while those with the highest scores had the most regression. Spirituality has also been found to be correlated to depression in patients with chronic heart failure. Depression is known to be associated with a variety of adverse health outcomes in cardiac patients, including poor quality of life, more frequent hospitalizations and higher mortality. In a study of outpatients with heart failure, Bekelman et al. (2007) found that greater spiritual well-being was strongly associated with less depression, thereby suggesting that spirituality may be a modifiable coping resource that potentially could reduce or prevent depression, and thus improve quality of life, among other outcomes. Not all studies, however, have reported consistent results in relating spirituality with positive health outcomes. In a study of 503 patients surviving an acute myocardial infarction, Blumenthal et al. (2007) found little evidence that self-reported spirituality, frequency of church attendance, or frequency of prayer was associated with cardiac morbidity or all-cause mortality in patients with depression and/or low perceived support.

There is a growing body of literature focused on the effects of intercessory prayer on health outcomes in patients with heart disease. The studies (Aviles et al. 2001; Benson et al. 2006; Byrd 1988; Harris et al. 1999; Krucoff, Crater, and Lee 2006) have varied considerably in methodological rigor, the populations studies, and the endpoints measured. While trends have been reported in the various studies, as a whole, the results have been inconclusive.

Assessing Spirituality

A spiritual assessment or screening can be conducted by a physician, nurse, spiritual care provider. or other health professional as a routine part of providing care. It is common for screening questions to be incorporated into standard health history interviews and forms. Table 7.2 provides an example of questions that may help to detect a spiritual need or issue.

The FICA interview guide (Puchalski and Romer 2000) is frequently used to obtain a spiritual history in clinical settings. FICA is an acronym that stands for faith, importance/ influence, community, and address. Within each of these four areas, there is a set of questions such as: What is your faith? How important is your faith? Are you part of a religious community? How would you like spiritual issues addressed in your care? A tool called Hope, developed by Anadarajah, Long, and Smith (2001), taps into four similar domains. Examples of questions in the interview guide include:

- H stands for sources of hope, meaning, comfort, strength, peace, love and connection
  - What do you hold onto in difficult times?
  - What sustains you and keeps you going?
- O stands for organized religion
  - Are you part of a spiritual or religious community?
  - What aspects of your religion are helpful or not so helpful to you?
- P stands for personal spirituality and practices
  - Do you have personal spiritual beliefs that are independent of your religion?
  - What spiritual practices do you find most helpful to you personally?

Table 7.2. Spiritual Screening Questions

What are your sources of hope, strength, comfort and peace?

Are you part of a religious or spiritual community?

What spiritual practices do you find most helpful to you personally?

Are there any specific practices or restrictions I should know about in providing your health care?

Leonard, B., and D. Carlson. 2003. Spirituality in Healthcare. www.csh.umn.edu/modules/index.html

- E stands for effects on medical care and end-of-life issues.
  - Has being sick affected your ability to do things that usually help you spiritually?

Beyond these tools, there are a growing number of standardized measures that have been developed to assess spiritual and religious beliefs and practices for the purpose of research and evaluation. The Spiritual Well-Being Scale (SWBS), developed by Paloutzian and Ellison (1983), measures both religious and existential well-being. Religious well-being refers to one's relationship with God or some higher power, and existential well-being refers to a sense of purpose in life and satisfaction with life. The Serenity Scale, developed by Roberts and Aspy (1993) and abbreviated by Kreitzer et al. (2009), focuses on a dimension of spirituality called serenity. Serenity is defined as being a spiritual experience of inner peace that is independent of external events.

Addressing Spiritual Issues

When patients develop heart disease, they may experience a number of physical symptoms including pain, shortness of breath, palpitations, lack of energy, sweating, nausea, dizziness, weakness, and edema. The predominant orientation of biomedicine is on curing—that is, diagnosing, treating, and repairing the broken or damaged part of the body. This requires technical competence on the part of the health care provider, as well as access to technology, and an environment in which care can be safely provided. Without a doubt, patients seek care to be cured, relieved of the burden of their illness or disease. The human experience, however, encompasses more than the physical symptoms that are often the stimulus for seeking care. A diagnosis of heart disease and its ensuing treatment may release a cascade of feelings and emotions ranging from anxiety and fear to profound sadness, depression, grief, loss, hopelessness, anger, isolation, or spiritual distress. As noted by Milstein (2005), the trauma of a diagnosis may shatter the person's beliefs about the predictability of the world and create a sense of meaninglessness. A critical task is to "make sense" of the loss and sort out its significance in the larger context of one's life. This is the work of spirituality and healing. Spirituality, as noted earlier, focuses on finding meaning, purpose, and connections. Healing is about restoring wholeness and integration and requires attending to the whole person—body, mind, and spirit. An integrative approach as described by Milstein includes a focus on curing and healing, on "being with" as well as "doing to."

"Being with" patients is a way for health care providers to more deeply connect with patients, and in doing so, provide spiritual support. This requires, however, cultivation of skills such as deep listening, compassion, and presence.

- Deep listening: Enables the health care provider to be alert for meanings, connections, and yearnings reflected in conversations. It is important to listen to both what is said as well as what is not said. Authenticity is critically important. Patients can sense when the listener is distracted or not really interested.
- Compassion: Cultivating compassion develops within us a consciousness of other's distress and suffering and a desire to alleviate it.
- Mindfulness: The skill of mindfulness enables us to be anchored in the present moment and free ourselves of reactive, habitual patterns of thinking, feeling, and acting.
- Presence: When we are truly present to another human being, we are intentionally choosing to be with another in a healing way. This requires more than just physical presence. In Western culture, there is a strong bias toward action. Health care providers too often feel that they are not effective unless they are doing something. Presence requires being, not doing. This may be especially challenging for providers during times of expressions of anger or anguish by patients or families. It is also difficult because in a fee-for-service environment, providers are paid to "do something" and are not paid for presence.

As noted by Anandarajah (2008), "The therapeutic intervention at this heart level is at once both simple and extremely difficult. It requires that health care professionals bring their humanity (?) to the medical encounter".

Health care providers need to recognize that at times, the person most able to meet the patient's needs is a professional trained in spiritual care, such as a chaplain or a community-based religious leader. This is particularly important if the patient is seeking support for specialized prayer, or ritual. While the chaplain or a religious leader may be the primary spiritual care provider, spiritual care can be effectively and interchangeably provided by multiple members of the care team.

In an exploratory study of spiritual care at the end of life, Daaleman and his colleagues (2008) identified barriers to and facilitators of spiritual care. Lack of sufficient time was a major barrier, as were institutional obstacles such as absence of privacy and lack of continuity of providers. Social, religious, or cultural discordance between caregivers and patients was another obstacle to care. Having ample time to foster relationships with a facilitator was important, as was effective communication among the caregivers and between the caregivers and the patient. Health care providers also noted that their personal experiences with serious illness and death helped them to more effectively provide spiritual care to patients.

Many patients engage in spiritual self-care practices that health care providers should be aware of which enhance their health, well-being, and ability to cope with illness. Commonly used spiritual practices include the following:

- Prayer: There are many forms of prayer. Prayer may be offered in words, song, sighs, cries, gestures, or silence. Prayer may be individual or communal, public or private. Prayers may be petitions or requests for healing, for peace, for safety, for acceptance, for strength to continue, as well as for courage. Prayer is a means of reaching out and connecting with a higher power.
- Meditation: Meditation is a self-directed practice for relaxing the body and calming the mind that has been used by people in many cultures since ancient times. Kabat-Zinn (2005) emphasizes that meditation is best thought of as a way of being, rather than a collection of techniques. Mindfulness expands the capacity for awareness and for self-knowing. When a mindful state is cultivated, it frees people from routinized thought patterns, senses, and relationships, and the destructive mind states and emotions that accompany them. When people are able to escape from highly conditioned, reactive, and habitual thinking, they are able to respond in more effective and authentic ways.
- Music, Art, and Nature: The arts are powerful healing tools that can help people explore feelings, gain new insights and perspectives, and enhance other spiritual practices. For some, being in nature is a powerful spiritual experience.
- Journaling: Journaling is both a way to record experiences and a way to get in touch with inner thoughts and feelings. People who journal on a regular basis often find it to be a way to measure progress in self-growth and attain a broader perspective on life and relationships.
- Walking a Labyrinth: A labyrinth is a circuitous path that leads to a center. It is different from a maze that has twists, turns, and blind alleys. A labyrinth has only one way in to the center and one way out. When people walk the labyrinth, they may pray, meditate, listen to music, or just observe nature. People report that when they walk a labyrinth, they gain insight or perspective. For some people, walking a labyrinth is both an actual physical experience as well as a metaphor for life's journey.
- Spiritual Direction or Counseling: Spiritual directors or counselors accompany people on their spiritual journeys. They help people

explore such spiritual issues as grief, loss, anger, and abandonment, as well as life challenges. They may offer guidance in prayer, journaling, and reading of sacred texts. Spiritual directors may also help explore how God or the divine is present and active in one's life. Spiritual directors are listeners and companions. Like other forms of counseling, spiritual directors do not give answers, but rather assist individuals in exploring questions, issues, and concerns in their lives. Spiritual directors are found at retreat centers and in private practice and may be employed by health care institutions or faith communities.

Spirituality of Physicians

Medicine's deepest roots spring from a spiritual foundation. Modern medicine evolved from the tradition and role of the spiritual healer. Whether in ancient Babylonia and Egypt (Jayne 2003) or in more contemporaneous tribal cultures (Aldridge 1991), the community healer utilized spiritual power to address the underlying spiritual issues thought to be at the basis of the patient's disease. Even today, many religious orders are deeply engaged in health care and offer a combination of biomedicine and spirituality (or religion) to address both the physical and spiritual needs of their patients.

The previous section documented the growing interest in, and extensive literature on, patient and family spiritual issues. The literature on nurse spirituality is also rich, in part due to the importance of spirituality in the practice of holistic nursing (3). In contrast to these voluminous literatures, the study of physician spirituality is conspicuous in its absence.

The perceived importance of physician spirituality has faded as medicine has become scientifically-based. The Western conception of the duality of body and spirit, combined with the spectacular successes that have accrued from considering disease as a biological disorder that can be understood through rational scientific inquiry, has led many to dismiss physician spirituality as a relic of a superstitious past.

However, relationships have symmetry, and it is fundamentally flawed to consider the impact of patient spirituality on the physician–patient relationship without also considering the impact of physician spirituality. Disregarding physician spirituality opens physicians up to the risk of misunderstanding a critical dimension of the physician–patient relationship, or missing chances to help patients cope with their fears and their pain; the physician may also miss opportunities to derive deep fulfillment from their professional work—perhaps the only source of true long-term satisfaction left in the modern practice of medicine. We consider each in order.

Physician Spirituality and the Physician–Patient Relationship

There appears to be general agreement that patient spirituality and religious issues are important determinants of decision-making and coping skills when dealing with illness, and thus deserve study and attention (Astro, Puchalski, and Sulmasy 2001; Mueller, Plevak, and Rummans 2001). These religious influences on the healthcare process are not confined to patients. Curlin and colleagues found that 55 percent of physicians agree with the statement, "My religious beliefs influence my practice of medicine" (2005).

However, as a group, physicians' religious characteristics are significantly different from the U.S. population as a whole. These differences include increased physician affiliation with religions that are underrepresented in the general population, an increased likelihood to consider themselves spiritual but not religious, and twice the likelihood of coping with major problems without relying on God (Curlin et al. 2005). These differences might be expected to have an impact on important components of the physician–patient relationship.

Sulmasy (1997)) has developed a four-quadrant model that explores physician–patient interactions categorized by the status of physician and patient religious beliefs. In one quadrant, both the patient and the physician believe in God. In this situation, there is the foundation for meaningful dialogue, tempered by the potential problem of different religious traditions. In the converse situation, neither the patient nor the physician believe in God. Here, religious or spiritual matters may not be important components of the relationship.

When the patient believes in God and the physician does not (statistically the most likely probability), the physician needs to know how best to respect the patient's beliefs within the context of his own belief system. In this statistically probable situation, it is important for physicians to be very clear on their own spiritual beliefs (or lack thereof) in order to feel comfortable and supportive interacting with a patient who just as firmly may feel very differently.

The last combination, and statistically the least probable, is for the physician to believe in God while the patient does not. Here the potential danger is for a physician, motivated by a desire to help a human being in distress, to inject religion or spirituality into the relationship when it is not desired. However, the normal process of obtaining a spiritual assessment serves to identify this potentially awkward situation and will guide the perceptive clinician appropriately. It is considered inappropriate for a physician to proselytize on behalf of his or her religious or spiritual beliefs.

Koenig (2008) has described seven reasons physicians may want to assess and address their patients' spiritual needs.

1. Many patients are religious, and many would like their faith to be a factor in their health care.
2. Religion influences patients' abilities to cope with their illnesses.
3. Religious beliefs and practices may influence health outcomes.
4. Patients may be isolated from their traditional sources of religious support.
5. Religious beliefs may impact medical decisions and choices of therapies.
6. Religious commitments may influence the type of follow-up care and support a patient receives after leaving the hospital.
7. The Joint Commission requires a spiritual history be taken and documented on every patient admitted to an acute care hospital.

Physician Spirituality and Compassion

Few, if any, physicians would challenge the proposition that compassion is a desirable trait in a physician. Yet few, if any, would disagree that compassion is in increasingly short supply in modern healthcare. Yet of the six "C" characteristics Emmanuel and Dubler (1995) defined as necessary in an ideal physician–patient relationship (choice, competence, communication, compassion, continuity, and [no] conflict of interest), compassion may be the only one not threatened by the effects of the changes sweeping across American healthcare.

In contrast to sympathy (sharing the feelings of another) or empathy (identifying with the feelings of another), compassion includes the desire to be of help and to alleviate the suffering of another. Sympathy and empathy may result from individual personality characteristics, or may be skills that can be taught in professional training (Burack et al. 1999; Carmer and Glick 1996; Pence 1983). Compassion, on the other hand, has traditionally been more closely associated with spirituality, particularly Buddhism and Christianity.

As described by Rinpoche and Shlim (2006), compassion is defined in Buddhism as the sincere desire to alleviate the suffering of another. Buddhists believe that people are fundamentally and inherently compassionate, but our compassion is masked by the distractions and fears created by our mind, particularly anger and attachment. Thus, in the Buddhist tradition, the way to cultivate compassion is to learn how to move beyond the mind-generated traps of anger and attachment. The tools used to do so include meditation, yoga, service to others, and the cultivation of a calm and detached mind.

The Christian canon has many references to the compassion of Jesus. In Matthew 20:34, Jesus is described as a compassionate healer: "So Jesus had compassion on them, and touched their eyes: and immediately their eyes received sight, and they followed him." Matthew 9:36 describes Jesus as a compassionate leader: "When he saw the crowds, he was deeply moved with compassion for them, because they were troubled and helpless, like sheep without a shepherd." Jesus as a compassionate healer is again referenced in Matthew 14:14: "When He went ashore, He saw a large crowd, and felt compassion for them and healed their sick."

Thus the pursuit and engagement of physician spirituality may be a powerful aid in fostering the development of physician compassion.

Physician Spirituality and Professional Satisfaction

There has been a profound increase in physician professional dissatisfaction over the past twenty years. In 1973, 15 percent of several thousand practicing physicians expressed any doubt that they had made the correct career choice. Surveys over the past 10 years have found that 30–40 percent of physicians now state they would not choose medicine as a career if starting out today. Many causes have been postulated, including managed care, the malpractice crisis, disparate expectations between what patients demand and what physicians can deliver, and lack of time (Zugler 2004). While improving physician satisfaction has obvious benefit to the physician and the profession, it also appears that patients of satisfied physicians are also more satisfied (Haas et al. 2000).

Physician stress and dissatisfaction are not limited to practicing physicians. Shanafelt et al. (2002) found that 76 percent of internal medicine residents met criteria for burnout, including high scores on depersonalization or emotional exhaustion subscales, leading one writer to ponder, "Who is sicker: patients—or residents?" (Clever 2002).

Sulmasy points out that illness, especially serious illness, is a spiritual event (1999). Patients must grapple with questions of a transcendent nature, including meaning, relationships, and ultimately life's value. It is these critical issues that constitute the spiritual aspects of health care, yet they are ignored and even disincentivized in our scientifically reductionist, industrialized medical culture.

Perhaps, then, the cause of this growing professional dissatisfaction is more fundamental than the environmental issues that have been proposed. Perhaps it falls more in line with Moore's plea: "I have plenty of machinery around me; what I really need is a more enchanting world in which to live and work" (1996).

As experienced physicians reflect back on their careers, they frequently recollect experiences that are more spiritual than technical. Lown muses, "No pleasure is quite akin to the joy of helping other human beings secure and lengthen their hold on life" (1999) Siegel states, "The healing I have done as a doctor has always come back to me tenfold. So who is the healer, who is the healed?" (1989). The compelling stories of medicine are filled with spiritual values and experiences that are outside of the narrow scope of technical biomedicine (Lacombe 1995).

Grubb (2003) pleads for a medicine "with a little more soul." He suggests that making a spiritual connection with patients will help physicians at least as much as patients. In a series of essays, Grubb has given us profound examples of experiencing the transcendent in the midst of normal medical practice, and the profoundly rewarding effect it has had on him as a physician and as an individual (Grubb 1998; 1999a; 1999b; 2000; 2002; 2003; 2005; 2006a; 2006b). He proposes that if physicians can reconceptualize themselves as healers who dedicate their lives to reducing human suffering, as opposed to being solely technicians, they will reconnect with the passion and dedication that initially directed them to medicine.

Conclusion

Spirituality and scientific biomedicine are not mutually exclusive. They deal with different components of the human being and the relationships between human beings. As Sulmasy (1999) observes, there is no reason that physicians can not practice excellent biomedicine and still be aware of the spiritual dimension of their work, and be responsive to the spiritual needs of their patients.

Yet these different components are interconnected and interwoven in both the physician and the patient in subtle but powerful ways. Many patients seem to do better physically when their spiritual needs are addressed (Siegel 1986). Similarly, physicians seem to be far more satisfied in their practice when they allow themselves to include both their patients' and their own spirituality in their work (Sulmasy 1997). The physician–patient relationship is strengthened. Physicians will find it easier to maintain a compassionate demeanor with their patients as they nurture their own spiritual dimension. Physicians may be able to rise above their profound dissatisfaction with the circumstances surrounding health care as they rediscover the deeper meaning of their work and its implications.

At the dawn of the twenty-first century, it may be that the most profound revolution awaiting Western biomedicine is not genomics, nanotechnology, or artificial organs, but rather the reintroduction of spirituality into the practice of medicine, resulting in extraordinary improvements in the satisfaction of patient and healer alike.

REFERENCES

Albaugh, J. A. 2003. Spirituality and life-threatening illness: A phenomenological study. *Oncology Nursing Forum* 30: 593–98.

Aldridge, D. 1991. Spirituality, healing and medicine. *British Journal of General Practice* 41: 425–27.

Ameling, A., and M. Povilonis. 2001. Spirituality, meaning, mental health, and nursing. *Journal of Psychosocial Nursing* 39: 14–20.

Anandarajah, G. 2008. The 3 H and BMSET models for spirituality in multicultural whole-person medicine. *Annals of Family Medicine* 6: 448–58.

Anadarajah, G., R. Long, and M. Smith. 2001. Integrating spirituality into the family medicine residency curriculum. *Academic Medicine* 76: 519–20.

Astro, A., C. Puchalski, and D. Sulmasy. 2001. Religion, spirituality, and health care: Social, ethical, and practical considerations. *American Journal of Medicine* 110: 283–87.

Aviles, J. S., E. Whelan, D. A. Hernke, B. A. Williams, K. E. Kenny, W. M. O'Fallon WM et al. 2001. Intercessory prayer and cardiovascular disease progression in a coronary care unit population: a randomized controlled trial. *Mayo Clinic Proceedings* 76: 1192–98.

Bekelman, B. D., D. M. Dy, D. M. Becker, I. S. Wittstein, D. E. Hendricks, T. E. Yamashita, and S. H. Gottlieb. 2007. Spiritual well-being and depression in patients with heart failure. *Journal of General Internal Medicine* 22: 470–77.

Benson, H., et al. 2006. Study of the therapeutic effects of intercessory prayer (STEP) in cardiac bypass patients: A multicenter randomized trial of uncertainty and certainty of receiving intercessory prayer. *American Heart Journal* 151: 934–42.

Blumenthal, J. A., M. A. Babyak, G. Ironso, et al. 2007. Spirituality, religion and clinical outcomes in patients recovering from an acute myocardial infarction. *Psychosomatic Medicine* 69: 501–08.

Burack, J. H., D. M. Irby, J. D. Carline, R. K. Root, and E. B. Larson. 1999. Teaching compassion and respect: attending physicians' response to problematic behavior. *Journal of General Internal Medicine* 14(1): 49–55.

Byrd, R. C. 1988. Positive therapeutic effects of intercessory prayer in a coronary care unit population. *Southern Medical Journal* 81: 826–29.

Carmel, S., and S. M. Glick. 1996. Compassionate-empathic physicians: personality traits and social-factors that enhance or inhibit this personality trait. *Social Science in Medicine* 43(8): 1253–61.

Chiu, L., J. D. Emblen, L. Van Hofwegen, R. Sawatzky, and H. Meyerhoff. 2004. An integrative review of the concept of spirituality in the health sciences. *Western Journal of Nursing Research* 26(4): 405–28.

Clever, L. H. 2002. Who is sicker: Patients—or residents? Residents' distress and the care of patients. *Annals of Internal Medicine* 136(5): 391–93.

Cohen, M. Z. 1993. Introduction: Spirituality, quality of life, and nursing care. *Quality of Life* 2 (3): 47–49.

Colliton, M. 1981. The spiritual dimensions of nursing. In *Clinical Nursing*, ed. E. Belland and J. Passos. New York: MacMillan.

Curlin, F. A., J. D. Lanton, J. C. Roach, et al. 2005. Religious characteristics of U.S. physicians: A national survey. *Journal of General Internal Medicine* 20: 629–34.

Daaleman, T. P., B. M. Usher, S. W. Williams, J. Rawlings, and L. C. Hanson. 2008. An exploratory study of spiritual care at the end of life. *Annals of Family Medicine* 6: 406–11.

Davidson, R. J. 2008. Spirituality and medicine: Science and practice. *Annals of Family Medicine* 6: 388–89.

Emanuel, E. J., and N. N. Dubler. 1995. Preserving the physician-patient relationship in an era of managed care. *JAMA* 273: 323–29.

Engel, G. L. 1977. The need for a new medical model: A challenge for biomedicine. *Science* 196: 129–36.

Fry, A. 1998. Spirituality, communication and mental health nursing: The tacit interdiction. *Australian and New Zealand Journal of Mental Health* 7: 25–32.

Golberg, B. 1998. Connection: An exploration of spirituality in nursing care. *Journal of Advanced Nursing* 27: 836–42.

Grubb, B. P. 1998. Cuando voy a morir? *PACE* 21: 268.

Grubb, B. P. 1999a. To save a life. *PACE* (Part 1) 22: 664.

Grubb, B. P. 1999b. The calling. *PACE* 22: 1542.

Grubb, B. P. 2000. The accident. *PACE* 23: 1431–32.

Grubb, B. P. 2002. Sunday in the park with George. *PACE* 25(2): 854–55.

Grubb, B. P. 2003. With a little more soul. *Cardiac Electrophysiology Review* 7: 85–87.

Grubb, B. P. 2005. Finding Private Reimer. *PACE* 28: 991–92.

Grubb, B. P. 2006a. The harvest. *PACE* 29: 905.

Grubb, B. P. 2006b. The sacrifice of Isaac. *PACE* 29: 1298.

Haas, J. S, E. F. Cook, L. Puopolo, et al. 2000. Is the professional satisfaction of general internists associated with patient satisfaction? *Journal of General Internal Medicine* 15: 122–28.

Harris, W.S.,M. Gowda, J. W. Kolb, C. P. Strychacz, J. L. Vacek, P. G. Jones, et al. 2001. A randomized controlled trial of the effects of remote, intercessory prayer on outcomes in patients admitted to the coronary care unit. *Archives of Internal Medicine* 159: 2273–78.

Hart, J. 2008. Spirituality and health. *Alternative and Complementary Therapies* 14: 189–93.

Haskell, W. 2003. Cardiovascular disease prevention and lifestyle interventions: Effectiveness and efficacy. *Journal of Cardiovascular Nursing* 18: 245–55.

Jayne, W. A. 2003. *Healing gods of ancient civilizations.* Whitefish, MT: Kessinger Publishing.

Joint Commission on Healthcare Organizations. 2008. Spiritual assessment. http://www.jointcommission.org/AccreditationPrograms/HomeCare/Standards/09_FAQs/PC/Spiritual_Assessment.htm

Kabat-Zinn, J. 2005. *Coming to our senses: healing ourselves and the world through mindfulness.* New York: Hyperion.

Koenig, H. G. 2008. *Medicine religion and health.* West Conshohocken, PA: Templeton University Press.

Kreitzer, M. J., C. R. Gross, O. Waleekhachonloet, M. Reilly-Spong, and M. Byrd. 2009. The brief serenity scale: A psychometric analysis of a measure of spirituality and well-being. *Journal of Holistic Nursing* 27: 7–16.

Krucoff, M. W., S. W. Crater, and K. L. Lee. 2006. From efficacy to safety concerns: A STEP forward or a step back for clinical research and intercessory prayer? The study of therapeutic effects of intercessory prayer (STEP). *American Heart Journal* 151: 762–64.

Lacombe, M. A., ed. 1995. *On being a doctor.* Philadelphia: American College of Physcians.

Larson, D. B., K. A. Sherrill, J. S. Lyons, F. C. Craigie Jr., S. B. Thielman, M. A. Greenwold, and S. S. Larson. 1992. Associations between dimensions of religious commitment and mental health reported in the American Journal of Psychiatry and Archives of General Psychiatry: 1978–1989. American Journal of Psychiatry 149: 557–59.

Legere, T. E. 1984. A spirituality for today. *Studies in Formative Spiritualit,* 5: 375–83.

Leonard, B. and D. Carlson. 2003. Spirituality in healthcare. www.csh.umn.edu/modules/index.html

Lown, B. 1999. *The lost art of healing: Practicing compassion in medicine.* New York: Random House.

Magyar-Russell, G., P. Fosarelli, H. Taylor, and D. Finkelstein D. 2008. Ophthalmology patients' religious and spiritual beliefs. *Archives of Ophthalmology* 126: 1262–65.

McCullough, M. E., W. T. Hoyt, D.B. Larson, H. G. Koenig, and C. Thoreson. 2000. Religious involvement and mortality: A meta-analytic review. *Health Psychology* 19: 211–22.

Milstein, J. 2005. A paradigm of integrative care: Healing with curing throughout life, "being with" and "doing to." *Journal of Perinatology* 25: 563–68.

Mische, P. 1982. Towards a global spirituality. In *Whole earth papers,* P. Mische. East Grange, New Jersey: Global Education Association.

Moore, T. 1996. *The Re-enchantment of everyday life.* Boston: GK Hall and Co.

Morris, E. L. 2001. The relationship of spirituality to coronary artery disease. *Alternative Therapies in Health and Medicine* 7: 96–98.

Mueller, P. S., D. J. Plevak, and A. T. Rummans. 2001. Religious involvement, spirituality, and medicine: Implications for clinical practice. *Mayo Clinic Proceedings* 76(12): 1225–35.

Murray, R. B., and J. P. Zentner. 1989. *Nursing concepts for health promotion.* London: Prentice Hall.

Nagai-Jacobson, M. G., and M. A. Burkhardt. 1989. Spirituality: Cornerstone of holistic nursing practice. *Holistic Nursing Practice* 3(3): 18–26.

Narayanasamy, A. 1999. A review of spirituality as applied to nursing. *International Journal of Nursing Studies* 36: 117–25.

Ornish, D. 1998. *Love and survival: The scientific basis for the healing power of intimacy.* New York: HarperCollins.

Pargament K. 1997. *The psychology of religion and coping: Theory, research, practice.* New York: Guilford Press.

Paloutzian, R. F., and C. W. Ellison. 1982. Loneliness, spiritual well-being and quality of life. In *Loneliness: a sourcebook of current theory, research and therapy,* ed. L. A. Peplau and D. Perlman., 224–37. New York: Wiley Interscience.

Pence, G. E. 1983. Can compassion be taught? *Journal of Medical Ethics* 9(4): 189–91.

Post, S. G., C. M. Puchalski, and D. Larson. 2000. Physicians and patient spirituality: Professional boundaries, competency and ethics. *Annals of Internal Medicine* 132: 578–83.

Puchalski, C., and D. B. Larson. 1998. Developing curricula in spirituality and medicine. *Academic Medicine* 73: 970–74.

Puchalski, C., and A. L. Romer. 2000. Taking a spiritual history allows clinicians to understand patients more fully. *Journal of Palliative Medicine* 3: 129–37.

Reed, P. G. 1992. An emerging paradigm for the investigation of spirituality in nursing. *Research in Nursing & Healt,* 15: 349–57.

Rinpoche, C. N., and D. R. Shlim. 2006. *Medicine and compassion.* Somerville, MA: Wisdom Publications.

Roberts, K., and C. Aspy. 1993. Development of the serenity scale. *Journal of Nursing Measurement* 1: 145–64.

Ruberman, W., J. Weinblatt, J. D. Goldberg, and B. S. Chaudhary. 1984. Psychological influences on mortality after myocardial infarction. *New England Journal of Medicine* 311: 552–59.

Shanafelt, T. A., K. A. Bradley, J. Wipf, and A. L. Back. 2002. Burnout and self-reported patient care in an internal medicine residency program. *Annals of Internal Medicine* 136: 358–67.

Siegel, B. S. 1986. *Love, medicine, and miracles.* New York: Harper and Row.

Siegel, B. S. 1989. *Peace, love, and healing.* New York: Harper and Row.

Sulmasy, D. P. 1999. Is medicine a spiritual practice? *Academic Medicine* 74(9): 1002–05.

Sulmasy, D. P. 1997. *The healer's calling.* Mahwah, NJ: Paulist Press.

Tanyi, R. A. 2002. Towards clarification of the meaning of spirituality. *Journal of Advanced Nursing* 39: 500–09.

Waldfogel, S. 1997. Spirituality in medicine. Primary care. *Clinics in Office Practice* 24: 963–76.

Williams, R. B., J. C. Barefoot, R. M. Califf, et al. 1992. Prognostic importance of social and economic resources among medically treated patients with angiographically documented coronary artery disease. *Journal of the American Medical Association* 267: 520–24.

Zugler, A. 2004. Dissatisfaction with medical practice. *New England Journal of Medicine* 350(1): 69–75.

8

Cardiac Behavioral Medicine: Mind–Body Approaches to Heart Health

KIM R. LEBOWITZ

KEY CONCEPTS

- Psychological distress, including depression, anxiety, and stress, is common among cardiac patients.
- The presence of psychological distress can interfere with a patient's ability to engage in healthy lifestyles and follow medical recommendations.
- Depression, anxiety, and stress have emerged as independent risk factors for the development of cardiac disease and are associated with an increased risk in cardiac morbidity and mortality.
- The causal mechanisms linking emotional health and cardiac outcomes remain unknown, but likely involve physiological and behavioral pathways.
- Cardiac patients should be routinely screened for emotional distress and referred for treatment when applicable.
- Treatment for psychological distress among cardiac patients is efficacious, safe, and has a positive impact on emotional functioning, quality of life, and lifestyle behaviors, although there is no research to indicate at present that treatment improves cardiac outcomes.

■

It was Hippocrates who commented, "You ought not to attempt to cure the body without the soul. The cure of many diseases is unknown to physicians because they disregard the whole." In the seventeenth century, William Harvey, one of the pioneers of cardiovascular physiology, observed a more specific connection between emotions and cardiovascular functioning, remarking that "a mental disturbance provoking pain, excessive joy, hope or anxiety extends to the heart where it affects temper and rate." (Harvey 1628, 109). The mind–body connection, as it relates specifically to cardiac health, has been the epicenter of empirical investigation for the past several decades in the emerging field of behavioral medicine. Cardiac behavioral medicine refers to a multidisciplinary approach to cardiac health that examines behavioral, social, and psychological factors that contribute to, maintain, or follow a cardiac diagnosis or event.

The origins of cardiac behavioral medicine lie within the traditional risk factors for cardiovascular disease. The field of cardiology provides a strong, direct link between individuals' behaviors and physical health. With the exception of age, sex, and family history, the traditional risk factors for cardiovascular disease are predominantly modifiable and reflect an individual's lifestyle behaviors, including smoking, diet, and activity. Cardiac behavioral medicine specialists—including psychologists, psychiatrists, social workers, physicians, dieticians, and exercise therapists—can work together to help individuals initiate and maintain behavior changes that can contribute to cardiac risk reduction and overall improvement in health.

Cardiac behavioral medicine also addresses the psychological component of cardiac health, which will be the focus of this chapter. Cardiac patients are at increased risk of experiencing emotional distress and impaired quality of life compared with the general population (Rozanski, Blumenthal, and Kaplan 1999; Skala, Freedland, and Carney 2005). For example, more than 30 percent of individuals with a recent myocardial infarction (MI) report significant depression (Lichtman et al. 2008; Skala, Freedland, and Carney 2005). This mind–body relationship is bidirectional; psychological disorders and personality characteristics also have been shown to have a negative impact on cardiac health, facilitating the development of cardiac disease and predicting increased morbidity and mortality following a cardiac event (Kubzansky and Kawachi 2000; Lichtman et al. 2008). A large multinational study (INTERHEART) demonstrated that psychosocial factors (including depression, stress, anxiety, anger, and social isolation) accounted for 32 percent of the risk for coronary artery disease (CAD). The magnitude of the risk conferred by psychosocial factors was equivalent to smoking and almost double the risk associated with hypertension (Rosengren et al. 2004; Yusuf et al. 2004). Psychological distress also can impede patients' ability to follow medical recommendations and reduce their cardiovascular risk through lifestyle modification (Carney et al. 2002). Assessment and treatment of mood and emotional distress should be integrated into cardiac care to optimize health, reduce cardiovascular risk, aid with adjustment to an illness, and enhance quality of life (Grissom and

Phillips 2005). This chapter will review depression, anxiety, and stress within the cardiac population, as these are the most common psychological antecedents and consequences of cardiac illness.

Depression

Clinical depression is a common sequelae of cardiac disease and cardiac surgery, impacting approximately 15 to 25 percent of cardiac patients, and up to double that in studies that include subclinical levels of depression. (Grissom and Phlllips, 2005; Lichtman et al. 2008; Rudisch and Nemeroff, 2003). Depression has drawn attention not only because of its prevalence in this population, but because depression has emerged as an independent risk factor for the development of CAD as well as a predictor of morbidity and mortality, especially among post-MI patients (Lichtman et al. 2008).

The prevalence of depression is 3 times higher among cardiac patients than it is in the general population.

Emotions represent a healthy form of expression and are a typical part of any significant event, including a medical diagnosis. Sadness, frustration, fear and even relief are commonly exhibited at various stages of medical treatment and are completely healthy. Emotions become problematic when they co-occur with a variety of other symptoms, last for a specific period of time, and either cause the individual distress or interfere with an individual's ability to function, at which point they constitute a syndrome or psychological disorder. Isolated symptoms or transient emotions are not to be confused with mental disorders. Tearfulness or sadness alone does not constitute depression.

Clinical depression (Major Depressive Disorder or MDD) is characterized by the presence of one or more major depressive episodes, each which requires the presence of depressed mood or markedly reduced interest in most activities for at least two weeks, plus the addition of at least four other depressive symptoms (American Psychiatric Association 2000; see Table 8.1). Symptoms of depression can be emotional, somatic, or cognitive in nature. Emotional symptoms include sadness, hopelessness, and anhedonia. Somatic symptoms involve change in body systems or routines and include change in appetite, weight change, sleep disturbances, psychomotor retardation or agitation, fatigue and loss of energy. Cognitive symptoms of depression include diminished memory or concentration, feelings of worthlessness, excessive guilt, and

Table 8.1. DSM-IV-TR Symptoms Of A Depressive Episode*

Emotional
- Depressed mood**
- Loss of interest in most activities**
- Increased tearfulness

Somatic
- Appetite or weight change
- Insomnia or hypersomnia
- Psychomotor agitation or retardation
- Fatigue or low energy

Cognitive
- Feelings of worthlessness or guilt
- Diminished concentration or decision-making
- Suicidal thoughts or behaviors

*Symptoms appear for at least two weeks and are associated with distress or impairment in functioning
**At least one of these symptoms must be present, plus at least four others

suicidal thoughts. The symptoms of depression must represent a change from the individual's baseline level of functioning and be severe enough to cause disability or interference in daily functioning. Many research studies in the cardiac arena examine the presence of depression several days after a cardiac event. As a result, the symptom duration criterion (2 weeks) is often disregarded. When symptoms of depression are present but the criteria for a major depressive episode are not met, other potential mood disorder diagnoses can include dysthymia (mild chronic depression), adjustment disorder, or minor depression (same criteria as major depression but only one to three additional symptoms are experienced per episode). Table 8.2 summarizes characteristics

Table 8.2. Factors Associated With An Increased Risk Of Developing Depression

- Female gender
- Younger age (diagnosis or symptom onset <60 years)
- Previous episodes of clinical depression
- Minimal social support
- Recent stressful life events
- Functional limitations in patients with heart failure*
- Family history of clinical depression

*With the exception of heart failure, disease status or severity does not predict depression.

in cardiac patients that are associated with an increased risk of developing depression.

DEPRESSION, COMPLIANCE, AND TRADITIONAL RISK FACTORS FOR CAD

Depression clusters with a majority of the established risk factors for heart disease and is associated with unhealthy lifestyle behaviors.

Smoking

A history of depression confers a three-fold increase in the likelihood of becoming a smoker (Breslau et al. 1998; Joynt, Whellan, and O'Connor 2003). The prevalence of smoking in the depressed population hovers around 49 percent. There is a dose-dependent relationship between depression and smoking, where more severe depression predicts a greater likelihood of smoking (Anda et al. 1990; Rudisch and Nemeroff 2003). Depression also impedes successful smoking cessation (Glassman et al. 1990). Depressed individuals are 40 percent less successful at quitting smoking, at least in part because they experience more physiological symptoms of withdrawal. The relationship between depression and smoking is bidirectional: smokers are at increased risk of developing clinical depression (Breslau et al. 1998).

Non-Adherence to Medical Recommendations

Depressed cardiac patients are less likely to adhere to medical recommendations and are more likely to drop out of cardiac rehabilitation (Blumenthal et al. 1982; Joynt et al. 2003; Rudisch and Nemeroff, 2003). Carney et al. (1995) tracked compliance to daily aspirin for 3 weeks in patients with CAD. Non-depressed patients were compliant with aspirin 69 percent of the time; clinically depressed patients exhibited a mere 45 percent compliance rate. Some studies suggest that noncompliance in and of itself (rather than to a specific treatment) is a prognostic indicator of poorer outcomes, as indicated by increased morbidity and mortality associated with noncompliance to a placebo (Granger et al. 2005;l McDermott, Schmitt, and Wallner 1997). The extent to which noncompliance is a marker of depression in these studies has not been examined.

Obesity

Several studies have found that obesity is associated with an increased risk of depression, with 25 percent of obese individuals meeting criteria for depression (Joynt et al. 2003; Simon et al. 2006). Depressed individuals have a greater BMI and present with increased central and whole-body adiposity compared with matched controls (Miller et al. 2002).

Diabetes

Depressed individuals are more than twice as likely to develop diabetes over a 13-year period, and diabetics are twice as likely to be depressed compared with the general population. Depression negatively influences glycemic control and increases risk of diabetic complications (Joynt et al. 2003).

Other Traditional Risk Factors

Depression is associated with an increase in homocysteine levels, with up to 50 percent of depressed individuals exhibiting levels that would confer an increased cardiac risk. Further, the use of folate to lower homocysteine levels has been found to have antidepressant properties (Joynt et al. 2003). Hypertension is more prevalent among depressed populations than healthy controls (Carney et al. 2002). Hypercholesterolemia is one of the only established risk factors for cardiovascular disease that is inversely correlated with depression. Depression is associated with low levels of serum cholesterol, and recovery from depression may be associated with an increase in cholesterol (Joynt et al. 2003). Physical activity and exercise tolerance are inversely related to symptoms of depression (Carney et al. 2002).

Cardiac risk reduction via behavior change can be challenging for most patients, but may be particularly daunting to an individual with clinical depression. Remember, depressed individuals are likely experiencing diminished motivation, apathy, and deficits in concentration and memory, not to mention possibly suicidal thoughts—each of which alone can be a major barrier to successfully executing lifestyle changes and appropriately following medical recommendations. Recognizing and addressing depression is an important first line of treatment for patients who require behavioral risk reduction.

Following the resolution of depression, patients are more likely to be involved and motivated members of the medical team, with more sufficient emotional and cognitive resources to successfully initiate and maintain lifestyle changes.

DEPRESSION AS A PREDICTOR OF MORBIDITY AND MORTALITY

The seminal studies of Frasure-Smith et al. (1993; 1995) evaluated the impact of MDD on survival among 222 post-MI patients. Depression emerged as an independent risk factor for mortality, conferring a risk equivalent to that of established risk factors, including left ventricular ejection fraction and previous MI. Those who were depressed in the hospital were four times more likely to die within 6 months, compared to those who were not depressed, regardless of disease severity and risks factors (Frasure-Smith et al. 1993). Mortality rates at an eighteen-month follow-up were 40 percent among those who experienced recurrent depression in the hospital (e.g., they were depressed in the hospital *plus* had a prior history of depression) compared with 7 percent for those who were non-depressed (Frasure-Smith et al. 1995). Investigations that did not formally assess for clinical depression have found associations between depressive symptoms and cardiac outcomes among post-MI patients, including increased mortality and repeat cardiac events (Rudish and Nemeroff 2003).

The relationship between depression and mortality has been most thoroughly investigated in the post-MI population, but depression also appears to predict cardiac and all-cause mortality among patients with unstable angina, CAD, congestive heart failure, individuals without coronary disease at the time of study enrollment, and among patients undergoing coronary artery bypass graft (CABG) and valve surgery (Blumenthal et al. 2003; Burg et al. 2003b; Carney and Freedland 2003; Ho et al. 2005; Jiang et al. 2001; van Melle et al. 2004).

The presence of MDD or subclinical depressive symptoms, particularly among patients with CAD and those undergoing CABG, has also been associated with morbidity and less favorable cardiac outcomes, including repeat hospitalizations, subsequent cardiac surgery, myocardial ischemia, MI, angioplasty, increased health care costs and utilization, failure to return to previous

There is a dose-dependent relationship between depression and mortality, where more severe depressive symptoms are associated with a greater risk of mortality. This relationship provides further support of a causal link between depression and cardiac outcomes.

activities, continued surgical pain, and diminished quality of life (Burg et al. 2003a; Carney et al. 1988; Carney and Freedland 2003; Frasure-Smith et al. 2000; Jiang et al. 2003; Mallik et al. 2005; van Melle et al. 2004).

DEPRESSION AND THE DEVELOPMENT OF CORONARY ARTERY DISEASE

Depression in otherwise healthy individuals predicts incident CAD and cardiac mortality even decades later. One study found a relative risk of 4.16 for incident CAD among community residents with MDD (Pratt et al. 1996). The consistent findings are impressive given the heterogeneity of the studies, which have varied with respect to depression severity (e.g., a clinical diagnosis of MDD versus current or previous depressive symptoms), symptom assessment (questionnaires versus clinical interview), age (ranging from individuals in their twenties to older adults at study onset), and length of follow-up (months to decades). A clinical diagnosis of depression appears to carry a greater risk than subclinical depressive symptoms (Carney and Freedland 2003).

MECHANISMS OF ACTION LINKING DEPRESSION AND CARDIAC OUTCOMES

Although the link between depression and poor cardiac outcomes is well established, the mechanisms of action are minimally understood. The most obvious explanation is behavioral. Given that depressed individuals are less physically active, more likely to smoke, less compliant with medical recommendations, and less likely to eat a heart- healthy diet, lifestyle behaviors seem to be the most plausible explanation for why depression can lead to the development of CAD or a poorer prognosis after a cardiac event. However, lifestyle behaviors account for no more than 50 percent of the variance in this relationship, and in most studies, depression remains a predictor of morbidity and mortality independent of these risk factors (Carney et al. 2002; Rudisch and Nemeroff 2003).

Physiological mechanisms must be involved as well, although there is minimal concrete empirical support for any particular pathophysiological mechanism at present. Despite depressed individuals appearing sluggish on the outside, there is evidence that depression is associated with physiological hyperarousal, either heightened sympathetic activity, diminished parasympathetic regulation, or both. Depression is associated with a high resting heart rate and decreased heart rate variability (Joynt et al. 2003; Rozanski, Blumenthal, and Kaplan 1999). Other hypothesized physiological pathways include inflammation that leads to endothelial damage, hypercoagulability as reflected by increased platelet activation in depressed individuals that may lead to thrombus formation, and rhythm disturbances that predispose depressed individuals to sudden cardiac death (Joynt et al. 2003; Rozanski, Blumenthal, and Kaplan 1999; Rudisch and Nemeroff 2003).

Anxiety

Anxiety disorders are the most common group of psychological disorders in the United States, affecting 25 percent of Americans across the lifespan (Kessler et al. 1994). Each of the different anxiety disorders share various symptoms of severe anxiety and carry a significant level of impairment. The specific symptoms, time frames, behaviors, and level of severity help to differentiate the various anxiety disorders (see Table 8.3). The prevalence of anxiety disorders and subclinical anxiety is greater among cardiac patients than in the general population. For example, 15 percent of patients presenting to the ED with noncardiac chest pain and up to 25 percent of patients seen in cardiology practices have panic disorder, which has a 0.9% prevalence rate in the general population (American Psychiatric Association 2000; Fleet et al. 1996; Janeway 2009). Cardiac patients often report anxiety following a cardiac diagnosis, after discharge of an implantable cardiac defibrillator (ICD), with symptom onset, or precipitating a cardiac procedure, including surgery. Among cardiac

Table 8.3. Psychological Disorders That Incorporate Anxiety as a Predominant Symptom

Generalized anxiety disorder

Panic disorder with or without agoraphobia

Agoraphobia without a history of panic

Specific phobia

Social phobia

Obsessive-compulsive disorder

Posttraumatic stress disorder

Acute stress disorder

Adjustment disorder with anxious mood

patients, anxiety can manifest itself as excessive worry, fear, phobias, panic attacks, agoraphobia, or increased health-checking behaviors.

Epidemiological data demonstrate an association between anxiety symptoms and CAD outcomes (Kubzansky et al. 1998; Kubzansky and Kawachi 2000). Several large-scale community-based longitudinal studies have demonstrated that anxiety disorders are associated with increased risk for the development of CAD, ventricular arrhythmias, coronary death, and sudden cardiac death. Specifically, the multivariate relative risk of fatal CAD among the most anxious in these studies ranged from 2.41 to 7.8, compared with those not presenting with anxiety (Kubzansky and Kawachi, 2000; Watkins et al. 2006). Furthermore, a dose-dependent relationship has been observed between anxiety symptoms and cardiac death (Rozanski, Blumenthal, and Kaplan 1999). Most of the longitudinal studies have examined men only, despite an increased prevalence of anxiety among women. One study that included women, the Framingham Heart Study, found anxious symptoms associated with increased MI and coronary death at a 20-year follow-up among homemakers, but not among women employed outside the home (Eaker, Pinsky, and Castelli 1992). Much less is known about the prevalence of anxiety in specific sub-cardiac populations, or the relationship between anxiety symptoms and disorders with the development or progression of non-CAD cardiac disorders.

Anxiety among cardiac patients can stem from patients' perceived inability to predict or control cardiac events, symptoms, or disease course. As human beings, we constantly search our surroundings for a sense of order and control. With any perceived loss of control or predictability, anxiety can result. In an effort to increase a sense of predictability, patients can become hypervigilant toward their surroundings and their bodies; they may start to avoid circumstances that they perceive as dangerous, and they may engage in health-checking behaviors or other safety behaviors to inflate their sense of safety.

PANIC

Panic disorder is characterized by recurrent panic attacks combined with concern about future attacks or the consequences of future attacks. A panic attack is a sudden episode of intense fear or discomfort that is associated with several cognitive and physical symptoms, several of which also are cardinal features of cardiac disease, including chest pain, palpitations, sweating, shortness of breath, sensations of choking, and hot flashes (American Psychiatric Association 2000; see Table 8.4 for diagnostic criteria). Panic attacks are often terrifying for the individual due to the intensity and sudden onset of symptoms, combined with a sense of danger. Because of the overlap of symptoms,

Table 8.4. DSM-IV-TR Symptoms of a Panic Attack*

Physical
* Palpitations or increased heart rate
* Sweating
* Trembling
* Shortness of breath
* Sensation of choking
* Chest pain or tightness
* Nausea or abdominal distress
* Dizziness, lightheadedness, or feeling faint
* Numbness or tingling sensations
* Chills or hut flashes

Emotional
* Fear of dying
* Fear of losing control or going crazy
* Feelings of detachment from oneself or feelings of unreality

*A panic attack requires at least 4 symptoms present during a discrete period of intense fear or discomfort. The onset of symptoms is abrupt and symptoms reach peak intensity within 10 minutes.

many patients with panic disorder present to the ED and often undergo costly and invasive cardiac testing, with normal results. In fact, panic disorder is 30 to 50 times more common among patients with noncardiac chest pain compared with the general population (Fleet, Lavoie, and Beitman 2000).

Among cardiac patients, anxiety often is related to physical health, resulting in increased awareness and perception of physical sensations, as if looking at one's body through a microscope. A cognitive model of panic asserts that misinterpreting a physical symptom as threatening will trigger fear and physiological arousal (hence, more physical symptoms), creating a self-sustaining downward spiral of anxiety and physical symptoms, resulting in a panic attack (Craske and Barlow 1993). See Figure 8.1 for an example of how catastrophic thoughts can trigger and sustain panic.

Following a new diagnosis, cardiac patients may have difficulty interpreting physical symptoms accurately due to limited experience with their new health condition, often leading to anxiety. For example, Michael was a 59-year-old professional Caucasian married male, newly diagnosed with atrial fibrillation. He became astutely aware of all symptoms in his body following this diagnosis, and he was uncertain how to determine which symptoms were benign and which warranted medical attention. As a result, he called his cardiologist every time he noticed a new symptom, which initially resulted in several urgent

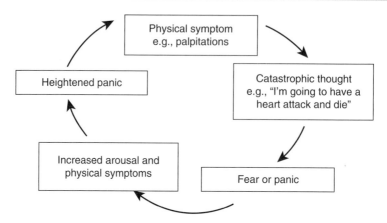

FIGURE 8.1. A model of the interactive cycle of physical symptoms, cognitive distortions, and emotions that can lead to panic.

phone calls per week. With education and more experience with his body, Michael became more adept at interpreting his symptoms more accurately. Additional information, often acquired through a combination of personal experience and medical feedback, will be sufficient for many patients to decrease their anxiety about their physical symptoms. This is comparable to having a new baby. At first, a new parent is unsure of which patterns or symptoms exhibited by the baby are benign versus problematic. First-time parents are more cautious and call their pediatrician's office more often than repeat parents, who have learned from firsthand experiences with their previous children. For many patients, a new diagnosis brings about a healthy increase in anxiety that will resolve with experience and increased comfort. For others, however, the panic becomes more frequent and disabling, leading to panic attacks.

AVOIDANCE

In an effort to predict cardiac events and control their health, anxious cardiac patients may start to avoid certain places or activities that they perceive as dangerous or embarrassing should they fall ill. Just as Pavlov's dogs learned to salivate by the sound of a bell, cardiac patients can develop learned responses based on their cardiac experiences. If Laura's ICD fired at the movie theater, she may start to avoid the movie theater in hopes of avoiding another discharge. After Ron experiences chest pain on the treadmill, he may choose to ignore exercising in an attempt to avoid similar symptoms. This logic works well when situational factors are responsible for cardiac events. In a majority of circumstances, however, the physiology has little to do with the logistics of the situation. Unfortunately, many individuals process the situational factors in an attempt to maintain some control and predictability over their health.

Avoidance is a key characteristic of anxiety disorders and is typically utilized to provide instant reduction or avoidance of anxiety. A child who is afraid of dogs may cross the street to avoid interacting with a dog. This behavior eliminates anxiety in the short term. However, in the long run, avoidance ends up maintaining and even strengthening a specific fear. Ultimately, exposing an individual to the feared stimuli (e.g., dogs, needles, exercising) can help the patient develop confidence and more accurate perceptions, leading to reduced anxiety in the long term (Craske and Barlow 1993).

> *Agoraphobia in cardiac patients refers to a marked anxiety in situations or places where escape would be difficult (or embarrassing) or help would be unavailable should panic symptoms or cardiac symptoms occur. This anxiety generally leads to pervasive avoidance of a variety of situations such as being alone, traveling in a bus or airplane, or being in an elevator.*

WORRY

Worry is the cognitive component of anxiety and refers to future-oriented thinking about possible negative outcomes to a situation—that is, the "what if's." Worry is healthy and is the driving force behind problem-solving and planning. For individuals with Generalized Anxiety Disorder, the worry becomes excessive and uncontrollable, causing distress and disability. Subclinical worry has been associated with an increased risk in developing CAD and experiencing cardiac mortality (Rozanski, Blumenthal, and Kaplan 1999). Cardiac patients, like many medical patients, experience worry about their health, mortality, finances, prognosis, test results, family relations, and coping resources. Table 8.5 lists some common worries among cardiac patients.

MECHANISMS OF ACTION LINKING ANXIETY
AND CARDIAC OUTCOMES

There remains much to learn about the association between anxiety and cardiac health, including gaining a better understanding of the potential pathways. Current theories suggest physiological and behavioral pathways. The increased

---

Table 8.5. Common Areas of Worry and Stress Among Cardiac Patients

---

- Fear of physical symptoms, such as fatigue, breathlessness, palpitations, or lightheadedness
- Body image concerns including surgical scars, implanted devices, or weight changes
- Lack of independence
- Fear of intubation with surgery
- Fear of ICD discharge or syncope
- Fear of death
- Fear that heart will stop (or will not restart after surgery)
- Fear of being a burden to others
- Worry about meeting financial obligations
- Fears about inability to caregive or parent effectively
- Worry about life expectancy and inability to meet goals
- Concern about treatment side effects
- Worry about test results and prognosis
- Fear of pain and inadequate pain management
- Concern of contributing to stress in the marriage or family

---

risk of cardiac death associated with anxiety is related to sudden cardiac death and not MI (Kubzansky et al. 1998; Rozanski, Blumenthal, and Kaplan 1999), suggesting that ventricular arrhythmias may be a possible mechanism (Watkins et al. 2006). Reduced heart rate variability further suggests abnormal autonomic control among anxious individuals. Alternate possibilities include the promotion of atherogenesis, perhaps through hypertension, and the triggering of coronary events, possibly through plaque rupture or coronary vasospasm. From a behavioral perspective, anxiety is associated with poor sleep, decreased activity, an unhealthy diet, increased smoking, and increased alcohol and drug use (Kubzansky et al. 1998; Kubzansky and Kawachi 2000). The extent to which these behaviors mediate the relationship between anxiety and CAD is unclear.

Stress

Stress is a common experience among cardiac patients and has been correlated with the development of CAD and the onset of acute cardiac events. Stress, unlike depression and anxiety, is not a diagnostic clinical syndrome, but rather a reaction to a real or perceived danger or challenge. Stress incorporates physical, emotional, cognitive, and behavioral symptoms, and can often lead to psychological disorders such as depression or anxiety (Baum, Gatchel, and Krantz 1997). One of the most predictable and prominent physiological

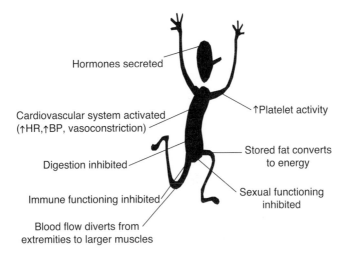

Hormones secreted

Cardiovascular system activated
(↑HR,↑BP, vasoconstriction)

Digestion inhibited

Immune functioning inhibited

Blood flow diverts from
extremities to larger muscles

↑Platelet activity

Stored fat converts
to energy

Sexual functioning
inhibited

FIGURE 8.2. The sympathetic nervous system: An overview of some physiological changes that occur when the "fight or flight" response is activated.

components of stress is the activation of the sympathetic nervous system, the body's "flight or flight" response, which mobilizes the body's resources to promote safety in the wake of an emergency. Figure 8.2 summarizes a few of the physiological changes that occur during the stress response. Although the body's stress response is a way to safe guard the body against danger, repeated or sustained activation of the fight or flight response (i.e., chronic stress) can cause wear and tear on various organ systems, leading to hypertension, atherosclerosis, immune dysfunction, digestive disorders, fertility problems, and depression (Baum, Gatchel, and Krantz 1997).

ACUTE STRESS AND CARDIAC EVENTS

Anecdotal reports and case studies have long speculated about an association between acute stress and cardiac events. Retrospective studies have found that up to one-quarter of heart attack patients report experiencing anger or upset in the hours prior to symptom onset (Krantz et al. 1996). Epidemiological studies have found increased cardiac events following large-scale acute stressors such as earthquakes and terrorist activity. On the day of the 1994 Los Angeles earthquake, the occurrence of sudden cardiac death rose from a daily average of 4.6 to 24 on the day of the earthquake (Leor, Poole, and Kloner 1996). Meisel et al. (1991) reported a sharp increase in myocardial infarction and a 2-fold increase in sudden cardiac death among residents near Tel Aviv during the initial days of the missile attacks during the 1991 Gulf War. Ventricular arrhythmias more than doubled among New York City residents with defibrillators in the month following September 11, 2001 (Steinberg et al. 2004).

Laboratory and observational studies have found that mental stress can trigger myocardial ischemia among patients with CAD, including those who do not have exercise-induced ischemia (Holmes et al. 2006; Ramachandruni et al. 2006). Mental-stress induced ischemia is predominantly silent and may occur in 40 to 70 percent of patients with CAD (Krantz et al. 1996). Laboratory studies have documented myocardial ischemia during mental stressors, including arithmetic tests, speech tasks, and when recalling a situation that previously made the patient angry (Holmes et al. 2006; Rozanski, Blumenthal, and Kaplan 1999). In addition to ischemic events, laboratory mental stressors have been found to trigger the onset of blood pressure increases (with relatively low heart rate increases), wall motion abnormalities, and acute drops in ejection fraction among individuals with CAD (Krantz et al. 1996). It is worth noting that the contrived laboratory stressors may underrepresent the potency of mental stress in real-life situations. Ambulatory monitoring found that emotional distress experienced during daily life among individuals with CAD more than doubled the likelihood of transient ischemia in the subsequent hour (Gullette et al. 1997).

CHRONIC STRESS AND THE DEVELOPMENT OF CAD

Chronic psychosocial stress has been implicated in the development of coronary atherosclerosis. Job strain is a well-studied chronic life stress often associated with CAD. Jobs with high demands and low decision latitude have been associated with a 4-fold increase in cardiac-related deaths across time (Karasek et al. 1981). Jobs with minimal control or insufficient rewards also have been related to cardiac events and progression of atherosclerosis (Rozanski, Blumenthal, and Kaplan 1999). Although some negative studies have been reported, a majority of the evidence points to a positive association between job stress and CAD risk. Chronic stress also has been examined in terms of recent life changes or culmination of life stressors. Although most of these studies are retrospective or rely on report bias, the majority of findings suggest an association between increased life stressors and cardiac morbidity and mortality (Baum, Gatchel, and Krantz 1997; Holmes et al. 2006; Krantz et al. 1996).

An extensive body of evidence from animal models nicely illustrates the impact of chronic social stress on atherosclerosis. Studies with cynomolgus monkeys, whose social organization is characterized by hierarchies of social dominance, generated chronic social stress by reorganizing groupings of monkeys and therefore causing unstable social groups. Compared with controls (who remained in a stable social group), the stressed monkeys experienced extensive coronary artery atherosclerosis, particularly the high ranking or dominant male monkeys (Manuck, Kaplan, and Matthews 1986). Studies of non-primates also have demonstrated effects of social stress on atherosclerotic changes of the coronary arteries and aorta (Manuck, Kaplan, and Matthews 1986). Cardiovascular hyperresponsivity during stress, as evidenced by stress-induced heart rate changes in monkeys, may account for some of the disease progression (Manuck, Kaplan, and Clarkson 1983).

MECHANISMS OF ACTION LINKING STRESS AND CARDIAC OUTCOMES

There is currently minimal direct evidence elucidating the pathophysiological processes that may promote stress-induced cardiac events. Hypothesized mechanisms include coronary vasoconstriction, autonomic dysfunction including cardiovascular reactivity, the promotion of plaque rupture and thrombus formation from endothelial dysfunction and prothrombotic responses, platelet aggregation, and electrical instability leading to ventricular arrhythmias (Bhattacharyya and Steptoe, 2007; Holmes et al. 2006; Rozanski, Blumenthal, and Kaplan 1999). Neuroendocrine changes also may be involved, as illustrated by changes in reproductive hormones among female monkeys at greater risk of atherosclerotic change (Manuck, Kaplan, and Matthews 1986). Psychosocial and behavioral pathways may be partly involved as well. Stress increases unhealthy behaviors such as smoking, alcohol consumption, inactivity, and a poor diet (Baum, Gatchel, and Krantz, 1997). Social support has a protective value and appears to diffuse the deleterious effects of stress, possibly by both behavioral and physiological pathways (Rozanski, Blumenthal, and Kaplan 1999; Skala, Freedland, and Carney 2005).

Treatment Modalities

Treatment goals for emotional distress in cardiac patients are multiple and include: 1) reducing emotional distress; 2) improving quality of life and patient functioning; and 3) enhancing the patient's ability to follow medical recommendations and engage in healthy behaviors. Ideally, a reduction in depression, anxiety, and stress also would translate into reduced cardiovascular risk, but large clinical trials to date have yet to show a significant treatment effect on cardiac outcomes (Lichtman et al. 2008; Writing Committee for the ENRICHD

Investigators 2003). Research examining specific mechanisms of action will hopefully lead to refined treatments targeted at physiological pathways implicated in the mind–body relationship. Current treatment options for depression, anxiety, stress, and poor adjustment to a cardiac event are varied and include pharmacotherapy, psychotherapy, stress management, relaxation therapy, physical activity, and less traditional options such as laughter, yoga, acupuncture, and massage. A majority of treatment outcome trials focus specifically on depression and primarily utilize the post-MI population.

PHARMACOTHERAPY

Safety considerations are a salient concern that may prevent some care providers from prescribing antidepressants or anxiolytics to cardiac patients. There are minimal clinical trials exploring the safety and efficacy of antidepressants in cardiac patients, but those limited trials have focused on post-MI patients. Results from these trials indicate that two selective serotonin reuptake inhibitor (SSRI) antidepressants are relatively safe for patients with CAD and are effective in treating moderate, severe, and recurrent depression: sertraline and citalopram (Glassman et al. 2002; Lespérance et al. 2007; Roose and Miyazaki 2005). These two SSRIs are considered the first-line antidepressant drugs for patients with CAD (Lichtman et al. 2008). The Sertraline Antidepressant Heart Attack Randomized Trial (SADHART) found sertraline to be more effective than placebo in reducing moderate and severe depression in 369 depressed post-MI patients who were randomized to treatment or placebo for 6 months. A non-significant trend favored sertraline over placebo in reducing severe adverse cardiovascular outcomes (Glassman et al. 2002). A post hoc analysis of the Enhancing Recovery in Coronary Heart Disease Patients (ENRICHD) study found that patients treated with an SSRI (non-randomized, but added in addition to cognitive behavioral therapy or usual care) had a 42 percent reduction in adverse cardiac outcomes, including recurrent MI and death, compared with depressed participants who did not receive antidepressants (Writing Committee for the ENRICHD Investigators 2003). SSRIs have no significant impact on blood pressure, heart rate, or cardiac conduction, making them a much safer and more favorable option over tricyclic antidepressants, which have been associated with antiarrhythmic properties, adverse side effects such as postural hypotension, and a less tolerable side effect profile (Glassman et al. 2002; Roose and Miyazaki, 2005). Less is known about antidepressants in non-CAD cardiac patients or about the safety and efficacy of anxiolytics in cardiac populations. The most common pharmacological treatment of anxiety includes benzodiazepines and SSRIs (Janeway 2009).

Many antidepressants have anxiolytic properties that can reduce the irritability and worry that often accompany anxiety.

Cardiotoxic side effects, adverse side effects, dependency (with benzodiazepines), and drug–drug interactions require careful consideration prior to beginning pharmacotherapy in cardiac patients. Education should always accompany prescriptions. Patients often are unaware of the side-effect profile of medications, or that these side effects usually diminish with time. They often misunderstand the delayed response associated with antidepressants and the importance of continuing the use of medication. Once started, cardiac patients should be monitored closely for the first two months and routinely thereafter to monitor suicidal risk, side effects, dosing titrations, and compliance with medication (Lichtman et al. 2008). Approximately 15 percent of patients discontinue antidepressant use within the first six months due to adverse side effects or lack of efficacy (Lespérance and Frasure-Smith 2000).

COGNITIVE BEHAVIORAL THERAPY

Although psychotherapy is effective in reducing emotional distress, minimizing relapse, improving quality of life, and enhancing motivation in depressive and anxious patients, only a few trials have examined the efficacy and safety of psychotherapy among cardiac patients. The most efficacious non-pharmacologic treatment for depression or anxiety among cardiac patients is cognitive behavioral therapy (CBT). (Lett, Davidson, and Blumenthal 2005; Skala, Freedland, and Carney 2005).

CBT operates on the premise that feelings and behaviors are dictated by thoughts, and that maladaptive thought patterns can be identified and changed to reduce psychological distress (Beck 1995). For example, an individual with depression may have the thought "I am worthless;" an individual with anxiety may have the thought "I am in danger;" and a stressed individual may have the thought "I have to be perfect." Therapy takes a direct approach to help the patient identify, test, and replace irrational beliefs, often by engaging in behavioral or cognitive exercises. The behavioral component of treatment may incorporate: increasing pleasurable activities, establishing daily routines, improving sleep patterns, facing feared situations, mobilizing social support, journaling daily thought patterns, increasing physical activity, or developing healthy responses to fears or emotions. CBT is an efficacious and empirically validated treatment for depression, anxiety, and numerous other psychological disorders.

A key component of the treatment of many anxiety disorders incorporates some form of exposure to the feared object, whether physical symptoms, situations, or places (Craske and Barlow 1993). CBT asserts that fear is maintained (and may increase) with avoidance, because avoidance *avoids* any opportunity to learn that the feared object may not be dangerous. Exposure provides learning opportunities to increase patients' sense of mastery and comfort in the face of a feared situation, and to help patients test and replace irrational beliefs related to their fears. Exposure can be imaginal or "in vivo" (real life). Regardless of which form exposure takes, exposure can be done *gradually*, whereby the therapist begins with a low-feared situation and slowly progresses to more-feared situations as the patient habituates. Exposure also can be done more abruptly, called *flooding*, where the therapist exposes the patient to the most-feared situation immediately. Although gradual (or graded) exposure is most common, both are effective. Table 8.6 outlines a graded exposure hierarchy for a cardiac patient who developed panic and agoraphobia after multiple syncopal episodes. The use of relaxation training often is utilized in

Table 8.6. Example of a Graded Fear Hierarchy for Exposure Treatment with a Cardiac Patient Exhibiting Panic and Agoraphobia After Multiple Syncope Episodes*

1. Sit in the therapist's office with only the therapist present (note: he initially required a friend to be present).
2. Sit in the waiting room for 10 minutes without my friend present.
3. Walk in place to get my heart rate up, with therapist present.
4. Close the bathroom door when showering or using the restroom (note: he initially required a friend to be present for fear of syncope).
5. Ride an elevator by myself.
6. Stand outside my house by myself for 10 minutes.
7. Walk down the street by myself for 15 minutes.
8. Eat a meal at home by myself.
9. Sit in my car by myself for 10 minutes.
10. Drive around the block by myself.
11. Stay at home alone for 1 hour.
12. Drive on the highway with a passenger present.
13. Drive on the highway for 2 exits (and back) by myself.
14. Stay at home alone all day by myself.
15. Drive myself to visit with friends at my old job.
16. Leave my house and walk to a restaurant or store by myself (gone 2 hours).
17. Drive on the highway at night and/or when raining.

*This graded hierarchy was created with direct input from the patient, based on his presenting fears and his degree of distress in certain circumstances, particularly those circumstances in which he was alone.

treatment for anxiety. Because anxiety and relaxation contradict each other, the body cannot be both relaxed and anxious at the same time.

To date, the ENRICHD trial is the only published randomized clinical trial that examined psychotherapy (CBT) for treatment of depression in patients with CAD. A total of 2,481 post-MI patients with either depression or low perceived support were randomized to six to twelve weeks of CBT or usual care, with patients receiving an SSRI when indicated for severe or persistent depression. At 6 months, CBT was favored over usual care in reducing depression, despite improvements in both groups. Although CBT was effective at reducing depressive symptoms, treatment had no impact on cardiac outcomes or survival (Writing Committee for the ENRICHD Investigator, 2003). Lespérance et al. (2007) recently evaluated the impact of short-term interpersonal psychotherapy (IP) plus simultaneous use of citalopram among clinically depressed individuals with CAD (the CREATE trial). Following twelve weeks of treatment, citalopram was superior to placebo in reducing depression. However, there was no additional benefit to IP above clinical management. Of note, the clinical management control consisted of weekly 25-minute sessions with a trained therapist who focused on education, support, encouragement of adherence to medication use, and problem-solving for side effects. These findings could suggest that the active problem-solving approach of clinical management (in some ways similar to CBT) may not be inert.

STRESS MANAGEMENT

Stress management is a nonspecific heterogeneous term that can encompass many treatment modalities, including cognitive behavioral strategies, education, and relaxation training. Stress management has been found to be effective in reducing headaches, cardiovascular reactivity, immune dysfunction, hypertension, and pain (Bernstein and Carlson 1993). Some studies have reported improved cardiac outcomes following stress management in patients with CAD (Blumenthal et al. 1997; Blumenthal et al. 2005). Blumenthal and colleagues (1997) found that a four-month stress management program for patients with CAD was successful in reducing mental stress-induced ischemia, ambulatory ischemia, and cardiac events at a three-year follow-up. The following components are often utilized in stress management.

Education

Patients typically benefit from information about stress, particularly about the physiological effects of stress on the body. Understanding the physiology behind their symptoms can offer relief and empowerment. Furthermore, awareness of the deleterious effects of stress on the body can improve patients' motivation to reduce stress and adopt healthier coping strategies.

The educational component also can address why stress is experienced. Lazarus (1966) describes the role of cognitive appraisals in stress. Specifically, stress occurs when a situation is perceived as dangerous, or when the resources to deal with the situation are perceived as insufficient. The balance of these appraisals can shift across time as information, coping skills, and personal abilities change. The essential component to this theory is that *appraisals* of a situation and internal resources dictate whether the stress response is activated. Altering those perceptions can be critical to reducing stress. Cognitive therapy can be used to address inaccuracies in someone's threat perceptions. A variety of tools can be used to increase someone's resources so they feel more adept at handling the situation at hand.

Protecting Healthy Behaviors

During stressful situations, many individuals are apt to forego healthy lifestyles and behaviors, which can be detrimental to healthy coping. Protecting sleep, exercising regularly, eating a well-balanced diet, and minimizing alcohol consumption are simple ways to reduce the effects of stress on the body and to increase the body's resources to cope with stressful events. Something as simple as poor sleep in the hospital can diminish someone's coping resources, so that events seem more overwhelming or challenging. Patients should be encouraged to protect their health by engaging in positive behaviors, particularly during stressful times.

Improving Coping Strategies

Coping refers to the behavioral or psychological strategies that are employed to tolerate or reduce a stressful situation. When coping skills and resources are healthy and intact, individuals are less likely to experience stress (Lazarus and Folkman 1984). Coping styles can generally be categorized as either problem-focused or emotion-focused. The former employs efforts to actively reduce the stressful situation, whereas the latter entails efforts to regulate or reduce the emotional consequences of the stressful event. Both types of coping are helpful, but coping may be most beneficial when the style of coping matches the level of control of a situation. When a stressful situation is perceived as less controllable (which is often the case with physical illness), emotion-focused coping may be preferable. Simply put, if the situation cannot be changed, an individual's reaction to that situation can always be controlled.

Even when the style of coping is well-matched to the situation's level of control, favored coping strategies can be inaccessible during illness, particularly when activity or independence are limited. For example, Veronica was a 35-year-old married female, employed full time, the mother of a toddler, who was hospitalized for valve replacement surgery. Veronica was emotionally healthy with no history of psychiatric distress. Her coping strategies were healthy and she typically coped with stress by running daily, practicing yoga weekly, remaining active, playing with her daughter, cooking, and maintaining control over her environment. During her hospitalization and recovery periods, Veronica's typical coping strategies were inaccessible to her, triggering emotional distress. Intervention with Veronica helped her develop coping strategies that were more accessible in the hospital and equally effective for her, such as imagery, listening to music, creating a recipe book, and updating her daughter's baby album. Veronica was able to sustain her emotional stability despite losing access to her typical coping strategies.

Relaxation

An important component of stress management (as well as a popular adjunct to other treatment modalities) is relaxation training, which aims to reduce or reverse the physiological effects of stress on the body and associated emotional distress. The relaxation response triggers activation of the parasympathetic nervous system, which works to restore physiological homeostasis following activation of the fight or flight response. Relaxation can come in many forms, including diaphragmatic breathing, progressive muscle relaxation (which involves the systematic tensing then releasing of muscle groups in the body), imagery, hypnosis, biofeedback, or a combination of the above. Among cardiac rehabilitation patients, progressive muscle relaxation has been associated with reductions in symptoms of depression, resting heart rate, and medication dosages (Collins and Rice 1997).

Another way to increase the relaxation response is to encourage patients to take a daily "time out" from stress. Protecting daily time for relaxation or a pleasurable activity can help reduce the emotional and physiological toll of stress. Pleasurable activities will vary by individual, but a time out may incorporate exercise, a bubble bath, reading a book, completing a crossword puzzle, having coffee with a friend, cooking a new recipe, gardening, listening to music, visiting a park, or getting a massage. As long as the activity is perceived as pleasurable, regardless of whether it is physically active or passive in nature, it can help protect the mind and body from the effects of daily stress.

Exercise

Increasing evidence points to exercise as an effective adjunct treatment for depression, anxiety, and stress (Barbour, Edenfield, and Blumenthal 2007). One longitudinal study found that a 4-month aerobic exercise program was as effective in treating MDD as sertraline. Furthermore, a 10-month follow-up revealed that patients in the exercise group had lower relapse rates than those in the medication group (Babyak et al. 2000; Blumenthal et al. 1999; Blumenthal et al. 2007). Controlled trials with cardiac patients are limited and many studies have methodological imitations, relying on self-report or lacking a control group. However, the few randomized controlled exercise trials among post-MI patients suggest that exercise is effective at reducing depressive symptoms across time compared with usual care, particularly when the exercise program is not home-based (Lett, Davidson, and Blumenthal 2005; Lichtman et al. 2008). Controlled trials are still needed to determine the impact of exercise on cardiac patients presenting with psychological disorders.

Other Therapeutic Modalities

The therapeutic modalities summarized in this chapter represent the most common and efficacious treatments for emotional distress and stress, but the most effective strategies for any given patient will be ones that take into account that particular patient's needs, resources, and preferences. For example, while efficacious, pharmacotherapy should not be the first line of treatment for a patient who is resistant to taking psychotropic medications. Similarly, exercise may not be an appropriate antidepressant for an angina patient with a positive stress test. Therefore, flexibility in treatment planning is imperative for cardiac patients, many of whom have barriers to engaging in traditional treatment, whether those barriers be physical, social, financial, geographical or time-based. Alternative approaches, such as online or telephone-based therapies, may help overcome some of these barriers; however, a lack of empirical investigations has made it difficult to determine the efficacy and safety of such approaches with cardiac patients.

The use of complimentary or alternative therapies also may be helpful adjuncts to treatment for cardiac patients. Although these approaches are less conventional treatments for psychological distress, they may be effective in helping to reduce physiological tension and emotional distress. An individual's emotional resources typically can be enhanced by engaging in any enjoyable activity, which can often take the form of a complementary modality, such as Qigong, yoga, Reiki, Healing Touch, massage, laughter, prayer, or acupuncture.

Role of the Medical Team: SERF

Given the prevalence of emotional distress in cardiac patients and its impact on morbidity and mortality, comprehensive cardiac care should incorporate assessment of emotional functioning (see Table 8.7). Emotional distress hinders patients' compliance, impedes their success at making lifestyle changes, contributes to a diminished quality of life, and predicts poorer cardiac outcomes. The accumulation of research findings within cardiac behavioral medicine emphasizes the importance of addressing emotional health routinely with cardiac patients, which was recognized by the American Heart Association in 2008 with their endorsement for the screening of depression in patients with coronary heart disease (Lichtman et al. 2008). A positive screen should result in a referral to a mental health professional and closer follow-up monitoring of patients' cardiac health (Lichtman et al. 2008). As a cardiac psychologist, I strongly encourage the medical team to SERF with their patients. This is a simple acronym I created based on a compilation of the existing research and suggested best practices to date, to provide professionals with an easy guide of how to incorporate emotional functioning into conventional clinical practice.

Table 8.7. The Role of the Medical Team in Addressing
Psychological Distress: SERF

SCREEN for depression and emotional distress
EDUCATE patients about the symptoms, prevalence, and cardiac risk related to depression, anxiety, and stress (and ENCOURAGE them to report symptoms)
REFER patients who screen positively to a mental health provider for comprehensive evaluation and/or treatment
FOLLOW depressed and distressed patients more closely to monitor their compliance and cardiac health

SERF STEP 1: SCREENING

There are no diagnostic tests for depression or anxiety. The only way to formally diagnose a patient with a psychological disorder is through clinical evaluation by a mental health professional. In lieu of comprehensive assessment, screening for emotional distress is gaining popularity in cardiac settings. In 2008, the American Heart Association formally recognized depression as a risk factor for morbidity and mortality among patients with coronary heart disease and called for routine screening of depression (Lichtman et al. 2008). Screening questions require minimal time or expense and can be completed in multiple settings and by a variety of team members. A positive screening will alert the medical team that a patient requires a referral to a mental health professional for a complete evaluation and possible treatment. Additionally, a positive screening will alert the medical team that a patient may be at increased risk of noncompliance, unhealthy lifestyle behaviors, morbidity, mortality, or the development of heart disease.

To determine whether an individual is at increased cardiac risk due to depression, a depression screening should incorporate the following three questions, at a minimum:

1. Have you ever been diagnosed with or treated for depression?
2. Have you been feeling sad, down, or hopeless for the past week or more?
3. Have you recently lost interest in activities that used to be pleasurable?

The following screening questions should be added to screen for nonspecific emotional distress:

1. Have you (or has anyone close to you) recently noticed a change in your mood or personality for the worse?
2. Have you been feeling anxious or stressed lately, to the point where your mood or routines have been affected?
3. Does everyday life seem harder to cope with lately?

SERF STEP II: EDUCATE

Patients often are upset to learn *afterwards* that their experience of depression following a cardiac event was not an isolated incident. Patients should be educated up front about the potential emotional consequences of a cardiac procedure or surgery in the same manner that they are educated about potential physical complications. At minimum, patients should be educated about the symptoms and prevalence of depression, especially after a heart attack and after cardiac surgery. Educating patients about depression, anxiety, and stress does not facilitate the development of these conditions, yet the information can provide relief and comfort if those symptoms arise. Furthermore, patients should be informed that depression and stress have a negative impact on their cardiac health so that patients respond appropriately to symptoms when they emerge. The negative stigma that often surrounds mental illness (and which can be a barrier to seeking treatment) can be reduced if the topic is addressed directly and proactively by the medical team.

SERF STEP III: REFER

Patients who screen positively for depression, or who acknowledge emotional distress, should be referred to a mental health provider for comprehensive evaluation, diagnosis, and treatment when applicable. In their editorial, Grissom and Phillips (2005) highlight the importance of education and referral, stating,

> When treatment [for depression] seems indicated, the physician's task is not necessarily to treat the patient, but instead, to motivate the patient to accept referral. Helping the patient to understand that depression commonly accompanies chronic illness, that it complicates treatment, and that, in most cases, it can successfully be treated can reduce the stigma and improve motivation. (pg. 1214)

Appropriate mental health referrals may include psychologists, psychiatrists, psychiatric nurses, social workers, or clinical counselors. Most academic medical centers or university settings have a department of psychiatry that will house resources for clinical evaluation or treatment, often with specialization in the growing field of behavioral medicine.

SERF STEP IV: FOLLOW

The presence of depression, anxiety, or stress should place a patient in an increased risk stratification. At this time, it is unclear whether treatment for psychological disorders translates into a reduction in cardiovascular risk. However, patients with depression, anxiety, or stress should be followed more closely than if they were not at increased cardiac risk. The frequency or form of follow-up best suited for distressed cardiac patients is unknown, but may include more frequent office visits, EKGs, or assessment of blood levels of medications.

Conclusions

Depression, stress, and anxiety are common experiences among cardiac patients. Unfortunately, their high prevalence often leads to a false conjecture on the part of the medical team that emotional distress is a "normal" or "healthy" reaction following a cardiac event. Psychological factors are far from benign healthy reactions, but play a significant role in the onset, course, and prognosis of cardiac disorders—perhaps almost as significant a role as traditional risk factors. Table 8.8 summarizes symptoms of emotional distress that may present in cardiac settings and have an impact on patients' emotional and

Table 8.8. Signs and Symptoms that a Patient may be
Depressed, Anxious, or Stressed

Symptom Presentation:
- Change in sleep (insomnia or hypersomnia)
- Change in weight without effort
- Increased irritability
- Sadness or tearfulness
- Minimal motivation
- Excessive fatigue or lack of energy
- Excessive worry about physical symptoms

Functional Impairment:
- Has not returned to previous levels of activity as expected
- Requests an extension of medical leave from work
- Unnecessary avoidance of certain activities or situations because of health concerns
- Poor hygiene
- Difficulty coping with medical status or life changes
- Reduced interest in previously pleasurable activities

Medical Management Challenges:
- Multiple visits to the ER or doctor's office for unexplained symptoms
- Difficulty complying with medication or treatment regimen
- Frequent phone calls to the medical team to seek reassurance or to report the same symptom without being asked
- Concern about symptoms or test results despite significant reassurance and information
- Multiple missed appointments

cardiovascular health. Although there are no consistent data to confirm whether psychological treatment can reduce cardiovascular risk, the treatments available for psychological disorders are efficacious, safe, and result in improved quality of life for cardiac patients. The incorporation of psychological health is a necessary component of comprehensive cardiac care.

REFERENCES

American Psychiatric Association. 2000. *Diagnostic and statistical manual of mental disorders.* 4th ed., text revision. Washington, DC: American Psychiatric Association.

Anda, R. F., D. F. Williamson, L. G. Escobedo, E. E. Mast, G. A. Giovino, and P. L. Remington. 1990. Depression and the dynamics of smoking. *Journal of the American Medical Association* 264: 1541–45.

Babyak, M., J. A. Blumenthal, S. Herman, P. Khatri, M. Doraiswamy, K. Moore, W. E. Craighead, T. T. Baldewicz, and K. R. Krishnan. 2000. Exercise treatment for major depression: Maintenance of therapeutic benefit at 10 months. *Psychosomatic Medicine* 62: 633–38.

Barbour, K. A., T. M. Edenfield, and J. A. Blumenthal. 2007. Exercise as a treatment for depression and other psychiatric disorders. *Journal of Cardiopulmonary Rehabilitation and Prevention* 27: 359–67.

Baum, A., R. J. Gatchel, and D. S. Krantz. 1997. *An introduction to health psychology.* 3rd ed. New York: The McGraw-Hill Companies, Inc.

Beck, J. 1995. *Cognitive therapy: Basics and beyond.* New York: The Guilford Press.

Bernstein, D. A, C. R. Carlson. 1993. Progressive relaxation: Abbreviated methods. In *Principles and practice of stress management.* 2nd ed., ed. P. M. Lehrer and R. L. Woolfolk, 53–87. New York: The Guilford Press.

Bhattacharyya, M. R. and A. Steptoe. 2007. Emotional triggers of acute coronary syndromes: strength of evidence, biological processes, and clinical implications. *Progress in Cardiovascular Diseases* 49: 353–65.

Blumenthal, J. A., S. Williams, A. G. Wallace, R. B. Williams, T. I. Needles. 1982. Physiological and psychological variables predict compliance to prescribed exercise therapy in patients recovering from myocardial infarction. *Psychosomatic Medicine* 44: 519–27.

Blumenthal, J. A., W. Jiang, M. A. Babyak, D. S. D. S. Krantz, D. J. Frid, R. E. Coleman, R. Waugh, M. Hanson, M. Appelbaum, C. O'Connor, and J. J. Morris. 1997. Stress management and exercise training in cardiac patients with myocardial ischemia: Effects on prognosis and evaluation of mechanisms. *Archives of Internal Medicine* 157: 2213–23.

Blumenthal, J. A., M. A. Babyak, K. A. Moore, W. E. Craighead, S. Herman, P. Khatri, R. Waugh, M. A. Napolitano, L. M. Forman, M. Appelbaum, P. M. Doraiswamy, and K. R. Krishnan. 1999. Effects of exercise training on older adults with major depression. *Archives of Internal Medicine* 159: 2349–56.

Blumenthal, J. A., H. S. Lett, M. A. Babyak, W. White, P. K. Smith, D. B. Mark, R. Jones, J. P. Mathew, M. F. Newman, and NORG Investigators. 2003. Depression as a risk factor for mortality after coronary artery bypass surgery. *The Lancet* 362: 604–609.

Blumenthal, J. A., A. Sherwood, M. A. Babyak, L. L. Watkins, R. Waugh, A. Georgiades, S. L. Bacon, J. Hayano, R. E. Coleman, and A. Hinderliter. 2005. Effects of exercise and stress management training on markers of cardiovascular risk in patients with ischemic heart disease: A randomized controlled trial. *Journal of the American Medical Association* 293: 1626–34.

Blumenthal, J. A., M. A. Babyak, M. Doraiswamy, L. Watkins, B. M. Hoffman, K. A. Barbour, S. Herman, W. E. Craighead, A. L. Brosse, R. Waugh, A. Hinderliter, and A. Sherwood. 2007. Exercise and pharmacotherapy in the treatment of major depressive disorder. *Psychosomatic Medicine* 69: 587–96.

Breslau, N., E. L. Peterson, L. R. Schultz, H. D. Chilcoat, and P. Andreski. 1998. Major depression and stages of smoking. A longitudinal investigation. *Archives of General Psychiatry* 55: 161–66.

Burg, M., M. C. Benedetto, R. Rosenberg, and R. Soufer. 2003b. Presurgical depression predicts medical morbidity 6 months after coronary artery bypass graft surgery. *Psychosomatic Medicine* 65: 111–18.

Burg, M., M. C. Benedetto, and R. Soufer. 2003a. Depressive symptoms and mortality two years after coronary artery bypass graft surgery (CABG) in men. *Psychosomatic Medicine* 65: 508–10.

Carney, R. M., and K. E. Freedland. 2003. Depression, mortality, and medical morbidity in patients with coronary heart disease. *Biological Psychiatry* 54: 241–47.

Carney, R. M., K. E. Freedland, S. A. Eisen, M. W. Rich, and A. S. Jaffe. 1995. Major depression and medication adherence in elderly patents with coronary artery disease. *Health Psychology* 14: 88–90.

Carney, R. M., K. E. Freedland, G. E. Miller, and A. S. Jaffe. 2002. Depression as a risk factor for cardiac mortality and morbidity: A review of potential mechanisms. *Journal of Psychosomatic Research* 53: 897–902.

Carney, R. M., M. W. Rich, K. E. Freedland, J. Saini, A. TeVelde, C. Simeone, and K. Clark. 1988. Major depressive disorder predicts cardiac events in patients with coronary artery disease. *Psychosomatic Medicine* 50: 627–33.

Collins, J. A., and V. H. Rice. 1997. Effects of relaxation intervention in phase II cardiac rehabilitation: replication and extension. *Heart & Lung: Journal of Acute and Critical Care* 26: 31–44.

Craske, M. G., and D. H. Barlow. 1993. Panic disorder and agoraphobia. In *Clinical handbook of psychological disorders*. 2nd ed., ed. D. H. Barlow, 1–47. New York: The Guilford Press.

Eaker, E. D., J. Pinsky, and W. P. Castelli. 1992. Myocardial infarction and coronary death among women: Psychosocial predictors from a 20-year follow-up of women in the Framingham Study. *American Journal of Epidemiology* 135: 854–64.

Fleet, R. F., G. Dupuis, A. Marchand, D. Burelle, A. Arsenault, and B. D. Beitman. 1996. Panic disorder in emergency department chest pain patients: prevalence, comorbidity, suicidal ideation and physical recognition. *American Journal of Medicine* 101: 371–80.

Fleet, R., K. Lavoie, and B. D. Beitman. 2000. Is panic disorder associated with coronary heart disease? A critical review of the literature. *Journal of Psychosomatic Research* 48: 347–56.

Frasure-Smith N, Lespérance F, Gravel G, Masson A, Juneau M, Talajic M, Bourassa MG. 2000. Depression and health-care costs during the first year following myocardial infarction. *Journal of Psychosomatic Research* 48: 471–478.

Frasure-Smith, N., F. Lespérance, and M.Talajic. 1993. Depression following myocardial infarction: Impact on 6-month survival. *Journal of the American Medical Association* 270: 1819–25.

Frasure-Smith, N., F. Lespérance, and M.Talajic. 1995. Depression and 18-month prognosis after myocardial infarction. *Circulation* 91: 999–1005.

Glassman, A. H., J. E. Helzer, L. S. Covey, L. B. Cottler, F. Stetner, J. E. Tipp, and J. Johnson. 1990. Smoking, smoking cessation, and major depression. *Journal of the American Medical Association* 264: 1546–49.

Glassman, A. H., C. M. O'Connor, R. M. Califf, K. Swedberg, P. Schwartz, J. T. Bigger Jr., K. R. Krishnan, L. T. van Zyl, J. R. Swensn, M. S. Fikel, C. Landau, P. A. Shaprio, C. J. Pepine, J. Mardekian, and W. M. Harrison. 2002. Sertraline treatment of major depression in patients with acute MI or unstable angina: Sertraline Antidepressant Heart Attack Randomized Trial. *Journal of the American Medical Association* 288: 701–09.

Granger, B. B., K. Swedberg, I. Ekman, C. B. Granger, B. Olofsson, J. J. V. McMurray, S. Yusuf, E. LL. Michelson, M. A. Pfeffer. 2005. Adherence to candesartan and placebo and outcomes in chronic heart failure in the CHARM programme: Double-blind, randomised, controlled clinical trial. *The Lancet* 366: 2005–12.

Grissom, G. R., and R. A. Phillips. 2005. Screening for depression: This is the heart of the matter. *Archives of Internal Medicine* 165: 1214–16.

Gullette, E. C., J. A. Blumenthal, M. Babyak, W. Jiang, R. A. Waugh, D. J. Frid, C. M. O'Connor, J. J. Morris, and D. S. Krantz. 1997. Effects of mental stress on myocardial ischemia during daily life. *Journal of the American Medical Association* 277: 1521–26.

Harvey, W. 1628. *Anatomical studies on the motion of the heart.* trans. C. D. Leake. Springfield, IL: Charles C. Thompson, 1928.

Ho, P. M., F. A. Masoudi, J. A. Spertus, P. N. Peterson, L. Shroyer, M. McCarthy Jr., F. L. Grover, K. E. Hammermeister, and J. S. Rumsfeld. 2005. Depression predicts mortality following cardiac valve surgery. *Annals of Thoracic Surgery* 79: 1255–59.

Holmes, S. D., D. S. Krantz, H. Rogers, J. Gottdiener, and R. J. Contrada. 2006. Mental stress and coronary artery disease: a multidisciplinary guide. *Progress in Cardiovascular Disease* 49: 106–22.

Janeway, D. 2009. An integrated approach to the diagnosis and treatment of anxiety within the practice of cardiology. *Cardiology in Review* 17: 36–43.

Jiang, W., J. Alexander, E. Christopher, M. Kuchibhatla, L. H. Gaulden, M. S. Cuffe, M. A. Blazing, C. Davenport, R. M. Califf, R. R. Krishnan, and C. M. O'Connor. 2001.

Relationship of depression to increased risk of mortality and rehospitalization in patients with congestive heart failure. *Archives of Internal Medicine* 161: 1849–56.

Jiang, W., M. A. Babyak, A. Rozanski, A. Sherwood, C. M. O'Connor, R. A. Waugh, R. E. Coleman, M. W. Hanson, J. J. Morris, and J. A. Blumenthal. 2003. Depression and increased myocardial ischemic activity in patients with ischemic heart disease. *American Heart Journal* 146: 5–61.

Joynt, K. E., D. J. Whellan, and C. M. O'Connor. 2003. Depression and cardiovascular disease: Mechanisms of interaction. *Biological Psychiatry* 54: 248–61.

Karasek, R. A., D. Baker, F. Marxer, A. Ahlbom, and T. Theorell. 1981. Job decision latitude, job demands, and cardiovascular disease: A prospective study of Swedish men. *American Journal of Public Health* 71: 694–705.

Kessler, R. C., K. A. McGonagle, S. Zhao, C. B. Nelson, M. Hughes, S. Eshleman, H. U. Wittchen, and K. S. Kendler. 1994. Lifetime and 12-month prevalence of DSM-III-R psychiatric disorder in the United States: Results from the National Comorbidity Survey. *Archives of General Psychiatry* 51: 8–19.

Krantz, D. S., W. J. Kop, H. T. Santiago, and J. S. Gottdiener. 1996. Mental stress as a trigger of myocardial ischemia and infarction. *Cardiology Clinics* 14: 271–87.

Kubzansky, L. D., and I. Kawachi. 2000. Going to the heart of the matter: Do negative emotions cause coronary heart disease? *Journal of Psychosomatic Research* 48: 323–37.

Kubzansky, L. D., I. Kawachi, S. T. Weiss, and D. Sparrow. 1998. Anxiety and coronary heart disease: A synthesis of epidemiological, psychological, and experimental evidence. *Annals of Behavioral Medicine* 20: 47–58.

Lazarus, R. S. 1966. *Psychological stress and the coping process.* New York: McGraw-Hill.

Lazarus, R. S., and S. Folkman. 1984. *Stress, appraisal, and coping.* New York: Springer.

Leor, J., W. K. Poole, and R. A. Kloner. 1996. Sudden cardiac death triggered by an earthquake. *New England Journal of Medicine* 334: 413–19.

Lespérance, F., and N. Frasure-Smith. 2000. Depression in patients with cardiac disease: a practical review. *Journal of Psychosomatic Research* 48: 379–91.

Lespérance F, N. Frasure-Smith, D. Koszycki, M. Laliberte, L. T. van Zyl, B. Baker, J. R. Swenson, K. Ghatavi, B. L. Abramson, P. Dorian, and M. C. Guertin. 2007. Effects of citalopram and interpersonal psychotherapy on depression in patients with coronary artery disease: The Canadian Cardiac Randomized Evaluation of Antidepressant and Psychotherapy Efficacy (CREATE) Trial. *Journal of the American Medical Association* 297: 367–79.

Lett, H. S., J. Davidson, J. A. Blumenthal. 2005. Nonpharmacologic treatments for depression in patients with coronary heart disease. *Psychosomatic Medicine* 67 (suppl): S58–S62.

Lichtman, J. H., J. T. Bigger Jr., J. A. Blumenthal, N. Frasure-Smith, P. G. Kaufman, F. Lespérance, D. Mark, D. S. Sheps, C. B. Taylor, and E. S. Froelicher. 2008. Depression and coronary heart disease. Recommendations for screening, referral and treatment. A science advisory from the American Heart Association Prevention Committee of the Council on Cardiovascular Nursing, Council on Clinical Cardiology, Council on Epidemiology and Prevention, and Interdisciplinary Council on Quality of Care and Outcomes Research. *Circulation* 118: 1768–75.

Mallik, S., H. M. Krumholz, Z. Q. Lin, S. V. Kasl, J. A. Mattera, S. A. Roumains, and V. Vaccarino. 2005. Patients with depressive symptoms have lower health status benefits after coronary artery bypass surgery. *Circulation* 111: 271–77.

Manuck, S. B., J. R. Kaplan, and T. B. Clarkson. 1983. Behaviorally induced heart rate reactivity and atherosclerosis in cynomolgus monkeys. *Psychosomatic Medicine* 45: 95–108.

Manuck, S. B., J. R. Kaplan, and K. A. Matthews. 1986. Behavioral antecedents of coronary heart disease and atherosclerosis. *Arteriosclerosis* 6: 2–14.

McDermott, M. M., B. Schmitt, and E. Wallner. 1997. Impact of medication nonadherence on coronary heart disease outcomes. A critical review. *Archives of Internal Medicine* 157: 1921–29.

Meisel, S. R., I. Kutz, K. I. Dayan, H. Pauzner, I. Chetboun, Y. Arbel, and D. David 1991. Effects of Iraqi missile war on incidence of acute myocardial infarction and sudden death in Israeli civilians. *The Lancet* 338: 660–61.

Miller, G. E., C. A. Stetler, R. M. Carney, K. E. Freedland, and W. A. Banks. 2002. Clinical depression and inflammatory risk markers for coronary heart disease. *American Journal of Cardiology* 90: 1279–83.

Pratt, L. A., D. E. Ford, R. M. Crum, H. K. Armenian, J. J. Gallo, and W. W. Eaton. 1996. Depression, psychotropic medication, and risk of myocardial infarction: Prospective data from the Baltimore ECA follow-up. *Circulation* 94: 3123–29.

Ramachandruni, S., R. B. Fillingim, S. P. McGorray, C. M. Schmalfuss, G. R. Cooper, R. S. Schofield, and D. S. Sheps. 2006. Mental stress provokes ischemia in coronary artery disease subjects without exercise- or adenosine-induced ischemia. *Journal of the American College of Cardiology* 47: 987–91.

Roose, S. P., and M. Miyazaki. 2005. Pharmacologic treatment of depression in patients with heart disease. *Psychosomatic Medicine* 67: S54–S57.

Rosengren, A., S. Hawken, S. Ounpuu, K. Sliwa, M. Zubaid, W. A. Almahmeed, K. N. Blackett, C. Sitthi-amorn, H. Sato, S. Yusuf, and INTERHEART investigators. 2004. Association of psychosocial risk factors with risk of acute myocardial infarction in 11,19 cases and 13,648 controls from 52countries (the INTERHEART study): Case-control study. *The Lancet* 364: 953–62.

Rozanski, A., J. A. Blumenthal, and J. Kaplan. 1999. Impact of psychological factors on the pathogenesis of cardiovascular disease and implications for therapy. *Circulation* 99: 2192–217.

Rudisch, B., and C. B. Nemeroff. 2003. Epidemiology of comorbid coronary artery disease and depression. *Biological Psychiatry* 54: 227–40.

Simon, G. E., M. Von Korff, K. Saunders, D. L. Miglioretti, P. K. Crane, G. van Belle, and R. C. Kessler. 2006. Association between obesity and psychiatric disorders in the US adult population. *Archives of General Psychiatry* 63: 824–30.

Skala, J. A., K. E. Freedland, and R. M. Carney. 2005. *Heart disease. Advances in psychotherapy: Evidence-based practice.* Cambridge: Hogrefe & Huber Publishers.

Steinberg, J. S., A. Arshad, M. Kowalski, A. Kukar, V. Suma, M. Vloka, F. Ehlert, B. Herweg, J. Donnelly, J. Philip, G. Reed, and A. Rozanski. 2004. Increased incidence of life-threatening ventricular arrhythmias in implantable defibrillator patients after the World Trade Center attack. *Journal of the American College of Cardiology* 44: 1261–64.

van Melle, J. P., P. de Jonge, T. A. Spijkerman, J. G. P. Tijssen, J. Ormel, D. J. van Veldhuisen, R. H. S. van den Brink, and M. P. van den Berg. 2004. Prognostic association of depression following myocardial infarction with mortality and cardiovascular events: A meta-analysis. *Psychosomatic Medicine* 66: 814–22.

Watkins, L. L., J. A. Blumenthal, J. R. T. Davidson, M. A. Babyak, C. B. McCants Jr., and M. H. Sketch Jr. 2006. Phobic anxiety, depression, and risk of ventricular arrhythmias in patients with coronary heart disease. *Psychosomatic Medicine* 68: 651–56.

Writing Committee for the ENRICHD Investigators. 2003. Effects of treating depression and low perceived social support on clinical events after myocardial infarction: The Enhancing Recovery in Coronary Heart Disease Patients (ENRICHD) randomized trial. *Journal of the American Medical Association* 289: 3106–16.

Yusuf, S., S. Hawken, S. Ounpuu, T. Dans, A. Avezum, F. Lanas, M. McQueen, A. Budj, P. Pais, J. Varigos, and L. Lisheng. 2004. Effect of potentially modifiable risk factors associated with myocardial infarction in 52 countries (the INTERHEART study): Case-control study. *The Lancet* 364: 937–52.

9

Energy Medicine

RAUNI PRITTINEN KING

KEY CONCEPTS

- Energy medicine is predicated on the concept that energy emanates from the body, and it can be influenced by skilled practitioners to promote health and healing.
- The human energy system has three components: meridians or energy tracts, chakras or energy centers, and auras or energy fields.
- Ancient cultures have been using energy healing modalities throughout history, including the Egyptians, Greeks, Chinese, the Indians, and Native Americans.

■

Energy Medicine

Energy medicine, also referred to as vibrational medicine, is the art and science of bringing balance and well-being into our lives. Our bodies are always looking to return to their natural state of health. The energy healing modalities are techniques to assist or enhance the process of healing.

For the body to function at its absolute peak of performance, all parts and processes must be interconnected by a system that delivers energy and information at the fastest possible speed available in nature. In the living body, each electron, atom, chemical bond, molecule, cell, tissue, and organ has its own vibratory character (Oschman 2000), as does the body as a whole. Energy medicine seeks to understand this vibratory energy, and to interact with it to facilitate healing (Gerber 1988).

When we are around other people, we are continuously interacting energetically, with words, sound vibrations, and our very acts of thinking. With healing intent we can enhance this interaction, and with a trained compassionate energy transfer from our hands, we have a very powerful yet subtle tool to alleviate suffering.

There are various hands-on healing studies that have looked at Therapeutic Touch, Qigong, and Healing Touch (Wind Wardell 2008,) but their exact mechanisms are still under investigation. It has been suggested that hands-on healers, through repeated practice of various techniques, might increase the size of their brain areas devoted to movement and finger sensitivity. This, in turn, could enhance the biomagnetic output from those areas of the brain, as it does in those who play stringed instruments. An increase in the strength of the brain waves would lead to a corresponding increase in the output from the fingers, as the brain waves are conducted to the fingers via the perineural and circulatory systems output from those areas (Oschman 2000).

Robert C. Beck's research on the brain wave activity of healers from a wide variety of subcultures around the world showed that all the healers produced similar brain wave patterns when they were in their "altered state" while performing a healing. Whatever their beliefs and customs, all healers registered brain wave activity averaging 7.8–8.0 cycles/second while in their healing state (Oschman 2000). This frequency is synchronized with the earth's geoelectric micropulsation, known as Schumann resonance. A Healing Touch practitioner is instructed to "find a quiet place within and center" before starting their hands-on healing. They are also instructed to connect to the earth's energy by grounding. This is combined with a healing intent for the client's or patient's highest good. Barbara Brennan, healer, author, and scientist writes,

> There is a vertical flow of energy that pulsates up and down the field in the spinal cord. It extends out beyond the physical body above the

---

Properties of Chakras

- We are energy or light beings as well as physical beings.
- Chakras are energy vortexes or wheels of spinning light that generate color.
- Chakras store information energetically, throughout our life.
- Chakras functions as our defense mechanism.
- The frequency of the spin generates the color.
- There are seven major chakras at the midline of the body.
- There are minor chakras in each joint, the palms of the hands, and the soles of the feet.

head and below the coccyx. I call this the main vertical power current. There are swirling cone-shaped vortexes called chakras in the field. Their tips point into the main vertical power current, and their open ends extend to the edge of each layer of the field they are located in. (Brennan 1987).

The healing power of touch dates back to Hippocrates, the Greek physician and father of modern medicine who noted that, "a force flowed from people's hands." Hippocrates used various words for this energy. Pythagoras, in Greece, referred to a "vital energy perceived as a luminous body that could produce cures." Paracelsus referred to a vital force and matter, calling it "illiaster." Today we call this "energy" flow. This energy has various names depending on the culture; *Chi* in China, *Prana* in India, *Ki* in Japan, or *Mana* in Polynesia, for example (Brennan 1993). Multicultural "bioenergy" healings have been reported throughout the history of humankind. Native Americans and aboriginal Australians, for example, have learned these techniques from their ancestors, as did the ancient Egyptians and Greeks (Bruyere 1989).

Dr. Valerie Hunt is internationally recognized for her pioneering research on human energy fields. She has discovered vibration patterns during pain, disease, and illness, and in various emotional and spiritual states. She has found scientific evidence of individualized field signatures and subtle energetic happenings between people and within groups (Hunt, 1995).

There are many paths to healing the body, mind and soul. Healing Touch and other energy-based therapies, including acupuncture, acupressure, Reiki, reflexology, Therapeutic Touch, and others, use the concept of the human energy system as the basis of their approaches.

Acupuncture

A tradition that is well over 2,500 years old, acupuncture represents one of the longest continuous forms of healing in existence. Acupuncture is based on important energy concepts, most notably *Qi* and *Yin/Yang*. Yin/Yang explores the important coexistence and necessary balance of opposites in the universe and within each individual (Stux 1998). Qi describes the vital force, or energy, that flows through each person. In a state of health, one's Qi circulate throughout the body in energy tracts known as meridians (Beinfield and Korngold 1992). Illness manifests as blockage or deficiency in one or more aspects of a meridian. Acupuncture techniques attempt to maintain balance and reduce illness by restoring the flow of Qi through the manipulation of acupuncture points and meridians (Kaptchuk, 2000).

Since the 1970s, when acupuncture first became popularized in the West, more than 1400 randomized controlled trials have been completed to examine its efficacy. A 1998 consensus statement by the National Institute of Health (NIH), as well as follow-up studies, endorsed the use of acupuncture for the adjunctive treatment of pain conditions (low back pain, fibromyalgia, tennis elbow, headache, osteoarthritis, carpal tunnel syndrome, etc.) as well as other conditions (including nausea from pregnancy, surgery or chemotherapy; hypertension, infertility, asthma, stomach disorders, and addiction). The NIH study concluded "further research is likely to uncover additional areas where acupuncture will be helpful" (1998) leading to more than 10 million treatments each year in the hope of maximizing the benefits of this positive, energy-based treatment (National Institutes of Health Consensus Conference 1998; White 1999).

Tai Chi and Qi Gong

Tai Chi and Qigong, the preeminent health practices developed in ancient China, are the major branches of modern Traditional Chinese Medicine. They consist of deep relaxation techniques for stress reduction, breathing exercises, visualizations to enhance mental acuity, self-massage, acupoint stimulation, and gentle fluid movements coordinated with the breath to release physical and emotional stress. All of these exercises promote the flow of bio-photon energy throughout the body known as "Qi" or "Chi." Qi Gong creates rather than exerts energy, so practitioners simultaneously feel completely relaxed and vitalized.

The unique contribution of Qi Gong to mind–body practice is the primary focus on the mind to guide the physical and emotional body. Techniques may be performed standing or in a seated position, so physically challenged individuals may experience the full benefit of the exercises. There are thousands of Qi Gong systems; the most popular in the West is the more physically oriented Tai Chi.

Taylor-Piliae and colleagues conducted a study to determine whether Tai Chi improves balance, muscular strength, endurance, and flexibility in patients with cardiac risk factors. Thirty-nine adults participated in a 60-minute Tai Chi exercise class three times per week. Statistically significant improvements were observed in all balance, muscular strength, and endurance and flexibility measures after six weeks with further improvement by week 12 (Taylor-Piliae et al. 2006). In 2004, Yeh and colleagues randomized 30 patients with congestive heart failure to 12 weeks of either Tai Chi or the standard care. Patients in the Tai Chi group demonstrated decreased levels of B-type natriuretic peptide, and improved 6-minute walk tests (Yeh et al. 2004). Multiple studies have demonstrated a reduction in blood pressure (Schaller 1996; Thornton, Sykes, and Tang 2004) and improvement in heart rate variability in patients taught Tai Chi and Qi Gong (Lee et al. 2002; Lu and Kuo 2003).

Since the 1950s, the Chinese government has conducted hundreds of scientific studies on the medical effectiveness of Qi Gong using Western medicine-approved measurements. The NIH has funded over 11 studies to date regarding Qi Gong's effectiveness in treating coronary disease, hypertension, fibromyalgia, chronic pain, basal cell carcinoma, geriatric health, and depression.

Reiki

Reiki is an ancient hands-on healing practice that originated in Japan with the spiritual teacher, Mikao Usui, a monk and educator who lived during the early twentieth century. The term "reiki," is derived from two Japanese words: *rei*, or universal, and *ki*, or life energy. Reiki is based on the belief that there is a universal energy source, and a person can be trained to access it to facilitate healing. The healing involves the transference of energy between practitioner and client. The practitioner places their hands lightly on or just above the person receiving treatment. The goal is to enhance the person's own healing response by restoring and realigning their biofield. Reiki is used to alleviate chronic pain, decrease anxiety, and promote deep relaxation. Reiki can be used as a self-care healing practice, or as a complementary therapy in a health care setting.

In 2002, a survey by the National Center for Health Statistics and the National Center for Complementary and Alternative Medicine (NCCAM) found that more than 2.2 million adults in the United States have used Reiki. Training in Reiki has three levels, each focusing on a different aspect of practice. Each level or degree includes one or more initiations or attunements. Mackay and colleagues evaluated autonomic changes during and after Reiki treatments. Although small in size, the researchers noted a significant reduction in heart rate and blood pressure compared to placebo and control groups (Mackay, Hansen, and McFarlane 2004). This study implies that Reiki impacts the autonomic nervous system and may offer a potential healing modality to alleviate stress and anxiety. NCCAM is currently conducting research to evaluate the effectiveness and safety of Reiki in patients with prostate cancer, fibromyalgia, and neuropathy.

Healing Touch

Healing Touch is an energy-based approach to health and healing. It is a collection of energy- based healing modalities from various cultures and healers, founded in the late 1980s by Janet Metgen, RN, for use by registered nurses and other health care professionals.

Healing Touch uses touch to influence the human energy system, specifically the energy field that surrounds the body, and the energy centers that control the energy flow from the energy field to the physical body. Disruption in the human energy system is viewed as a blockage of energy flow. The blockages can lead to illness or be the result of illness.

Healing Touch utilizes the hands to clear, energize, and balance the human and environmental energy fields, thus affecting physical, emotional, mental and spiritual health. Therapy is based on a heart-centered, caring relationship, in which the practitioner and client come together energetically to facilitate the client's health and healing. The goal in Healing Touch is to restore harmony and balance in the energy system, placing the client in the best state possible to self-heal. Healing Touch complements conventional health care and is used in collaboration with other approaches to health and healing (Healing Touch Certification Program, Healing Touch International, Inc. 1996).

The human energy system includes energy tracts (meridians), energy centers (chakras), and energy fields (auras). "Chakra" is a Sanskrit word meaning wheels of spinning light (Bruyere 1989). The frequency of the chakra spin generates its color. Chakras store information energetically, throughout a person's life. Chakras also function as defense mechanisms. The human energy body has seven major chakras in the midline of the body. Energy centers are also

Table 9.1. The Seven Major Chakras

Chakra	Function	Gland	Color	Sound	Musical Key of
One	Physical	Adrenal	Red	Lam	C
Two	Emotional	Gonads	Orange	Vam	D
Three	Mental/Self	Pancreas	Yellow	Ram	E
Four	Love/Forgiveness	Thymus	Green	Yam	F
Five	Expression	Thyroid	Blue	Ham	G
Six	Intuition	Pituitary	Indigo	Am	A
Seven	Spiritual	Pineal	Lilac/White	Om	B

located in each joint. The largest are in the shoulders, hips, and knees. Smaller energy centers are located in the palms of our hands and soles of our feet. (Hover-Kramer 2002). The first major chakra is located at the base of the spine (root), second below the naval (sacral), third above the naval (solar plexus), fourth at the mid chest (heart), fifth at the lower part of the throat (throat), sixth in the forehead just above the eyebrow (third eye) and seventh on top of the head (crown). These chakras work with the endocrine glands to provide continuous communication with the physical body. Each of the major chakras has a color and sound vibration.

The first chakra, or root, is at a lower vibration, creating a red color. The sacral or second is orange, the solar plexus chakra is yellow, the fourth or heart chakra is green, the fifth or throat chakra is sky blue, and the sixth chakra is indigo. The seventh chakra has the highest vibration and gives the color of white with a hue of lilac. This is the same prism of color seen in the rainbow. Therefore, we are light beings as well as physical beings.

Healing Touch training is organized in five levels of workshops. Certification as a practitioner is available to those who meet eligibility requirements and have successfully completed Levels 1–5 as taught by a certified Healing Touch

Table 9.2. Journey to Self-Healing with Chakras

First or Root Chakra (Physical): Color Red, Gland Adrenal, Sound Lam, Note C
In Balance: Profound connection to nature and understanding of its flow. Grounded.
Imbalance: Inability to trust nature. Focus on material possessions. Fear and need to satisfy own desires and wishes. Ungrounded.

Second or Sacral Chakra (Emotional): Color Orange, Gland Gonads, Sound Vam, Note D
In Balance: A considerate, friendly, kind, and open person.
Imbalance: Unstable, unsure in sexual and emotional matters. Guilt and cannot express feelings. Suppresses natural needs.

Third or Solar Plexus (Mental/Self): Color Yellow, Gland Pancreas, Sound Ram, Note E
In Balance: Feeling of inner calm, peace, and wholeness. Logical thinking. Inner acceptance and tolerance of others. A balance of the spiritual and material worlds. Healthy self esteem.
Imbalance: No trust in natural flow. Shame and need to dominate. Great need for material security. Poor self esteem.

Fourth or Heart Chakra (Love and Forgiveness): Color Green, Gland Thymus, Sound Yam, Note F
In Balance: Feeling of wholeness. Acceptance of the flow of life and relationships. Able to love.
Imbalance: Love given is not sincere. Cannot accept love given by others. Looks for rewards. Grief.

(continued)

Table 9.2. (Continued)

Fifth or Throat Chakra (Self Expression): Color Blue, Gland Thyroid/Parathyroid, Sound Ham, Note G
In Balance: Speaking one's own truth. Knows balance of silence and speech. Self-expression and creativity. Trusts intuition, knows how to listen to the "inner voice."
Imbalance: Cannot find expression despite much talking. Unable to express ones truth, lies. Fearful of being judged and rejected. Afraid of silence.

Sixth or Third Eye Chakra (Intuition): Color Indigo, Gland Pituitary, Sound Am, Note A
In Balance: Awareness of spiritual side of being. Inner awareness and knowing in everyday life. Dreams and Wisdom. Connects to the universe.
Imbalance: Rejects spiritual aspects of self and others. Illusions. Focus on science and intellect. Only sees obvious, surface moving. Afraid of intuition.

Seventh or Crown Chakra (Spiritual): Color White/Lilac, Gland Pineal, Sound Om, Note B
In Balance: Living with the knowledge of unity. Knowing that the self reflects in the divine. Abandon individual ego for universal ego.
Imbalance: Unable to let go of anxiety, fear, and attachment. Unable to imagine cosmic unity. Unsatisfied and depressed.

instructor. This organized infrastructure and credentialing makes this energy healing modality easy to implement in any healthcare setting.

Healing Touch in Clinical Practice

PREOPERATIVE AND POSTOPERATIVE

The goal of preoperative Healing Touch is to decrease anxiety and pain by opening the energy centers, or chakras, and balancing the energy fields. The patient is prepared to enter surgery with the best possible outcome. The treatment goal for postoperative Healing Touch is also to affect the energy system and open closed chakras. Cardiac patient undergoing coronary stenting or open-heart surgery at the Scripps Clinic and the Scripps Green Hospital receive pre- and postoperative Healing Touch and guided imagery treatments. A protocol is in place for open-heart surgery patients to have an integrative service coordinator, who is a nurse, provide Healing Touch. Patients are provided with guided imagery CDs and a portable CD player to prepare them psychologically and emotionally for their upcoming surgery. When the patient returns to the intensive care unit after surgery, they receive another Healing Touch treatment and guided imagery CD, which focuses on pain management.

Additionally, it is my experience that Healing Touch, guided imagery, and hypnosis are wonderful ways to prepare patients for cardiac transplantation.

VASCULAR DISEASE

The sympathetic nervous system, when unchecked, leads to the outpouring of stress hormones—most notably adrenaline, aldosterone, noradrenaline, and cortisol. These hormones lead to platelet aggregation, hypertension, hyperlipidemia, arrhythmia, central obesity, and immune system suppression. The cardiovascular literature reports an increased risk of acute coronary syndrome and myocardial infarction during times of stress.

Various energy healing techniques can be employed to decrease stress hormones, such as adrenalin and noradrenalin, thereby decreasing sympathetic tone. While working in the coronary care unit (CCU) or in the cardiac catheterization laboratory, these techniques can often calm and relax a patient while waiting for medication to take effect. These techniques are not a substitute for conventional care but a perfect complement to it as they place the patient in a relaxed parasympathetic state.

Simple energy healing techniques can be used with and taught to patients and caregivers to help with peripheral vascular disease. It is important to keep in mind that your intent to heal is as important as the techniques you use.

Spiritual Crises, Death, and Dying

When a person is admitted to a critical care unit, they are not only in physical crisis, but in emotional and spiritual crisis as well. They are afraid of pain, potential disability, and dying. A holistic approach requires listening to those concerns and finding an opening to discuss difficult topics. I instruct my students of Healing Touch (many of them nurses and doctors) to introduce Healing Touch as a stress reduction technique. For the anxious and worried patient, less information is often more. If the patient wants to have more details frequently they will ask for them.

Since Healing Touch works on all levels—body, mind, emotions, and spirit—the patient will usually easily express their fears and concerns. Energy healing is also a wonderful way to ease the dying process, whether it is in the hospital, hospice, or a home setting. Healing Touch has techniques that relax the body, allowing pain, anxiety and even struggled breathing to ease. When curing is not possible, healing can still take place. Very frequently a dying person will want to heal life issues such as troubled relationships. During a treatment they may "experience" their deceased loved ones' presence. The Healing Touch provider may be totally unaware of this communion.

Frequently, family members present during the Healing Touch treatment find the environment to be very healing for them. This is due to the calm energy that is created by the grounded provider of Healing Touch. After all the emotional turmoil loved ones have gone through, whether this is a sudden death or the result of a prolonged illness, the emotional exhaustion and letting go is often appreciated.

What a Clinician should know before making Energy Medicine Referrals

If you work in a health care setting, find an individual certified to provide energy healing for your patients. Your healer must be familiar with conventional medicine and how it functions. For example, an ICU can be an intimidating place to a non-medical Healing Touch provider. The energy healer must "speak the language" of a health care provider to ensure accurate communication. The allopathically trained healer may pick up problems during the healing sessions, such as low oxygenation, hemodynamic changes (if the patient is monitored), and sleep apnea. There are so many issues and events that happen in the health care setting that you can "bypass" potential problems by choosing a healer that is familiar with health care practice regulations. Make sure that your healer is certified in their field, ideally by an accredited organization, such as a Certified Healing Touch Practitioner (CHTP) by Healing Touch International or the Healing Touch Program, which are sponsored by the American Holistic Nurses Association (AHNA). Be aware of the fact that there may be certification programs that are less well known. Become familiar with a program and its certification policies before referring patients. It is also a good idea to obtain several professional and personal recommendations.

When making a referral for an energy medicine consultation, it is important to clearly express to the referring practitioner your reason for referral and desired outcome. For example, the CAM practitioner may be a Doctor of Oriental Medicine (OMD) or a doctor of Naturopathy (ND). The patient may not know the difference between these doctors and allopathic physicians. It is also good to keep in mind (and address any related issues immediately if needed) that the CAM practitioner in a health care setting always aligns himself or herself with the health care model. It is important that the CAM practitioner does not advise the patient to replace traditional medicine with complementary therapies, but rather understands the supportive and complementary role that integrative medicine plays.

REFERENCES

Beinfield, H., and Korngold, E. 1992. *Between heaven and earth: A guide to Chinese medicine.* New York: Ballantine Books.

Brennan, B. 1987. *Hands of light.* New York: Pleiades Books.

Brennan, B. 1993. *Light emerging: The journey of personal healing.* New York: Bantam Books.

Bruyere, R. 1989. *Wheels of light: A a study of the chakras, vol. 1.* Sierra Madre, CA: Bon Productions.

Gerber, R. 1988. *Vibrational medicine: New choices for healing ourselves.* Santa Fe: Bear.

Healing Touch International, Inc. 1996.

Hover-Kramer, D. 2002. *A healing touch: A guidebook for practitioners, 2nd ed.* Albany, NY: Delmar.

Hunt, V. 1995. *Infinite mind: The science of human vibrations.* Malibu, CA: Malibu Publishing Co.

Kaptchuk, T. J. 2000. *The web that has no weaver: Understanding Chinese medicine.* Chicago, IL: Contemporary (McGraw-Hill).

Lee, M. S., H. J. Huh, B. G. Kim, et al. 2002. Effects of Qi-training on heart rate variability. *American Journal of Chinese Medicine* 30(4): 363–70.

Lu, W. A., and C. D. Kuo. 2003. The effect of Tai Chi Chuan on the autonomic nervous modulation in older persons. *Medicine and Science in Sports and Exercise* 35(12): 1972–76.

Mackay, N., S. Hansen, and O. McFarlane. 2004. Autonomic nervous system changes during Reiki treatment: A preliminary study. *Journal of Alternative and Complementary Medicine* 10(6): 1077–81.

National Institutes of Health Consensus Conference. 1998. Acupuncture. *Journal of the American Medical Association.* 280(17): 1518–24.

Oschman, J. L. 2000. *Energy medicine: The scientific basis.* London: Churchill-Livingstone.

Schaller, K. J. 1996. Tai Chi Chih: An exercise option for older adults. *Journal of Gerontological Nursing* 1996 22(10): 12–17.

Stux, G., and B. Pomerantz. 1998. *Basics of acupuncture.* New York: Springer Publishing, (1998).

Taylor-Piliae, R. E., W. L. Haskell, N. A. Stotts, and E. S. Froelicher. 2006. Improvement in balance, strength, and flexibility after 12 weeks of Tai chi exercise in ethnic Chinese adults with cardiovascular disease risk factors. *Alternative Therapies in Health and Medicine* 12(2): 50–58.

Thornton, E. W., K. S. Sykes, and W. K. Tang. 2004. Health benefits of Tai Chi exercise: improved balance and blood pressure in middle-aged women. *Health Promotion International* 19(1): 33–38.

White, A., and E. Ernst. 1999. *Medical acupuncture: A western scientific approach.* Edinburgh: Churchill Livingstone.

Wind Wardell, D. 2008. *Healing touch research survey, 9th ed.* Denver: Healing Touch International, Inc.

Yeh, G. Y., M. J. Wood, B. H. Lorell, et al. 2004. Effects of tai chi mind-body movement therapy on functional status and exercise capacity in patients with chronic heart failure: A randomized controlled trial. *American Journal of Medicine* 117(8): 541–48.

II

Integrative Approaches to Cardiovascular Disease

10

Integrative Approaches to Preventive Cardiology

STEPHEN DEVRIES

KEY CONCEPTS

- Nutritional strategies emphasizing a Mediterranean-style diet can have therapeutic benefit at least as potent as lipid management, yet are not typically emphasized in conventional cardiology.
- Exercise improves heart health in a dose-response relationship: as little as 30 minutes of walking per day is helpful. Longer/more intensive workouts can result in up to a 40 percent reduced risk of heart disease.
- Conventional measurement with a standard cholesterol panel is an incomplete assessment; serious heart risks, often inherited, can be uncovered by evaluation of LDL particle size and number, HDL, Lp(a), and high sensitivity CRP.
- Intolerance to prescription statin therapy is common and can be overcome with many effective strategies.
- Several supplements have potent lipid altering properties and should be considered as therapeutic options, including red yeast rice, fish oil, niacin, soy, fiber, and stanols/sterols.
- Emotional health, especially stress level, is a major determinant of heart health.

■

Cardiologists are typically regarded as disaster relief specialists. It all begins with their training. Most young physicians enter the field of cardiology with the anticipation of caring for patients in the throes of a life-threatening emergency. The molding of cardiologists as high-tech emergency specialists is further reinforced in their hospital-based training programs.

Training rotations are typically divided into segments defined either by procedures (cardiac catheterization, electrophysiology, or echocardiography, for example) or by inpatient clinical service (coronary care unit or telemetry unit, for example). It is no wonder when, at the completion of training, most newly minted cardiologists gravitate toward managing patients with advanced cardiovascular disease.

The focus of most cardiologists, based both on interest and expertise, is to work with patients with advanced disease. Patients, on the other hand, are increasingly focused in a different direction—one emphasizing prevention and self-care. Based on the nature of their training, it is not surprising that most cardiologists feel ill prepared when it comes to prevention.

A growing segment of the public seeks to become more proactive in their health care. Patients are asking questions about how they can best protect their health. They want to know about diets, exercise and, in many cases, they want to explore all options available to them—including the use of nonprescription therapy. Unfortunately, cardiologists are typically poorly prepared to address these therapies. Patients tell me that they have rarely received helpful dietary information from physicians. Occasionally, referrals are made to a dietitian or exercise specialist, but patients often perceive that these referrals are made without the gravitas associated with other "high-tech" prescriptions. When patients inquire about supplements, they are often met with ridicule or, at best, a lack of information. Because training in medical school and beyond typically does not include discussion of nonprescription therapeutics, physicians often cannot help their patients in sorting through the potential role of therapies other than pills and procedures.

Moreover, when pills are used—whether they are prescription or over-the-counter—they are an incomplete solution at best. For example, prescription statins have been shown to provide no more than a one-third reduction in the risk of future cardiac events. Although this is a powerful and important treatment, it still leaves two-thirds of the risk on the table—a risk that a more comprehensive approach to prevention can address. It is in this gap that an integrative approach to preventive cardiology is born.

An integrative approach to preventive cardiology is the intelligent combination of a wide variety of therapies combining conventional and alternative strategies. The foundation of an integrative approach rests on lifestyle changes incorporating nutrition, exercise, and mind/–body connections. These interventions are highly effective, cheap, and offer myriad benefits extending far beyond the promotion of cardiovascular health. For those with several risk factors or with established heart disease, the "foundations" of lifestyle changes are conjoined with the best that science has to offer, including conventional medication and procedures. In this chapter, the palette that makes up this integrative approach to preventive cardiology will be explored, with an emphasis on practical strategies that can be readily incorporated into practice.

Nutrition for Heart Health

Most health professionals intuitively understand the value of diet in maintaining good health. However, while the importance of diet is generally understood, the power of dietary interventions is not adequately recognized. The following discussion will focus on a "Mediterranean-style" diet. Although a wide range of diet strategies have been proposed for promotion of cardiovascular health, including ultra-low-fat and ultra-low carbohydrate diets, the Mediterranean-style approach has the advantage of the best supporting evidence focused primarily on cardiovascular benefits, but extending far beyond. The Mediterranean diet emphasizes three key nutritional strategies proven to be beneficial: 1) substitution of polyunsaturated fat for saturated and trans fats, 2) consumption of omega-3 fatty acids from fish or plant sources and 3) focus on a diet rich in vegetables and fruit that emphasizes whole grains and is low in refined carbohydrates (Hu and Willett 2002).

The Lyon Diet Heart study (de Lorgeril et al. 1994) was a landmark trial that was the first to demonstrate the potency of a Mediterranean-style diet for prevention of heart disease. This study of myocardial infarction survivors evaluated the impact of dietary changes on cardiovascular events and death. Patients in the experimental group were advised to adopt a Mediterranean-style diet including more vegetables, more fish, and less red meat. Butter and cream were replaced with a canola-based margarine. Patients were advised to use this spread or olive oil as their sole cooking and food preparation oil. They were also advised to reduce their consumption of refined grains and to choose whole grain products. The control group followed a "prudent" diet and received advice from a hospital dietitian or attending physician advising the American Heart Association Step I diet, emphasizing reduction of total fat, saturated fat, and cholesterol.

This test of the Mediterranean diet was intended to run for five years. However, an intermediate analysis by the oversight committee halted the study after a mean follow-up of 27 months due to the finding of significant early benefit in the Mediterranean diet group. A striking 73 percent risk reduction was observed for the combined end points of cardiac death and non-fatal myocardial infarction.

Five years after the publication of the initial study, findings from an extended follow-up of the Lyon Diet Heart Study were reported (de Lorgeril 1999). This follow-up study demonstrated that the considerable early benefit of the Mediterranean diet group was maintained: the composite end point of cardiac deaths and nonfatal myocardial infarction was reduced by 72 percent (p<0.0001).

> **Diet is a form of "interventional cardiology:"** The Mediterranean Diet has been shown to reduce the risk of a cardiac event by 73 percent, a therapy more potent than any other treatment in cardiology.

Although the study design of the Lyon trial did not specify the quantity of any particular food item to be eaten, a diet history was recorded at the completion of the trial to better understand what was actually consumed (Simopoulos and Visioli 2000). For example, the intake of fresh vegetables in the Mediterranean diet group was 427 ± 222 [SD] g vs 340 ± 203 g in the controls, p<0.005; fresh fruit in the Mediterranean diet group was 271 ± 218 g vs 214 ± 201 g in the controls, p = 0.05.

The dramatic decrease in cardiovascular events associated with the Mediterranean-style diet is not surprising in light of subsequent studies demonstrating benefit from its constituent parts. In a combined analysis from the Nurses' Health Study and the Health Professionals' follow-up study, each serving of fruit or vegetables was associated with a 4 percent reduction in the risk of coronary disease (Joshipura et al. 2001). Of particular note, each daily serving of green leafy vegetables was associated with a 23 percent reduction in the risk of coronary disease. Similarly, in a trial examining the use of fish oil in survivors of myocardial infarction, a 53 percent reduction in the risk of sudden death was noted as early as four months after one gram per day of fish oil was started (Marchioli et al. 2002).

The Lyon diet study was performed in Europe, raising questions about the reproducibility of the findings to other regions and cultures. An Indian study performed in 2002 examined 1000 participants either with coronary artery disease or at high risk for heart disease. Individuals were encouraged to eat large amounts of fruit, vegetables, nuts, and whole grains. Mustard seed oil or soybean oil were used in place of olive oil due to accessibility and local preference. High intake of foods rich in omega-3 was encouraged and sources were largely from mustard or soybean oil, walnuts, grains, and vegetables rather than from fish. After two years of follow-up, there was a 52 percent reduction in total cardiovascular end points in the Mediterranean-style diet group compared to controls (Singh et al. 2002).

Since the Lyon Diet Heart Study and the Indo–Mediterranean diet study were published, several retrospective analyses have been performed demonstrating benefits of the Mediterranean style diet extending beyond the cardiovascular system.

One of the most intriguing benefits of the Mediterranean-style diet is the associated reduced risk of cancer—a finding identified in the original Lyon study and reproduced in subsequent trials. Although the Lyon study was not intended to evaluate the impact on cancer, the adjusted cancer risk in the Mediterranean diet group compared to controls was 61 percent (p =0.05). A subsequent metaanalysis of a Mediterranean-style diet compared 12,000 individuals with cancer to 10,000 healthy controls and identified a 70 percent reduction in the risk of cancer for those individuals consuming the highest versus lowest percentile of vegetable (Gallus, Bosetti, and La Vecchia 2004).

The NIH–AARP Diet and Health study performed in the United States followed over 380,000 individuals with no known history of cancer or heart disease (Mitrou et al. 2007). In this investigation, the reduction in cancer mortality in those with high versus low conformity to a Mediterranean diet was 17 percent in men (p<0.001) and 12 percent (p<0.05) for women. Similarly, cardiovascular mortality was reduced in the high versus low Mediterranean diet adherence groups by 22 percent in men (p<0.001) and 19 percent in women (p<0.02). Most importantly, high adherence to a Mediterranean-style diet was associated with a reduction in all cause mortality of 21 percent in men and 20 percent in women (p<0.001 for both). A larger analysis of over 514,000 patients demonstrated an inverse association between adherence to a Mediterranean diet and death (Sofi et al. 2008). Increasing adherence to a Mediterranean-style diet showed incremental reduction of total mortality, as well as cardiovascular and cancer death, as previously demonstrated.

In addition to reducing the risk of death from heart disease and cancer, the Mediterranean diet appears to reduce the risk of developing other conditions that impact on quality of life, including Parkinson's disease and Alzheimer's disease (Scarmeas et al. 2009; Sofi et al. 2008).

The mechanism of benefit of the Mediterranean-style diet is not completely understood. Surprisingly, the potent benefits of the Mediterranean diet are not associated with a significant improvement in standard lipid values (de Lorgeril 1999). There was no significant change in total cholesterol, LDL cholesterol, HDL cholesterol, or triglycerides between the Mediterranean-style diet group and controls.

What factors could account for the observed benefits? Most evidence suggests that the Mediterranean-style diet is antiinflammatory (Esposito et al. 2004; Giugliano, Ceriello, and Esposito 2006), although there is some evidence to the contrary (Michalsen et al. 2006). The Mediterranean diet improves endothelial function (Esposito et al. 2004), and decreases the likelihood of developing the metabolic syndrome (Esposito et al. 2004). The impact of a Mediterranean-style diet on the metabolic syndrome is appreciable. In a study of 180 patients with metabolic syndrome randomized to either a "prudent" or a Mediterranean diet, 56 percent of those in the Mediterranean diet group lost their diagnosis of metabolic syndrome, while only 13 percent in the prudent diet group did so (p<0.001).

With regards to weight loss, the Mediterranean-style diet appears to be more effective than a low-fat diet, and especially helpful for glucose control. A two-year trial of 322 moderately obese individuals compared three diets: low carbohydrate, low-fat, and Mediterranean. Among the 36 patients with diabetes, only the Mediterranean-style diet group was shown to lower fasting plasma glucose level (Shai et al. 2008). The Mediterranean-style diet group had a 33 mg/dL decrease in glucose. Surprisingly, this improvement in glucose level was far greater than that seen in the low carbohydrate diet group.

The benefits of a Mediterranean-style diet are unequivocal. The challenge for health providers is to learn how to counsel patients to adopt the diet and reap the multifold benefits. Based on the diet consumed in the Lyon study, a simple daily diet prescription can be advised:

- *vegetables*: 1 colorful side salad with both lunch and dinner every day and a side of vegetables with dinner
- *fruit*: berries with breakfast and an apple or orange later in the day
- *fish*: 2 fish dinners per week
- *grains*: minimize refined carbohydrates and emphasize "whole" grains
- *oil*: exclusive use of olive or canola
- *red meat*: minimize

The gulf between the typical Western diet and the Mediterranean-style "ideal" diet is wide, and many patients will not be able to consistently adhere to the optimal levels of intake. Fortunately, benefits can still be accrued by incremental adherence, as there exists a "dose-response" relationship between adherence and benefit. Both the NIH–AARP (Mitrou et al. 2007) and the 514,000 patient metaanalysis (Sofi et al. 2008) demonstrated clear incremental benefit with increasing degrees of adherence to a Mediterranean-style diet. Therefore, if a patient currently is consuming one serving of vegetable or fruit per day, clear benefit would be expected from an incremental change, by even as little as one additional daily serving of vegetable, fruit, and fish.

Exercise

In addition to diet, exercise is among the most potent interventions available for prevention of heart disease. The benefits of exercise extend far beyond cardiovascular health and include longevity. For example, performance of moderate intensity physical activity, including brisk walking at 3–4 mph for five days per week, results in up to a 30 percent reduction in all cause mortality (Lee and Skerrett 2001). Unfortunately, the potential benefits of exercise are rarely realized. Health care professionals are often pessimistic regarding the capacity of their patients to adopt an exercise program. This attitude can become a self-fulfilling prophecy, as the likelihood of patient success is related, in part, to the patient's perception of how important exercise is to the health care professional.

How much exercise is required in order to obtain benefit? Although there appears to be a dose-response relationship between exercise and all cause mortality, even modest levels of exercise are beneficial. In a group of over 44,000 men enrolled in the Health Professionals Follow-Up Study, as little as thirty minutes per day of brisk walking was associated with an 18 percent reduction in the risk of coronary heart disease (Tanasescu et al. 2002). More intensive exercise, including running one hour or more per week, resulted in greater benefit, with a 42 percent risk reduction. In a study of over 73,000 post-menopausal women enrolled in the Women's Health Initiative Observational Study, even women with a relatively low level of exercise (median of 4.2 MET-hr/week) experienced a 27 percent reduction in risk of coronary heart disease (Manson et al. 2002). Again, more active women, who exercised 10.0 MET-hr/week or 32.8 MET-hr/week, had successively greater risk reductions of 31 percent and 53 percent, respectively.

The mechanism of benefit from exercise for the prevention of heart disease is multifaceted. Exercise is clearly beneficial in reducing hypertension, improving dyslipidemia (reducing LDL cholesterol, reducing triglycerides, and increasing HDL cholesterol), improving glycemic control, and reducing stress. Exercise has also been shown to be a powerful mediator of endothelial function (Hambrecht et al. 2000).

Although aerobic exercise is typically recommended for cardiovascular health, resistance training confers additional benefit, including a favorable influence on blood pressure and glycemic control (Braith and Stewart 2006). In men, resistance training is associated with a reduction in the risk of coronary heart disease. Men who trained with weights for 30 minutes or more per week had a 23 percent reduced risk of heart disease compared to no resistance training (Tanasescu et al. 2002).

A common dilemma for the practitioner is whether or not to proceed with stress testing in a sedentary, but asymptomatic, individual prior to beginning an exercise program. The rationale to do so is supported by a study demonstrating that the relative risk of cardiac arrest during exercise in a previously sedentary individual is as high as 56-fold compared to the risk at rest (Siscovick et al. 1984). The ACC/AHA Exercise Guidelines do not recommend routine

Practical tips: the goal of exercise for primary prevention of heart disease should include, as a minimum, 30 minutes of moderate intensity exercise on most days. A simple strategy of brisk walking for 30 minutes per day, broken into 10–15 minute blocks if necessary, is an excellent start. More intensive exercise sessions for longer duration appeared to be of additional benefit and should be encouraged as a goal. The addition of resistance training to an aerobic program has added benefit, not only for general fitness, but also for cardiovascular health. These recommendations are in accordance with American Heart Association Guidelines for primary prevention of cardiovascular disease (Pearson et al. 2002).

screening of asymptomatic individuals, but do acknowledge potential benefit of stress testing sedentary individuals with multiple cardiovascular risk factors prior to beginning an exercise program as a Class IIb indication, where "conflicting evidence" in which the "usefulness/efficacy is less well established by evidence/opinion" (Gibbons et al. 2002). The practitioner should take into account the number and extent of cardiovascular risk factors, especially diabetes, in making a decision about proceeding with stress testing individuals prior to beginning an exercise program.

Cholesterol

Cholesterol management is often the focal point of efforts to prevent heart disease. On closer inspection, a more balanced emphasis may be appropriate. As many as one-third of individuals with myocardial infarction have a total cholesterol level in the "normal range" of under 200 mg/dl. Similarly, many individuals with elevated cholesterol levels never develop cardiac events.

A balanced view, supported by the literature, clearly demonstrates that cholesterol is only one of many important factors in the development of heart disease. A wealth of information exists in both primary and secondary prevention trials demonstrating the value of cholesterol reduction with statin therapy. The risk reduction most commonly observed in these trials is approximately one-third. In this chapter, strategies will be discussed to maximize opportunities for treatment of cholesterol disorders, with an emphasis on integrative approaches.

Traditionally, the primary target of lipid therapy is the cholesterol content of low-density lipoprotein (LDL). The emphasis on LDL is well-placed, based on outcomes data from LDL lowering clinical trials. Conventional guidelines for treatment of LDL, along with the rationale for therapy, are carefully summarized in the Adult Treatment Panel guidelines (Grundy et al. 2004).

Despite the clear importance of LDL, there is considerable controversy that this marker may not be the best indicator of LDL-related risk. Conventional lipid tests measure the cholesterol content in LDL. Interestingly, the cholesterol content of LDL particles can vary substantially from person to person. The explanation for this is that some individuals have a predominance of small, dense LDL particles. For others, the LDL cholesterol exists as larger, more buoyant particles. Smaller particles are associated with greater risk, as they are more easily oxidized and are mechanically better able to intercalate within the plaque (Tribble et al. 1992).

If the LDL particles are small and, therefore, carry less cholesterol per particle, any given LDL cholesterol concentration will be associated with a greater number of LDL particles. Therefore, two individuals can have the same LDL cholesterol level, yet have a very different number of atherogenic LDL particles and, consequently, very different risks.

Interestingly, the risk of cardiovascular events is more closely linked to the number of LDL particles than to their cholesterol content, with higher risk closely linked to a higher number of atherogenic particles (Barter et al. 2006). For that reason, many lipidologists argue that a test of the number of atherogenic particles is a more useful gauge of risk, and a superior end point to therapy, than the LDL cholesterol.

A useful, and simple, indicator of the number of atherogenic particles is the calculation of non-HDL cholesterol. This term is obtained from the standard lipid panel, and can by calculated by subtracting HDL cholesterol from the total cholesterol. Non-HDL cholesterol has been found to more closely correlate with cardiac risk than LDL-C, especially in situations where triglycerides are > 200 mg/dl (Packard and Saito 2004).

An alternative measurement of the number of LDL particles (LDL-P) is a nuclear magnetic resonance test. This is a proprietary test that typically is reported bundled with an assessment of LDL size, and is a better predictor of cardiovascular risk better than LDL cholesterol (Hsia et al. 2008).

Arguably the most robust measurement of atherogenic particle burden is Apolipoprotein B (ApoB). The value of ApoB as a marker of risk is the convenient fact that each atherogenic particle, including low density lipoprotein, very low density lipoprotein, intermediate density lipoprotein, and lipoprotein (a), contain one and only one molecule of ApoB. Therefore, ApoB can be considered an aggregate marker of the overall risk of atherogenic particles. This is a relatively cheap and reproducible test demonstrated to correlate with cardiovascular risk to a degree similar to LDL-P and superior to non-HDL cholesterol (Sniderman 2005).

Table 10.1. Comparison of Methods to Measure Atherogenic Cholesterol

	50th percentile	*20th percentile*	*2nd percentile*
LDL Cholesterol (mg/dL)	130	100	70
Non-HDL Cholesterol (mg/dL)	153	119	83
LDL Particle (nmol/L)	1440	1100	720
ApoB (mg/dL)	97	78	54

Adapted from et al. 2009.

Interpretation of the results of these new measurements relative to the traditional LDL-C test can be challenging. A recent study demonstrates a cross comparison of these tests from data gleaned from the Framingham study (Contois et al. 2009). For example, the fiftieth percentile for LDL-C =130 mg/dl; for non-HDL= 153 mg/dl; for LDL-P = 1440 nmol/L; and for ApoB = 97 mg/dl. The twentieth percentile for LDL-C = 100 mg/dl; for non-HDL = 119 mg/dl; for LDL-P = 1100 nmol/L; for ApoB 78 mg/dl. The second percentile for LDL-C = 70 mg/dl; for non-HDL= 83 mg/dl; for LDL-P = 720 nmol/L; for ApoB = 54 mg/dl.

Based on this data, aggressive control of LDL-related risk for those at highest risk of vascular disease could be accomplished by ensuring that the following criteria are met: LDL-C <70 mg/dl and ApoB < 60 mg/dl or LDL-P < 700 nmol/L.

It is likely that future versions of the cholesterol treatment guidelines will incorporate some measurement of atherogenic particle number for both diagnostic purposes, as well as to better define an end point for therapy.

Treatment of Elevated LDL

As previously noted, the cornerstone of prevention in general, including treatment of cholesterol disorders, rests in diet and exercise. When therapy is required beyond lifestyle measures, a variety of options exist—both prescription and over the counter.

Many hundreds of over-the-counter products have been proposed for reduction of LDL cholesterol. Data for many of these products, however, is conflicting and demonstrates a modest impact at best. Moreover, some over the counter products have substantial cholesterol lowering value and may be an ideal solution under certain circumstances. Therefore, it is incumbent on the clinician interested in integrative approaches to acquire a thorough understanding of the science behind the use of supplements.

As an introduction to this topic, it is important to make note of supplements commonly mentioned for treatment of cholesterol that are not particularly helpful for that purpose. Commonly used supplements with little or no significant benefit for cholesterol management include garlic (Khoo and Aziz 2009), gugulipid (Szapary et al. 2003), and policosanol (Dulin et al. 2006).

Over-the-counter products shown to have the greatest potency for LDL reduction include: soluble fiber, plant stanols/sterols, soy, niacin, and red yeast rice.

FIBER

The water-soluble portion of fiber has been shown to both reduce the intestinal absorption of cholesterol as well as decrease hepatic synthesis. Each daily gram of soluble fiber intake can decrease LDL-C by 2.2 mg/dL (Brown et al. 1999). Rich dietary sources of soluble fiber include: kidney beans (6 grams/cup), oatmeal (2 grams/cup), oat bran (2 grams/cup), orange (2 grams/whole fruit), broccoli 2 grams/cup), and apples (1 gram/whole fruit). Fiber supplements added to dietary sources of fiber can have additional benefit. Twice daily use of psyllium 5-gram supplement results in a 7 percent reduction in LDL-C, as well as a reduction in glycemic measures (Anderson et al. 2000).

STANOLS/STEROLS

Mammalian cells contain cholesterol. Plants have no cholesterol but contain small quantities of phytosterols and their saturated derivatives, plant stanols. Both sterols and stanols reduce the intestinal absorption of cholesterol by competing with dietary and biliary sources of cholesterol for production of micelles. Intake of 1.8 to 2.6 grams per day of stanols supplemented in margarine reduces LDL cholesterol by 14 percent (Miettinen et al. 1995) A single daily dose of stanols-enriched margarine has been shown to be as effective as divided doses (Plat et al. 2000). Stanols can be added to ongoing statin therapy for an additional 10 percent reduction of LDL-C reduction (Blair et al. 2000).

More recently, stanols and sterols have been incorporated into a wide range of foods. The type of food to which stanols/sterols are added may influence the degree of cholesterol reduction. One convenient method of enhancing dietary intake is through stanol-enhanced yogurt. Consumption of 1 g per day of stanol introduced into a low-fat yogurt resulted in a 13.7 percent reduction in LDL cholesterol (Mensink et al. 2002). Maximal benefit was noted after one week of daily intake. Stanols/sterols are also widely available in pill form, but data is lacking regarding efficacy of stanols and sterols in pill form.

SOY PROTEIN

In a metaanalysis of 38 controlled trials in which soy protein intake averaged 47 g/day (range 17 to 124), soy reduced total cholesterol by 9.3 percent, LDL by 12.9 percent, and triglycerides by 10.5 percent, with no significant increase in HDL (Anderson, Johnstone, and Cook-Newell 1995). The mechanism of benefit is not completely defined, but likely includes an increase in hepatic LDL receptors (Erdman, 2000). Soy contains isoflavones, a form of phytoestrogen. The degree to which isoflavone content in soy contributes to cholesterol reduction is unclear. A metaanalysis of 10 studies showed no independent effect of isoflavone concentration on lipid changes (Weggemans and Trautwein 2003). The American Heart Association Nutrition Committee has concluded that 25 g/day of soy protein is effective for improving lipid profiles (Erdman 2000). Soy intake of 25 to 50 g/day would be expected to lower LDL by 4 to 8 percent (Erdman 2000).

COMBINATION OF FIBER, SOY, ALMONDS, AND STEROLS ("PORTFOLIO DIET")

A low-saturated-fat diet concentrated with fiber, soy, sterols, and almonds, referred to as the "Portfolio Diet," has been shown in a four-week trial to lower LDL by 29 percent and C-reactive protein by 28 percent, values similar to those achieved with a low fat diet and lovastatin 20 mg (Jenkins et al. 2003). The diet contained approximately 2 g/day of plant sterols from a sterol enhanced margarine, 20 gram per day of soluble fiber from oats, barley, and psyllium, 50 g/day of soy protein from soy milk and soy meat substitute, and 30 g/day of almonds. Of note, this was a four-week study in which only 40 percent of the study participants judged the Portfolio Diet to be "acceptable."

NIACIN

Niacin, available over the counter as well as by prescription, is unique in that it improves a broader range of lipid parameters than with any other lipid therapy: it lowers LDL, shifts LDL particle size to the more favorable larger forms, lowers triglycerides, reduces Lp(a), and raises HDL. Niacin reduces the mobilization of free fatty acids from the periphery, thereby reducing the production of VLDL and LDL.

The benefits of niacin are dose-dependent, with LDL reduction in the range of 3–17 percent with doses ranging from 500 to 2000 mg per day. Reductions of cardiovascular events with niacin have been reported when used as monotherapy (Canner et al. 1986), as well as in combination therapy with other lipid lowering agents. The combination of over-the-counter niacin and simvastatin resulted in an 89 percent event reduction in the HDL Atherosclerosis Treatment Study (Brown et al. 2001).

> *Be aware that "no-flush" and "flush-free" niacin are ineffective for lipid management.*

Immediate release products (available over the counter) and intermediate release versions (available by prescription) are both effective. Nonprescription forms are cheaper, and may be preferred by patients seeking to avoid prescriptions, but have the disadvantage of uncertainty in content. The major limitation of niacin is the annoying but harmless side effect of flushing.

Of note, several forms of "no-flush" niacin are available which appear attractive choices, but should not be used due to poor efficacy. "Flush-free" and "no-flush" niacin are inositol hexaniacinate, a bound form of niacin, which requires an esterase for release of the active, free niacin. Because this reaction is very limited in most individuals, minimal free niacin is produced and, consequently, "no-flush" or "flush-free" niacin are generally ineffective for lipid management (Meyers et al. 2003).

Successful Strategies for Reducing Flushing Associated with Niacin

1. Take niacin with food—ideally with dinner (avoid taking niacin on an empty stomach). Alternatively, take niacin with applesauce in the evening.
2. Take aspirin or a non-steroidal antiinflammatory with niacin.
3. Avoid alcohol and spicy foods at the time niacin is taken
4. Avoid "no-flush" or "flush-free" brands due to poor efficacy.

RED YEAST RICE

Red yeast rice is the most potent over the counter therapy available for reduction of LDL cholesterol. This is a fermentation product which results from growing the yeast Monascus purpureus on rice. Red yeast rice contains monacolins, constituents that are HMG-CoA reductase inhibitors, or statins. Analysis of red yeast rice reveals nine monacolins; the one present in greatest concentration is monacolin K, also known as lovastatin (Heber et al. 1999). The monacolin content and, therefore, the cholesterol lowering properties, vary greatly between different brands of red yeast rice (Gordon et al. 2009). Need for caution exists, as some brands have been found to contain citrinin, a nephrotoxic substance that should be removed during the fermentation process (Gordon et al. 2009).

If red yeast rice is a form of a statin, why recommend it instead of prescription statins? There are two reasons to consider doing so: 1) patients who are philosophically opposed to taking prescription medication for cholesterol reduction; 2) patients who have experienced adverse reactions to prescription statins (particularly myalgias).

A growing body of literature supports the use of red yeast rice. Reductions in LDL cholesterol season with red yeast rice are typically in the range of 20 to 30 percent (Becker et al. 2009; Heber et al. 1999; Lin, Li, and Lai 2005). A 12-week study of red yeast rice prescribed at 2400 mg per day resulted in a decrease in LDL cholesterol of 23 percent, a decrease in triglycerides of 15 percent, and no significant change in HDL cholesterol. Of note, no myalgias were reported among patients in this study (Heber et al. 1999).

Red yeast rice may be better tolerated than prescription statins; some patients who have experienced adverse reactions with multiple prescription statins, even at low dosages, have been able to take red yeast rice, with excellent results.

A study of 62 individuals with a history of needing to discontinue therapy with prescription statins due to severe myalgias were randomized to red yeast rice at 1800 mg per day or placebo, for 6 months. In the group receiving red yeast rice, only 2 of 29 (7 percent) of previously statin intolerant patients needed to discontinue treatment with red yeast rice because of myalgias, with the benefit of a 21 percent decrease in LDL from baseline at week 24 (Becker et al. 2009).

Table 10.2. Supplements to Lower LDL

Supplement	LDL Reduction
Red yeast rice	20–30%
Niacin	10–20%
Plant stanols/sterols	5–15%
Soluble fiber	5–10%
Soy protein	5–10%

The potency of a nonprescription approach to the patient with dyslipidemia was demonstrated in a trial comparing a moderate dose of a statin with an "alternative approach" combining over-the-counter supplements and lifestyle changes (Becker et al. 2008). In this study, patients were randomized to receive either receive simvastatin at 40 mg per day along with AHA handouts on diet and exercise, or a combination of red yeast rice (2400–3600 milligrams per day), fish oil (3.8 g per day), and weekly lifestyle counseling. At the completion of the three-month study period, both the prescription and the "alternative" groups had striking, yet similar, reduction in LDL cholesterol: 40 percent for the simvastatin group and 42 percent for the alternative group, p=ns. The alternative group had a significantly greater reduction in triglycerides, however, of 29 percent versus 9 percent in the simvastatin group, p<0.005.

Most importantly, there is outcomes data with red yeast rice showing improvement in both cardiovascular end points, as well as total mortality. A study of 4870 individuals with myocardial infarction randomized to placebo or red yeast rice 1200 mg per day for 4.5 years demonstrated a 45 percent decrease in the primary end point of a major coronary event in the group receiving a red yeast rice. Moreover, a reduction in total mortality of 33 percent in the treatment group was observed (p < 0.0005) (Lu et al. 2008). The red yeast rice used in this study contained a daily total of lovastatin 10–12 mg, and the LDL reduction was 18 percent. It is interesting to speculate that other constituents of red yeast rice may contribute to the outcome benefits, which appear disproportionate to the lipid lowering effect.

Patients with Intolerance or Philosophical Opposition to Prescription Statins

Managing lipids in patients who are either intolerant of prescriptions statins or philosophically opposed to their use is one of the most challenging of all prevention scenarios. Most clinicians have encountered patients who refuse to take prescription statins. They often avoid medication for fear of adverse reactions, as well as a general sense that prescriptions are associated with an increased risk of harm. Others are quite willing to take prescription cholesterol medication but have been intolerant to them, often despite trying multiple agents, even at low dosages.

STATIN INTOLERANCE

Although patients often fear liver toxicity from statins, the adverse reaction most likely to trigger discontinuation of therapy is muscle pain. The package insert for most prescription statins lists the incidence of myalgias as being 3–5%. Based on personal communications from primary care physicians, this number is likely a considerable underestimate. Determination of a causal relationship between statin use and muscle complaints can be perplexing, as muscle pain is ubiquitous and distinguishing baseline muscle aches and pains from those related to statin use can be difficult. Relying on serum CK levels to gauge a cause and effect relationship between myalgias and statins is problematic, as histologically proven muscle inflammation related to statin use may exist in the absence of elevated circulating CK (Phillips et al. 2002).

Dealing with statin intolerance is frustrating for both patients and medical providers. Doctors may suspect that adverse reactions are experienced as a type of "self-fulfilling prophecy," in which patients, reluctant to have initiated statins in the first place, seemingly will themselves into an adverse reaction. In response, many patients report that their complaints of muscle aches after starting statin therapy are minimized by their health care providers, who often advise patients to "tough it out" and continue taking their statin.

In order to maximize the chance for patients to distinguish statin-related myalgias from everyday muscle pain, I always have a discussion with patients prior to beginning statin therapy. I ask them to make a mental note of muscle pains they experience from time to time and suggest that similar discomfort should not trigger alarm after beginning statin therapy. If a new pattern or increased severity of muscle discomfort should develop, this could be a warning sign of an adverse reaction and should be considered as a possible adverse reaction. Based on the severity of symptoms, I advise patients to either lower the dose or discontinue the statin.

Although psychological factors undoubtedly play a role in some patients with statin intolerance, there is a growing understanding of the biochemical basis for statin-related myalgias, including insights into genetic predisposition. A unique single nucleotide polymorphism has been associated with a

17-fold increase in the risk of statin-related myalgias (Link et al. 2008). A more complete understanding of genetic determinants of statin-related myalgias could allow for prediction of individuals best suited for lower dosages or alternative treatments.

In patients with statin intolerance, a search should be made for reversible factors that can predispose individuals to adverse reactions. Metabolic causes of statin intolerance include: 1) hypothyroidism, and 2) low vitamin D level. All patients with dyslipidemia should be screened for hypothyroidism, because it can be a contributing factor in the development of dyslipidemia, as well as lower the threshold for statin-related myalgias (Antons et al. 2006).

Low-circulating Vitamin D has also been implicated as a trigger for statin intolerance, with an association noted between statin-related myalgias and vitamin D 25 (OH) levels below 30 (Duell and Connor 2008) and 32 ng/ml (Ahmed et al. 2009). Furthermore, statin-related myalgias in patients with vitamin D deficiency may improve with vitamin D replacement therapy (Ahmed et al. 2009; Duell and Connor 2008).

Once metabolic impairments have been excluded, tolerance to prescription statins may be enhanced by changes in the method of statin administration. Variations in statin administration can include: choosing a different brand of statin; decreasing the daily dose; or decreasing the dosing frequency. Many patients intolerant of one or two brands of statins will have no problem with a different brand. There is a theoretical rationale for believing that the more lipid-soluble statins may have a lower risk of myalgias, but this relationship has not been proven. Regardless of the statin chosen, the use of the lowest possible dose will increase the likelihood of tolerance.

Some of the most potent statins can be given at even one-half or one-quarter of the lowest pill strength with upward titration as tolerated. For example, rosuvastatin at a dose of 1 mg, which is less than one-quarter of the lowest strength tablet available, has been shown to reduce LDL by 34 percent (Olsson et al. 2001). Appreciation of the potency of even extremely low statin dosages is enhanced by the knowledge that a 50 percent reduction in dosage would be expected to reduce LDL cholesterol lowering by only 7 percent (Roberts 1997).

In addition to using a different statin at a lower dose, lengthening the dosing interval may be useful. Significant LDL reduction has been noted with statin dosing frequencies ranging from one to three times a week (Gadarla, Kearns, and Thompson 2008; Mackie et al. 2007; Ruisinger et al. 2009). In the study of twice a week statin dosing, 40 patients previously intolerant of at least one statin were given rosuvastatin 5 or 10 mg (Gadarla, Kearns, and Thompson 2008). A 26 percent reduction in LDL cholesterol was observed over the 8-week study period. Over the 8-week study, 80 percent of patients were able to continue therapy without adverse reactions. Extending the dosing interval to once-a-week rosuvastatin at a mean dose of 10 mg led to a 23 percent reduction of LDL, with 74 percent of patients able to continue therapy throughout the 4-month study (Ruisinger et al. 2009).

If changes to the type, dosage, or frequency of administration of the prescription statin are not successful in avoiding adverse reactions, one might consider redirecting therapy to include nonprescription options including soluble fiber, sterols/stanols, and red yeast rice.

COENZYME Q10

Coenzyme Q10 is a fat-soluble substance involved in electron transport in the mitochondria during oxidative phosphorylation. Supplementing coenzyme Q10 in patients receiving statins has long been proposed as a treatment to reduce the risk of adverse reactions from statins. The relationship between coenzyme Q10 and adverse reactions from statins, however, is controversial. What is clear is that that the circulating level of coenzyme Q10 is reduced during therapy with statins (both prescription statins as well as red yeast rice) (Folkers et al. 1990). As coenzyme Q10 is required for cellular energy production, and since levels drop during therapy with statins, it can be logically concluded that coenzyme Q10 levels should be restored with exogenous supplements during statin treatment.

On the other side of the argument is that fact that the circulating level of coenzyme Q10 may not reflect the more important tissue level. Of note, reduction in the blood level of coenzyme Q 10 with statin therapy is largely due to the fact that up to 50 percent of circulating coenzyme Q 10 is contained in the LDL particle (Tomasetti et al. 1999). The role of coenzyme Q10 in statin-related myalgias is further obscured by inconsistency in the impact of statins on tissue levels, with one study showing no change in skeletal muscle levels of coenzyme Q10 (Laaksonen et al. 1996), in contrast to other data indicating as much as a 34 percent reduction in tissue levels (Paiva et al. 2005).

Two randomized clinical trials have evaluated the benefit of coenzyme Q10 on statin-related myalgias. In one study, patients were randomized to coenzyme Q10 (200 mg or placebo) and studied for 12 weeks during upward titration of simvastatin. No improvement in myalgias or tolerance of statins was observed in the group receiving coenzyme Q10 (Young et al. 2007). In the second study, after 30 days of treatment with coenzyme Q10 at 100 mg per day, the severity of muscle pain decreased by 40 percent (p <0.001) and the occurrence of pain interfering with daily activities decreased by 38 percent (p <0.02), with no improvement noted in the placebo group (Caso et al. 2007).

Therefore, although the rationale behind coenzyme Q10 appears sound, the clinical data regarding improvement of coenzyme Q10 on statin-related myalgias is conflicted. Nevertheless, the safety profile of coenzyme Q10 is excellent (Hathcock and Shao 2006). Based on available information, coenzyme Q10 doses in the range of 100 to 200 mg/day may be considered in an effort to reduce the risk of myalgias.

The role of coenzyme Q10 in cardiology extends beyond its use in patients treated with statins, to include patients with congestive heart failure (Molyneux et al. 2008) and hypertension (Rosenfeldt et al. 2007) as well. These areas are discussed in detail in the chapters on metabolic cardiology, congestive heart failure, and hypertension.

Strategies for Statin Intolerance

- Evaluate for hypothyroidism with TSH level.
- Evaluate for vitamin D deficiency with 25 (OH) level. Goal is > 30 ng/ml.
- Add Coenzyme Q10 200 mg per day.
- Switch to a low dose of an alternative statin (ie. rosuvastatin 1.25–2.5 mg, lovastatin 10 mg, simvastatin 10 mg, or atorvastatin 5 mg) or decrease the frequency of doses (ranging from every other day to once a week).
- Consider red yeast rice at 1200 to 2400 mg per day.
- Add plant sterols/stanols and soluble fiber for additional LDL lowering.

STRATEGIES FOR THE PATIENT UNWILLING TO TAKE PRESCRIPTION STATINS

For the patient who is philosophically opposed to the use of prescription cholesterol agents, several approaches may be helpful. Many individuals have an inordinate fear of the risk associated with statin medications and, on occasion, a discussion with the patient describing the actual, minor risk of adverse reactions may be helpful. Patients typically fear permanent damage to their liver, which, fortunately, is extremely rare. For example, in my 20 years of practice, I have not personally had a single patient experience severe or permanent liver damage related to cholesterol therapy.

Nevertheless, if patients adamantly refuse to use prescription cholesterol therapy, over-the-counter products may be considered. For such patients, the lowest risk (and lowest potency) option could include the addition of soluble fiber, as well as the plant stanols or sterols. This strategy could be expected to lower LDL cholesterol in the range of 10–20 percent. If additional LDL lowering is required, red yeast rice could be recommend. The combination of fiber, plant stanols, and red yeast rice may lower LDL cholesterol between 30 and 40 percent. If HDL cholesterol needs to be increased, over-the-counter niacin can be added.

Author's Recommendation

In my experience, most patients who initially express a desire to avoid prescription cholesterol medication are ultimately open to using prescription medication if initial therapy with diet, exercise, and over-the-counter supplements fail to achieve the desired goal. I believe that many of these patients are asking nothing more than to be listened to, and to have their preferences incorporated into the decision-making process.

Since cholesterol control is rarely required on an urgent basis, I see no reason not to make at least an initial attempt at therapy that is most congruent with the patient's belief system. For example, if a patient is adamant about trying a nonprescription approach even when I would prefer a more potent prescription treatment, I will often express my preference to the patient, but will typically accede to their wishes if strongly held. In this way, I believe that a true partnership is established that will keep the patient motivated to engage in a long-term relationship directed at maximizing opportunities for prevention.

If therapy using a nonprescription approach achieves the desired goals, the initial strategy can be considered a success. If not, I emphasize to my patients that I am goal oriented, and that I believe we should move on to a prescription treatment—often at a low dosage, if appropriate. I have found that most patients, despite their initial reluctance, will be inclined to proceed with a prescription approach once they feel they have been listened to and that nonprescription alternatives have been exhausted.

The Role of HDL

HDL cholesterol has several beneficial functions, including the "reverse transport" of LDL cholesterol out of the plaque, as well as potent antioxidant capabilities. Low levels of HDL are associated with increased risk of vascular disease. Interestingly, there are gender differences in normal HDL levels, with higher values expected in women. Normal values for men are 40–45 mg/dL and for women, 50–55 mg/dL. Consequently, HDL levels associated with increased risk are gender dependent: < 40 mg/dL for men and <50 mg/dL for women. Population studies show an increase in cardiovascular risk for individuals with low HDL, even if LDL is well controlled (deGoma, Leeper, and Heidenreich 2008).

Relative to our understanding of the benefits of treating LDL, the impact of HDL-raising therapy is lacking. One prospective HDL-raising trial, the VA–HIT study, demonstrated an approximately 2 percent lower cardiovascular risk for each 1 mg/dL increase in HDL (Robins et al. 2001). More studies are needed to determine the conditions and agents most likely to achieve clinical benefit from raising HDL.

In any effort to optimize HDL, the first strategy is to remove influences known to depress levels. Factors that decrease HDL include: smoking, high glycemic load diet, and the use of a wide range of medication including beta blockers and thiazide diuretics. When such medication is used in those with low HDL, consideration should be given to determine if acceptable substitutes are available.

Lifestyle measures are fundamental to raising HDL levels, with particular impact resulting from reducing glycemic load in the diet, weight loss, and aerobic exercise. Carbohydrate intake, especially that contained in high-glycemic-load food, stimulates a decrease in HDL, paired with an increase in triglycerides (Liu et al. 2001). Emphasizing low-glycemic-load food choices, as well as foods rich in monounsaturated fat, can be effective in raising HDL. Reducing the intake of foods such as bread, chips, rice, potatoes, and sweets and replacing them with fruit, vegetables, and nuts is a key strategy for raising HDL. These measures typically have the added benefit of weight loss, which also raises HDL (Dattilo and Kris-Etherton 1992).

Aerobic exercise can also be useful in raising HDL, but relatively high amounts are needed for significant improvement. Running for 45 minutes four days per week, covering 4.5 miles/session, was associated with a 4 mg/dL increase in HDL (Kraus et al. 2002). Although both intensity and duration of exercise influence the degree of HDL increase, the number of minutes per week of exercise appeared to be the strongest determinant of change in HDL. A metaanalysis suggests that the minimal energy expenditure to raise HDL is approximately 900 kcal, or 2 hours of exercise per week (Kodama et al. 2007). The mean increase in HDL observed with exercise was 2.5 mg/dL. A dose-response relationship was suggested with each additional 10 minutes of exercise per workout session associated with a 1.4 mg/dL increase in HDL. In this analysis, the total number of minutes exercised per week was more influential for raising HDL than the frequency or intensity of exercise.

Pharmacologic therapy for HDL includes alcohol, fibrates, niacin, and insulin-sensitizing agents. Alcohol intake is associated with up to a 55 percent reduced risk of myocardial infarction in those with the highest consumption of alcohol (three or more drinks per day) compared to those with less than one

Table 10.3. Strategies to Raise HDL

	HDL Increase
Niacin 2000 mg/day	10mg/dL
Low glycemic load diet	6 mg/dL
Alcohol: 1 glass wine/day	5 mg/dL
Pioglitazone	5 mg/dL
Aerobic exercise 3 hrs/week	4 mg/dL
Fibrates	4 mg/dL

alcoholic drink per month (Gaziano et al. 1993). Consumption of 1 glass of wine every one to two days would be expected to increase HDL by 3 mg/dL in men and 7 mg/dL in women (Gaziano et al. 1993).

Fibrates, including gemfibrozil and fenofibrate, raise HDL an average of 4 mg/dL, or 10 percent (Birjmohun et al. 2005). Niacin is the most potent agent available to raise HDL, at an average of 7 mg/dL, or 16 percent (Birjmohun et al. 2005). The increase in HDL associated with extended-release niacin (22 percent) and immediate release (23 percent) is greater than that observed with slow-release niacin (13 percent). As previously noted, "flush-free" or "no-flush" niacin are bound forms of niacin with minimal therapeutic efficacy. Therapies that target insulin resistance, especially the thiazolidinedione or TZD class of agents, are also effective at raising HDL (Deeg et al. 2007) Pioglitazone has been shown to increase HDL by approximately 5 percent, and rosiglitazone by approximately 2 percent (Deeg et al. 2007) Statins can raise HDL, but increases are more modest, generally in the range of 3–10 percent.

The Role of Triglycerides

Although historically controversial, it appears increasingly clear that elevated triglycerides are an independent risk factor for vascular disease. Interestingly, elevated levels are more closely linked to risk in women than in men (Hokanson and Austin 1996). An optimal level for both genders is <100 mg/dL. At a minimum, fasting levels should be < 150 mg/dL, with levels over 200 mg/dL considered to be significantly elevated. The mechanism of increased risk attributed to triglycerides is unclear but appears rooted, in part, to the predominance of small dense LDL associated with elevated triglycerides (Mudd et al. 2007).

The initial treatment of elevated triglycerides is to reduce the stimulus for triglyceride production from other medical conditions or medication. Obesity, impaired fasting glucose, diabetes, hypothyroidism, and liver disorders can contribute to elevated triglycerides. B-blockers, thiazides, oral contraceptives, hormone replacement therapy (oral but not topical), retrovirals and Accutane (isotretinoin) often lead to elevated triglycerides.

Similar to measures that favorably impact HDL, weight loss, adoption of a diet with low glycemic load (Liu et al. 2001; Pelkman 2001), and aerobic exercise are all helpful at lowering triglycerides. Of particular note, alcohol is one of the most potent stimulants for triglycerides; therefore, its use should be minimized when triglycerides are significantly elevated.

Prescription agents that lower triglycerides include statins (up to 25 percent reduction), fibrates (55 percent), niacin (35 percent), and fish oil (50 percent). These agents can be used as monotherapy for patients with isolated hypertriglyceridemia, or in combination with statins for those with mixed dyslipidemia.

FISH OIL

Fish oil has long been associated with cardiovascular health. It has potential beneficial antiinflammatory, anticoagulant, antihypertensive, and antiarrhythmic properties (Kris-Etherton, Harris, and Appel 2002; Maki et al. 2008). In addition, fish oil is an extremely effective therapy for reduction of triglycerides, but it is not particularly effective at raising HDL or lowering LDL. Nevertheless, fish oil is useful in favorably altering the type of LDL, assisting in the conversion of the more risky small, dense particles into the more desirable larger, buoyant forms (Maki et al. 2008).

Fish and fish oil have been shown to be protective against cardiac events, although the data is stronger for secondary than primary prevention. Benefit of fish for secondary prevention has been shown in the Diet and Reinfarction Trial (DART), in which men with prior MI who consumed 2–3 fish meals per week had a 29 percent reduction in all cause mortality, mostly due to a lower rate of coronary death (Burr et al. 1989). In the GISSI trial, post-MI patients were randomized to fish oil containing EPA 465 mg and DHA 375 mg (total EPA and DHA of 840 mg) or placebo, with the result of a 53 percent reduction in sudden cardiac death by 4 months in the group receiving fish (Marchioli et al. 2002).

The active ingredients in fish oil are EPA and DHA. Accordingly, recommendation for fish oil dosage should include a specific daily total of EPA and DHA, as opposed to the total content of omega-3. For prevention, the recommended daily total of EPA and DHA is 840 mg. For treatment of elevated triglycerides, a dose range between 1000 and 4000 mg of EPA and DHA per day may be helpful.

Over-the-counter products vary greatly in their concentration of EPA and DHA. Despite containing a total omega-3 content of 1000 mg, the total EPA and DHA per pill can range from 100 to 500 mg. Over-the-counter fish oil preparations can be excellent choices, as long as they provide the desired daily total of EPA and DHA. A prescription version of fish oil is also available, Lovaza™, which contains 840 mg of combined EPA and DHA per tablet, the exact content of the omega-3 used in the GISSI trial.

Vegetarians can find non-fish sources of DHA in pill form derived from algae. Flax seed and flax oil are alternative, but less efficient, sources of omega-3. Flax is rich in alpha linolenic acid but contains no DHA or EPA. Conversion of alpha-linolenic acid to the active DHA and EPA requires enzymes that function poorly in most individuals. Therefore, only approximately 5 percent of alpha-linolenic acid is converted into EPA, and less than 1 percent into DHA (Plourde and Cunnane 2007).

> *The active ingredients in fish oil are EPA and DHA. Accordingly, recommendation for fish oil dosage should include a specific daily total of EPA and DHA (typically listed on the back of the supplement bottle), as opposed to the total content of fish oil (listed on the front of the bottle). For prevention purposes, the recommended daily total of EPA and DHA is 840 mg. For treatment of elevated triglycerides, a range of 1000 to 4000 mg of EPA and DHA per day may be helpful.*

RISK FACTORS BEYOND LDL: LP(a)

Lp(a) is a glycoprotein that is produced in the liver by combining an LDL molecule with apo(a). Apo(a) is structurally similar to plasminogen, thereby acting as a molecular decoy in the coagulation cascade, promoting thrombosis. As expected, Lp(a), as a dual lipid and procoagulant molecule, has been strongly correlated with the development of coronary heart disease and stroke (Danesh, Collings, and Peto 2000; Schaefer et al. 1994).

Lp(a) exists in different sizes, with individual variations dictated by the number of repeating units, referred to as "kringles" in apo(a). Available immunologic assays target different portions of this molecule, with errors in measurement introduced by some assays that target the kringle repeat regions. The number of repeat regions also impacts atherogenic risk; those with fewer repeat units (smaller isoforms) are associated with higher risk (Emanuele et al. 2004; Kronenberg et al.1999).

Lp(a) can accompany elevated LDL-C or, alternatively, may be markedly elevated in the face of a desirable appearing standard lipid profile. Clinical situations where evaluation for Lp(a) may be especially relevant are those in which the patient has a personal or family history of premature atherosclerotic disease (Bostom et al. 1996; Genest et al. 1992). The risk of Lp(a) appears to be linked to the circulating level. Given a reference range of Lp(a) of < 30 mg/dL, adjusted risk increases from 1.7-fold for levels over 30 mg/dL, to 3.6-fold for levels in excess of 120 mg/dL (Kamstrup et al. 2008).

Lp(a) levels are not appreciably influenced by diet, exercise, or administration of statins. Niacin is the only agent in common use for treatment of dyslipidemia that reduces the level of Lp(a), up to 39% at dose of niacin 2,000 mg per day (Capuzzi et al. 1998). The highest risk of elevated Lp(a) levels appears to be in those with concomitant increased levels of LDL-C (Maher et al. 1995; Suk Danik 2006) and, therefore, another approach to treatment is to reduce LDL-C. To date, however, there has not been a prospective Lp(a) intervention study, and the optimal approach to treatment has not been identified. In high-risk individuals, some experts suggest intensive treatment of LDL-C (no data to guide how aggressive to be, but in practice, levels are often reduced to at least< 100 mg/dL, with more aggressive goals set by some to 60-80 mg/dL). A second approach is to treat Lp(a) itself with niacin in maximally tolerated doses up to 2,000 mg. The most aggressive treatment of Lp(a), again without supporting data, is to give a statin to lower LDL-C to a value between 60–80 mg/dL, in addition to a maximally tolerated dose of niacin up to 2,000 mg. An alternative approach, for those who refuse or do not tolerate prescription medication, includes the use of red yeast rice to lower LDL-C, combined with over-the-counter niacin.

RISK FACTORS BEYOND LDL: *hs-CRP*

The long-held view of coronary syndromes as evolving from a slow progression of gradual plaque buildup has been uprooted by the recognition of the role of inflammation in the development of atherosclerotic plaque. Active atherosclerotic disease appears to be closely related to the degree of local inflammatory cell infiltration, as well as circulating measures of inflammation. The best-studied of the circulating inflammatory markers is high sensitivity C-Reactive Protein (CRP). CRP is produced in the liver and by vascular smooth muscle. Incremental risk associated with elevated high sensitivity CRP has been shown to be in excess of 2-fold (Danesh et al. 2000), and is one of the strongest predictors of death from coronary disease, even after adjustment for

Framingham risk score (Boekholdt et al. 2006). A link exists between CRP and the metabolic syndrome, as the level of CRP rises incrementally with the number of criteria for metabolic syndrome—up to an increase of 6-fold for individuals with 5 criteria (Rutter et al. 2004).

Levels of high-sensitivity CRP associated with low risk are < 1 mg/L, neutral values between 1.0 and 3.0 mg/L, and elevated levels > 3 mg/L (Yeh and Willerson 2003).

Although there appears to be an association between high levels of CRP and the incidence of coronary disease, no studies have been performed to determine whether CRP reduction, as a goal of therapy, is associated with improved outcome. Nevertheless, it is interesting to note that lifestyle measures known to improve cardiovascular outcome also reduce CRP. Diet is one of the most potent interventions for reducing CRP, with a significant reduction accompanying weight loss(Selvin, Paynter, and Erlinger 2007). Other dietary measures associated with reduced CRP include: lower glycemic load diets (Liu et al. 2002), reduction in trans fats (Lopez-Garcia et al. 2005), and adoption of a Mediterranean-style diet(Church et al. 2002; Esposito et al. 2004). Aerobic exercise also leads to reduced markers of inflammation, regardless of body mass index (Church et al. 2002).

In addition to lifestyle changes, statins also have been known to dramatically decrease CRP, with reductions of 30–40 percent noted with both prescription statins (Ballantyne et al. 2003) as well as with red yeast rice (Li et al. 2005). Other agents that lower CRP include omega-3 fatty acids(Lopez-Garcia et al. 2004) and probiotics (Kekkonen et al. 2008).

RISK FACTORS BEYOND LDL: *HOMOCYSTEINE*

Homocysteine has long been linked to the development of atherosclerosis, with evidence suggesting an association of homocysteine with inflammation, thrombosis, and endothelial dysfunction. Levels exceeding 10 μmol/liter are associated with increased risk, with incrementally greater risk associated with higher levels (Wald, Law, and Morris 2002). Folic acid, vitamin B6, and vitamin B12 have all been demonstrated to lower homocysteine level. Therefore, homocysteine-lowering therapy with these nutrients has been studied to determine if treatment would reduce the risk of cardiovascular disease.

Large, randomized clinical trials in patients with vascular disease or diabetes have been conducted using high-dose folic acid, vitamin B6, and vitamin B12, with primary ends point of stroke reduction (Toole et al. 2004) and reduction of cardiovascular events in the HOPE-2 and NORVIT trials (Bonaa et al. 2006, Lonn et al. 2006). In each of these studies, combined multivitamin therapy was successful in lowering homocysteine levels but, paradoxically, no clinical benefit was observed, and the primary end points were not achieved. In fact, the NORVIT study of multivitamin therapy in patients with diabetes or vascular disease demonstrated a trend toward harm in the active treatment group. Of note, mean plasma homocysteine levels were not severely elevated at baseline in either the HOPE-2 or NORVIT trials (12.2 and 13.1 μmol/liter, respectively).

The failure of homocysteine reduction with folic acid, vitamin B6, and vitamin B12 for secondary prevention is puzzling. Explanations include the possibility that homocysteine is a marker rather than a trigger for atherosclerosis, as well as the possibility that high-dose multivitamin therapy may have adverse consequences that offset the benefits of homocysteine reduction. Folic acid stimulates cell proliferation and, perhaps, accelerates growth of constituents within the atherosclerotic plaque.

Much remains unknown about the role of homocysteine and its treatment. Unresolved issues include: the role of vitamin therapy to lower homocysteine levels for primary prevention; the preventive value of multivitamin therapy in selected patients with extremely high homocysteine levels; and the potential benefit of therapies other than folic acid, B6, and B12. Betaine (trimethylglycine) has been shown to reduce homocysteine (Schwab et al. 2002), but no outcomes data is available using this agent.

> *Elevated homocysteine is associated with increased cardiovascular risk, and multivitamin therapy with folic acid, B6, and B12 is effective at reducing levels. Nevertheless, no studies have demonstrated cardiovascular benefit from lowering homocysteine. Although there is no support for high-dose folic acid supplementation, increasing the intake of vegetables rich in folate is associated with remarkable cardiovascular protection.*

At the present time, my own practice is to advise most patients to take no more than 400 mcg of folic acid in supplements (typically this amount is contained in multivitamins) and to further increase folate intake through increased consumption of vegetables. Increased intake of green leafy vegetables, rich in folate, has been linked to reduced cardiovascular events, with each daily serving of green leafy vegetables associated with a 23 percent reduction in the risk of coronary heart disease (Joshipura et al. 2001). Exceptional patients, however, may require individualized assessment, including high-risk individuals with markedly elevated homocysteine levels.

RISK FACTORS BEYOND LDL: *LOW VITAMIN D*

There is mounting evidence that low levels of vitamin D contribute to cardio-vascular disease. Vitamin D receptors are found in both vascular smooth muscle and in the heart, where activation leads to favorable changes, including reduced secretion of rennin (Li et al. 2002), suppression of smooth muscle cell proliferation, and inhibition of cytokine release from lymphocytes(Rigby, Denome, and Fanger 1987).

Low vitamin D is associated with up-regulation of the renin-angiotensin system, and restoration of normal levels to individuals with low vitamin D by either nutritional supplementation or by UVB exposure has been shown to decrease blood pressure by 6 mmHg (Krause et al. 1998; Li 2003).

Vitamin D deficiency is also linked to insulin resistance and the metabolic syndrome, with supplementation of 800 IU per day shown to decreased the risk of type 2 diabetes by one-third (Pittas et al. 2006). Assuring normal Vitamin D levels in infancy may have profound implications for the future development of diabetes. A metaanalysis of five observational studies evaluating the impact of vitamin D supplementation in infancy demonstrated a 29 percent reduction in the development of type I diabetes in infants supplemented with vitamin D, compared to those who were not treated (Zipitis and Akobeng 2008).

Apart from increasing the incidence of atherosclerotic risk factors, mounting clinical evidence suggests an association between low vitamin D and increased likelihood of cardiovascular disease (Poole et al. 2006; Scragg et al. 1990). Initial observations were confirmed in a larger study of 1,739 individuals from the Framingham Offspring Study, in which a 25-OH vitamin D level <15 ng/ml was associated with a 62 percent increased risk of a cardiovascular event. This extremely low level of vitamin D is relatively common, with levels <15 ng/ml found in 28 percent of the study population (Wang et al. 2008). Increased risk was found primarily in hypertensive individuals, with a 2.1x hazard ratio in patients with both low Vitamin D and hypertension.

What is the optimal serum level of Vitamin D? Serum levels of 25(OH) D of > 30 ng/ml are considered ideal (Bischoff-Ferrari et al. 2006). Some experts suggest that even higher levels are best, but there is general agreement that a value of at least 30 ng/ml should be targeted. Epidemiologic data suggests that levels greater than 100 ng/ml are to be avoided, with levels exceeding 150 ng/ml associated with hypercalcemia. Among healthy young adults, the prevalence of vitamin D inadequacy is 36 percent, and rises to 41 percent in middle-age and older outpatients (Holick 2006). Factors associated with low vitamin D levels include: living in cold climates with decreased sun exposure; darkly pigmented skin; obesity; and advanced age. On average, levels in most individuals tent to be about one-third lower in the winter compared to the summer (Tangpricha et al. 2002).

How can Vitamin D levels be increased? The body's primary source of vitamin D is internal production stimulated by sun exposure. Exposure of arms and legs to midday sun for 5 to 30 minutes (depending on skin pigment, age, and geography) twice a week has been estimated to be sufficient to maintain healthy vitamin D levels (Holick 2007).

Dietary sources of vitamin D include fish and dairy products. Wild salmon is among the richest whole food dietary sources of vitamin D, with 360 IU per 3.5 oz serving. Cod liver oil contains 1,360 IU per tablespoon. Vitamin D-fortified skim milk has approximately 100 IU per cup (2009, Dietary Supplement Fact Sheet).

Beyond nutritional sources, supplemental vitamin D is often required to replenish severely depleted levels. Vitamin D can be administered by prescription in the form of vitamin D_2 50,000 IU pills, which are typically taken once every one to two weeks. Alternatively, over the counter vitamin D_3 can be prescribed in dosages of 1,000 to 5,0000 IU per day. Either strategy is effective, and vitamin D levels should be checked 2–3 months after beginning therapy.

Mind/Body Interventions

None. That is the amount of time dedicated in my cardiology training to the study of the impact of thoughts and emotions on heart health. No wonder that the bidirectional mind–body path remains one that few cardiologists travel. How could it be otherwise, when physicians have been trained to restrict attention to "objective" measures that lend themselves to diagnostic studies? Chest pain may be evaluated with a stress test or even an angiogram, then dismissed when no "objective" abnormalities are uncovered. The fact that the patient lost his job, is having a difficult personal relationship, or is feeling sad about his life situation is often lost in the analysis—yet may be the most critical element of the evaluation.

Studies are clear on this point: mental stress can induce the same demand on the heart as physical stress, often with severe consequences. A study of patients with established heart disease has demonstrated that mental anxiety can produce scintigraphic evidence of ischemia to a degree indistinguishable from that produced with exercise (Dimsdale 2008).

The mere act of a health care professional inquiring about, and acknowledging, the emotional state of the patient during the clinical encounter is healing.

An extreme manifestation of stress on the heart is a newly described syndrome of stress heart failure, or Takotsubo cardiomyopathy. This cardiac emergency is a condition in which the development of severe cardiac dysfunction is triggered by stress. Overdrive of the autonomic system leads to a curious pattern of left ventricular wall motion abnormalities in which the apical segments become akinetic with preserved function in basal regions. Cardiac dysfunction leads to shock and possibly death if not properly supported (Wittstein et al. 2005).

Interestingly, the antecedent stressors associated with this catastrophic cardiac condition are often less than dramatic, including stress related to: a class reunion; a surprise party; public speaking; or fear of a medical procedure (Wittstein et al. 2005). If these stressors, common to everyone's life experiences, are capable of evolving into a cardiac emergency, what other less dramatic manifestation of cardiac disease may be missed in our daily outpatient evaluations?

An integrative approach to prevention demands inquiry into emotional influences that can color, and possibly trigger, a wide range of cardiovascular conditions, including hypertension, lipid disorders, arrhythmias, angina, heart failure, and myocardial infarction. It is my belief that the mere act of a health care professional inquiring about, and acknowledging, the emotional state of the patient during the clinical encounter is healing. Moreover, emotional discovery is the critical step needed for the health care provider to initiate referral of patients for appropriate help when stress, anxiety, or depression becomes problematic.

Conventional options for referral of such patients include psychologists and psychiatrists—two outstanding choices. An integrative approach to mind–body interactions in cardiology, however, expands the options for healing. Additional options within the integrative framework include: Healing Touch; biofeedback; acupuncture; and Reiki. Matching the patient with the modality is much more of an art than a science, incorporating the severity of the condition, the patient's prior health care experience, personal preference, as well as local availability and expertise. It is my belief that the inquiry and open exploration is far more important than the particular modality chosen.

The critical area of emotional influences on the heart are more fully evaluated by John Longhurst in Chapter 6 (Acupuncture in Cardiovascular Medicine),by Mary Jo Kreitzer in Chapter 7 (Spirituality and Heart Health), by Kim R. Lebowitz in Chapter 8 (Cardiac Behavioral Medicine: Mind–Body Approaches to Heart Health), and by Rauni Prittinen King in Chapter 9 (Energy Medicine).

Conclusion

Most of us begin life with a healthy heart. As we enter middle age and beyond, heart disease becomes so common that we can mistakenly believe it is inevitable. To the contrary, heart disease is largely preventable. In this chapter, I have attempted to illustrate the many ways we can act to maintain heart health, including the use of strategies that are not often included in physician training. For example, the fact that nutritional therapy is one of the most powerful interventions in cardiology is a concept foreign to many. Or, that a mind–heart pathway, although largely out of view, can frighten us to death if provoked, or lower our blood pressure and relieve chest pain if soothed.

This chapter has explored a wide range of tools at our disposal for prevention of heart disease including exercise, nutrition, supplements, mind–body paths, and medication. The integrative practitioner seeks to expand the conventional view and to explore as many opportunities as possible to promote heart health.

REFERENCES

Ahmed, W., Khan, C. J. Glueck, S. Pandey, P. Wang, N. Goldenberg, M. Uppal, and S. Khanal. 2009. Low serum 25 OH vitamin D levels <32 ng/mL are associated with reversible myositis-myalgia in statin-treated patients. *Transl Re,* 153: 11–16.

Anderson, J. W., M. H. Davidson, L. Blonde, W. V. Brown, W. J., Howard, H. Ginsberg, L. D. Allgood, and K. W. Weingand. 2000. Long-term cholesterol-lowering effects of psyllium as an adjunct to diet therapy in the treatment of hypercholesterolemia. *Am J Clin Nutr* 71: 1433–38.

Anderson, J. W., B. M. Johnstone, and M. E. Cook-Newell. 1995. Meta-analysis of the effects of soy protein intake on serum lipids. *N Engl J Me,* 333: 276–82.

Antons, K. A., C. D. Williams, S. K. Baker, and P. S. Phillips. 2006. Clinical perspectives of statin-induced rhabdomyolysis. *Am J Med* 119: 400–09.

Ballantyne, C. M., J. Houri, A. Notarbartolo, L. Melani, L. J. Lipka, R. Suresh, S. Sun, A. P. Lebeaut, P. T. Sager, and E. P. Veltri. 2003. Effect of ezetimibe coadministered with atorvastatin in 628 patients with primary hypercholesterolemia: a prospective, randomized, double-blind trial. *Circulation* 107: 2409–15.

Barter, P. J., C. M. Ballantyne, R. Carmena, M. Castro Cabezas, M. J. Chapman, P. Couture, J. De Graaf, P. N. Durrington, O. Faergeman, J. Frohlich, C. D. Furberg,

C. Gagne, S. M. Haffner, S. E. Humphries, I. Jungner, R. M. Krauss, P. Kwiterovich, S. Marcovina, C. J. Packard, T. A. Pearson,K. S. Reddy, R. Rosenson, N. Sarrafzadegan, A. Sniderman, A. F. Stalenhoef, E. Stein, P. J. Talmud, A. M. Tonkin, G. Walldius, and K. M. Williams. 2006. Apo B versus cholesterol in estimating cardiovascular risk and in guiding therapy: report of the thirty-person/ ten-country panel. *J Intern Med* 259: 247–58.

Becker, D. J., R. Y. Gordon, S. C. Halbert, B. French, P. B. Morris, and D. J. Rader. 2009. Red yeast rice for dyslipidemia in statin-intolerant patients: a randomized trial. *Ann Intern Med* 150: 830–39, W147–49.

Becker, D. J., R. Y Gordon, P. B. Morris, J. Yorko, Y. J. Gordon, M. Li, and N. Iqbal. 2008. Simvastatin vs therapeutic lifestyle changes and supplements: randomized primary prevention trial. *Mayo Clin Proc* 83: 758–64.

Birjmohun, R. S., B. A. Hutten, J. J. Kastelein, and E. S. Stroes. 2005. Efficacy and safety of high-density lipoprotein cholesterol-increasing compounds: a meta-analysis of randomized controlled trials. *J Am Coll Cardiol* 45: 185–97.

Bischoff-Ferrari, H. A., E. Giovannucci, W. C. Willett, T. Dietrich, and B. Dawson-Hughes. 2006. Estimation of optimal serum concentrations of 25-hydroxyvitamin D for multiple health outcomes. *Am J Clin Nutr* 84: 18–28.

Blair, S. N., D. M. Capuzzi, S. O. Gottlieb, T. Nguyen, J. M. Morgan, and N. B. Cater. 2000. Incremental reduction of serum total cholesterol and low-density lipoprotein cholesterol with the addition of plant stanol ester-containing spread to statin therapy. *Am J Cardiol* 86: 46–52.

Boekholdt, S. M., C. E. Hack, M. S. Sandhu, R. Luben, S. A. Bingham, N. J. Wareham, R. J. Peters, J. W. Jukema, N. E. Day, J. J. Kastelein, and K. T. Khaw. 2006. C-reactive protein levels and coronary artery disease incidence and mortality in apparently healthy men and women: the EPIC-Norfolk prospective population study 1993-2003. *Atherosclerosis* 187: 415–22.

Bonaa, K. H., I. Njolstad, P. M. Ueland, H. Schirmer, A. Tverdal, T. Steigen, H. Wang, J. E. Nordrehaug, E. Arnesen, and K. Rasmussen, K. 2006. Homocysteine lowering and cardiovascular events after acute myocardial infarction. *N Engl J Med* 354: 1578–88.

Bostom, A. G., L. A. Cupples, J. L. Jenner, J. M. Ordovas, L. J. Seman, P. W. Wilson, E. J. Schaefer, and W. P. Castelli. 1996. Elevated plasma lipoproteina and coronary heart disease in men aged 55 years and younger. A prospective study. *JAMA* 276: 544–48.

Braith, R. W., and K. J. Stewart. 2006. Resistance exercise training: its role in the prevention of cardiovascular disease. *Circulation* 113: 2642–50.

Brown, B. G., X. Q. Zhao, A. Chait, L. D. Fisher, M. C. Cheung, J. S. Morse, A. A. Dowdy, E. K. Marino, E. L. Bolson, P. Alaupovic, J. Frohlich, and J. J. Albers. 2001. Simvastatin and niacin, antioxidant vitamins, or the combination for the prevention of coronary disease. *N Engl J Med* 345: 1583–92.

Brown, L., B. Rosner, W. W. Willett, and F. M. Sacks. 1999. Cholesterol-lowering effects of dietary fiber: a meta-analysis. *Am J Clin Nutr* 69: 30–42.

Burr, M. L., A. M. Fehily, J. F. Gilbert, S. Rogers, R. M. Holliday, P. M. Sweetnam, P. C., Elwood, and N. M. Deadman. 1989. Effects of changes in fat, fish, and fibre intakes on death and myocardial reinfarction: diet and reinfarction trial DART. *Lancet* 2: 757–61.

Canner, P. L., K. G Berge, N. K. Wenger, J. Stamler, L. Friedman, R. J. Prineas, and W. Friedewald. 1986. Fifteen year mortality in Coronary Drug Project patients: long-term benefit with niacin. *J Am Coll Cardiol* 8: 1245–55.

Capuzzi, D. M., J. R. Guyton, J. M. Morgan, A. C. Goldberg, R. A. Kreisberg, O. Brusco, and J. Brody. 1998. Efficacy and safety of an extended-release niacin Niaspan: a long-term study. *Am J Cardiol* 82: 74U–81U; discussion 85U–86U.

Caso, G., P. Kelly, M. A. Mcnurlan, and W. E. Lawson. 2007. Effect of coenzyme q10 on myopathic symptoms in patients treated with statins. *Am J Cardiol* 99: 1409–12.

Church, T. S., C. E. Barlow, C. P. Earnest, J. B. Kampert, E. L. Priest, and S. N. Blair. 2002. Associations between cardiorespiratory fitness and C-reactive protein in men. *Arterioscler Thromb Vasc Biol* 22: 1869–76.

Contois, J. H., J. P. Mcconnell, A. A. Sethi, G. Csako, S. Devaraj, D. M. Hoefner, and G. R. Warnick. 2009. Apolipoprotein B and cardiovascular disease risk: position statement from the AACC Lipoproteins and vascular diseases division working group on best practices. *Clin Chem* 55: 407–19.

Danesh, J., R. Collins, and R. Peto. 2000. Lipoproteina and coronary heart disease. Meta-analysis of prospective studies. *Circulation* 102: 1082–85.

Danesh, J., P. Whincup, M. Walker, L. Lennon, A. Thomson, P. Appleby, J. R. Gallimore, and M. B. Pepys. 2000. Low grade inflammation and coronary heart disease: prospective study and updated meta-analyses. *BMJ* 321: 199–204.

Dattilo, A. M., and P. M. Kris-Etherton. 1992. Effects of weight reduction on blood lipids and lipoproteins: a meta-analysis. *Am J Clin Nutr* 56: 320–28.

De Lorgeril, M., S. Renaud, N. Mamelle, P. Salen, J. L. Martin, I. Monjaud, J. Guidollet, P. Touboul, and J. Delaye. 1994. Mediterranean alpha-linolenic acid-rich diet in secondary prevention of coronary heart disease. *Lancet* 343: 1454–59.

Deeg, M. A., J. B. Buse, R. B. Goldberg, D. M. Kendall, A. J. Zagar, S. J. Jacober, M. A. Khan, A. T. Perez, and M. H. Tan. 2007. Pioglitazone and rosiglitazone have different effects on serum lipoprotein particle concentrations and sizes in patients with type 2 diabetes and dyslipidemia. *Diabetes Care* 30: 2458–64.

Degoma, E. M., N. J. Leeper, and P. A. Heidenreich. 2008. Clinical significance of high-density lipoprotein cholesterol in patients with low low-density lipoprotein cholesterol. *J Am Coll Cardiol* 51: 49–55.

Delorgeril, M. 1999. Mediterranean diet, traditional risk factors, and the rate of cardiovascular complications after myocardial infarction: final report of the Lyon diet heart study. *Circulation* 99: 779–85.

Dietary Supplement Fact Sheet: Vitamin D. Office of Dietary Supplements, NIH Clinical Center, National Institutes of Health. 2009 Available at: http://ods.od.nih.gov/Health_Information/VitaminD_Fact_Sheet_Options.aspx Accessed May 29, (2010).

Dimsdale, J. E. 2008. Psychological stress and cardiovascular disease. *J Am Coll Cardiol* 51: 1237–46.

Duell, P. B., and W. E. Connor. 2008. Vitamin D deficiency is associated with myalgias in hyperlipidemic subjects taking statins. *Circulation* 118: S470.

Dulin, M. F., L. F. Hatcher, H. C. Sasser, and T. A. Barringer. 2006. Policosanol is ineffective in the treatment of hypercholesterolemia: a randomized controlled trial. *Am J Clin Nutr* 84: 1543–48.

Emanuele, E., E. Peros, P. Minoretti, A. D'angelo, L. Montagna, C. Falcone, and D. Geroldi. 2004. Significance of apolipoproteina phenotypes in acute coronary syndromes: relation with clinical presentation. *Clin Chim Acta* 350: 159–65.

Erdman, J. W., Jr. 2000. AHA Science Advisory: Soy protein and cardiovascular disease: A statement for healthcare professionals from the Nutrition Committee of the AHA. *Circulation* 102: 2555–59.

Esposito, K., R. Marfella, M. Ciotola, C. Di Palo, F. Giugliano, G. Giugliano, M. D'armiento, F. D'andrea, and D. Giugliano. 2004. Effect of a mediterranean-style diet on endothelial dysfunction and markers of vascular inflammation in the metabolic syndrome: a randomized trial. *JAMA* 292: 1440–46.

Folkers, K., P. Langsjoen, R. Willis, P. Richardson, L. J. Xia, C. Q. Ye, and H. Tamagawa. 1990. Lovastatin decreases coenzyme Q levels in humans. *Proc Natl Acad Sci U S A* 87: 8931–34.

Gadarla, M., A. K. Kearns, and P. D. Thompson. 2008. Efficacy of rosuvastatin 5 mg and 10 mg twice a week in patients intolerant to daily statins. *Am J Cardiol* 101: 1747–48.

Gallus, S., C. Bosetti, and C. La Vecchia. 2004. Mediterranean diet and cancer risk. *Eur J Cancer Prev* 13: 447–52.

Gaziano, J. M., J. E. Buring, J. L. Breslow, S. Z. Goldhaber, B. Rosner, M. Vandenburgh, W. Willett, and C. H. Hennekens. 1993. Moderate alcohol intake, increased levels of high-density lipoprotein and its subfractions, and decreased risk of myocardial infarction. *N Engl J Med* 329: 1829–34.

Genest, J. J., Jr., S. S. Martin-Munley, J. R. Mcnamara, J. M. Ordovas, J. Jenner, R. H. Myers, S. R. Silberman, P. W. Wilson, D. N. Salem, and E. J. Schaefer. 1992. Familial lipoprotein disorders in patients with premature coronary artery disease. *Circulation* 85: 2025–33.

Gibbons, R. J., G. J. Balady, J. T. Bricker, B. R. Chaitman, G. F. Fletcher, V. F. Froelicher, D. B. Mark, B. D. Mccallister, A. N. Mooss, M. G. O'Reilly, W. L. Winters, Jr., E. M. Antman, J. S. Alpert, D. P. Faxon, V. Fuster, G. Gregoratos, L. F. Hiratzka, A. K. Jacobs, R. O. Russell, and S. C. Smith, Jr. 2002. ACC/AHA (2002) guideline update for exercise testing: Summary article: A report of the American College of Cardiology/American Heart Association Task Force on Practice Guidelines Committee to Update the (1997) Exercise Testing Guidelines. *Circulation* 106: 1883–92.

Giugliano, D., A. Ceriello, and K. Esposit. 2006. The effects of diet on inflammation: Emphasis on the metabolic syndrome. *J Am Coll Cardiol* 48: 677–85.

Gordon, R., W. Obermeyer, T. Cooperman, and D. Becker. 2009. Marked variability of monacolin and citrinin content of 12 readily available red yeast rice formulations. *J Am Coll Cardiol* 53: A198.

Grundy, S. M., J. I. Cleeman, C. N. Merz, H. B. Brewer, Jr., L. T. Clark, D. B. Hunninghake, R. C. Pasternak, S. C. Smith, Jr., and N. J. Stone. 2004. Implications of recent clinical trials for the National Cholesterol Education Program Adult Treatment Panel III guidelines. *Circulation* 110: 227–39.

Hambrecht, R.,A. Wolf, S. Gielen, A. Linke, J. Hofer, S. Erbs, N. Schoene, and G. Schuler. 2000. Effect of exercise on coronary endothelial function in patients with coronary artery disease. *N Engl J Med* 342: 454–60.

Hathcock, J. N. and A. Shao. 2006. Risk assessment for coenzyme Q10 Ubiquinone. *Regul Toxicol Pharmacol* 45: 282–88.

Heber, D., I. Yip, J. M. Ashley, D. A. Elashoff, R. M. Elashoff, and V. L. Go. 1999. Cholesterol-lowering effects of a proprietary Chinese red-yeast-rice dietary supplement. *Am J Clin Nutr* 69: 231–36.

Hokanson, J. E., and M. A. Austin. 1996. Plasma triglyceride level is a risk factor for cardiovascular disease independent of high-density lipoprotein cholesterol level: a meta-analysis of population-based prospective studies. *J Cardiovasc Risk* 3: 213–19.

Holick, M. F. 2006. High prevalence of vitamin D inadequacy and implications for health. *Mayo Clin Proc* 81: 353–73.

Holick, M. F. 2007. Vitamin D deficiency. *N Engl J Med* 357: 266–81.

Hsia, J., J. D. Otvos, J. E. Rossouw, L. Wu, S. Wassertheil-Smoller, S. L. Hendrix, J. G. Robinson, B. Lund, and L. H. Kuller. 2008. Lipoprotein particle concentrations may explain the absence of coronary protection in the women's health initiative hormone trials. *Arterioscler Thromb Vasc Biol* 28: 1666–71.

Hu, F. B., and W. C. Willett. 2002. Optimal diets for prevention of coronary heart disease. *JAMA* 288: 2569–78.

Jenkins, D. J., C. W. Kendall, A. Marchie, D. A. Faulkner, J. Wong, R. De Souza, A. Emam, T. L. Parker, E. Vidgen, K. G. Lapsley, E. A. Trautwein, R. G. Josse, L. A. Leiter, and P. W. Connelly. 2003. Effects of a dietary portfolio of cholesterol-lowering foods vs lovastatin on serum lipids and C-reactive protein. *JAMA* 290: 502–10.

Joshipura, K. J., F. B. Hu, J. E. Manson, M. J. Stampfer, E. B. Rimm, F. E. Speizer, G. Colditz, A. Ascherio, B. Rosner, D. Spiegelman, and W. C. Willett. 2001. The effect of fruit and vegetable intake on risk for coronary heart disease. *Ann Intern Med* 134: 1106–14.

Kamstrup, P. R., M. Benn, A. Tybaerg-Hansen, and B. G. Nordestgaard. 2008. Extreme lipoproteina levels and risk of myocardial infarction in the general population: The Copenhagen City Heart Study. *Circulation* 117: 176–84.

Kekkonen, R. A., N. Lummela, H. Karjalainen, S. Latvala, S. Tynkkynen, S. Jarvenpaa, H. Kautiainen, I. Julkunen, H. Vapaatalo, and R. Korpela. 2008. Probiotic intervention has strain-specific antiinflammatory effects in healthy adults. *World J Gastroenterol* 14: 2029–36.

Khoo, Y. S., and Z. Aziz. 2009. Garlic supplementation and serum cholesterol: A meta-analysis. *J Clin Pharm Ther* 34: 133–45.

Kodama, S., S. Tanaka, K. Saito, M. Shu, Y. Sone, F. Onitake, E. Suzuki, H. Shimano, S. Yamamoto, K. Kondo, Y. Ohashi, N. Yamada, and H. Sone. 2007. Effect of aerobic exercise training on serum levels of high-density lipoprotein cholesterol: A meta-analysis. *Arch Intern Med* 167: 999–1008.

Kraus, W. E., J. A. Houmard, B. D. Duscha, K. J. Knetzger, M. B. Wharton, J. S. Mccartney, C. W. Bales, S. Henes, G. P. Samsa, J. D. Otvos, K. R. Kulkarni, and C. A. Slentz. 2002. Effects of the amount and intensity of exercise on plasma lipoproteins. *N Engl J Med* 347: 1483–92.

Krause, R., M. Buhring, W. Hopfenmuller, M. F. Holick, and A. M. Sharma. 1998. Ultraviolet B and blood pressure. *Lancet* 352: 709–10.

Kris-Etherton, P. M., W. S. Harris, and L. J. Appel. 2002. Fish consumption, fish oil, omega-3 fatty acids, and cardiovascular disease. *Circulation* 106: 2747–57.

Kronenberg, F., M. F. Kronenberg, S. Kiechl, E. Trenkwalder, P. Santer, F. Oberhollenzer, G. Egger, G. Utermann, and J. Willeit. 1999. Role of lipoproteina and apolipoproteina phenotype in atherogenesis: prospective results from the Bruneck study. *Circulation* 100: 1154–60.

Laaksonen, R., K. L. Jokelainen, J. Laakso, T. Sahi, M. Harkonen, M. J. Tikkanen, and J. J. Himberg. 1996. The effect of simvastatin treatment on natural antioxidants in low-density lipoproteins and high-energy phosphates and ubiquinone in skeletal muscle. *Am J Cardiol* 77: 851–54.

Lee, I. M., and P. J. Skerrett. 2001. Physical activity and all-cause mortality: what is the dose-response relation? *Med Sci Sports Exerc* 33: S459–71; discussion S493–94.

Li, J. J., S. S. Hu, C. H. Fang, R. T. Hui, L. F. Miao, Y. J. Yang, and R. L. Gao. 2005. Effects of xuezhikang, an extract of cholestin, on lipid profile and C-reactive protein: a short-term time course study in patients with stable angina. *Clin Chim Acta* 352: 217–24.

Li, Y. C. 2003. Vitamin D regulation of the renin-angiotensin system. *J Cell Biochem* 88: 327–31.

Li, Y. C., J. Kong, M. Wei, Z. F. Chen, S. Q. Liu, and L. P. Cao. 2002. 1,25-Dihydroxyvitamin D3 is a negative endocrine regulator of the renin-angiotensin system. *J Clin Invest* 110: 229–38.

Lin, C. C., T. C. Li, and M. M. Lai. 2005. Efficacy and safety of Monascus purpureus Went rice in subjects with hyperlipidemia. *Eur J Endocrinol* 153: 679–86.

Link, E., S. Parish, J. Armitage, L. Bowman, S. Heath, F. Matsuda, I. Gut, M. Lathrop, and R. Collins. 2008. SLCO1B1 variants and statin-induced myopathy A genomewide study. *N Engl J Med* 359: 789–99.

Liu, S., J. E. Manson, J. E. Buring, M. J. Stampfer, W. C. Willett, and P. M. Ridker. 2002. Relation between a diet with a high glycemic load and plasma concentrations of high-sensitivity C-reactive protein in middle-aged women. *Am J Clin Nutr* 75: 492–98.

Liu, S., J. E. Manson, M. J. Stampfer, M. D. Holmes, F. B. Hu, S. E. Hankinson, and W. C. Willett. 2001. Dietary glycemic load assessed by food-frequency questionnaire in relation to plasma high-density-lipoprotein cholesterol and fasting plasma triacylglycerols in postmenopausal women. *Am J Clin Nutr* 73: 560–66.

Lonn, E., S. Yusuf, M. J. Arnold, P. Sheridan, J. Pogue, M. Micks, M. J. Mcqueen, J. Probstfield, G. Fodor, C. Held, and J. Genest, Jr. 2006. Homocysteine lowering with folic acid and B vitamins in vascular disease. *N Engl J Med* 354: 1567–77.

Lopez-Garcia, E., M. B. Schulze, J. E. Manson, J. B. Meigs, C. M. Albert, N. Rifai, W. C. Willett, and F. B. Hu. 2004. Consumption of n-3 fatty acids is related to plasma biomarkers of inflammation and endothelial activation in women. *J Nutr* 134: 1806–11.

Lopez-Garcia, E., M. B. Schulze, J. B. Meigs, J. E. Manson, N. Rifai, M. J. Stampfer, W. C. Willett, and F. B. Hu. 2005. Consumption of trans fatty acids is related to plasma biomarkers of inflammation and endothelial dysfunction. *J Nutr* 135,: 562–66.

Lu, Z., W. Kou, B. Du, Y. Wu, S. Zhao, O. A. Brusco, J. M. Morgan, D. M. Capuzzi, and S. Li. 2008. Effect of Xuezhikang, an extract from red yeast Chinese rice, on coronary events in a Chinese population with previous myocardial infarction. *Am J Cardiol* 101: 1689–93.

Mackie, B. D., S. Satija, C. Nell, J. Miller, III, and L. S. Sperling. 2007. Monday, Wednesday, and Friday dosing of rosuvastatin in patients previously intolerant to statin therapy. *Am J Cardiol* 99: 291.

Maher, V. M., B. G. Brown, S. M. Marcovina, L. A. Hillger, X. Q. Zhao, and J. J. Albers. 1995. Effects of lowering elevated LDL cholesterol on the cardiovascular risk of lipoproteina. *JAMA* 274: 1771–74.

Maki, K. C., J. M. McKenney, M. S. Reeves, B. C. Lubin, and M. R. Dicklin. 2008. Effects of adding prescription omega-3 acid ethyl esters to simvastatin 20 mg/day on lipids and lipoprotein particles in men and women with mixed dyslipidemia. *Am J Cardiol* 102: 429–33.

Manson, J. E., P. Greenland, A. Z. Lacroix, M. L. Stefanick, C. P. Mouton, A. Oberman, M. G. Perri, D. S. Sheps, M. B. Pettinger, and D. S. Siscovick. 2002. Walking compared with vigorous exercise for the prevention of cardiovascular events in women. *N Engl J Med* 347: 716–25.

Marchioli, R., F. Barzi, E. Bomba, C. Chieffo, D. Di Gregorio, R. Di Mascio, M. G. Franzosi, E. Geraci, G. Levantesi, A. P. Maggioni, L. Mantini, R. M. Marfisi, G. Mastrogiuseppe, N. Mininni, G. L. Nicolosi, M. Santini, C. Schweiger, L. Tavazzi, G. Tognoni, C. Tucci, and F. Valagussa. 2002. Early protection against sudden death by n-3 polyunsaturated fatty acids after myocardial infarction: time-course analysis of the results of the Gruppo Italiano per lo Studio della Sopravvivenza nell'Infarto Miocardico GISSI-Prevenzione. *Circulation* 105: 1897–903.

Mensink, R. P., S. Ebbing, M. Lindhout, J. Plat, and M. M. Van Heugten. 2002. Effects of plant stanol esters supplied in low-fat yoghurt on serum lipids and lipoproteins, non-cholesterol sterols and fat soluble antioxidant concentrations. *Atherosclerosis:* 160: 205–13.

Meyers, C. D., M. C. Carr, S. Park, and J. D. Brunzell. 2003. Varying cost and free nicotinic acid content in over-the-counter niacin preparations for dyslipidemia. *Ann Intern Med* 139: 996–1002.

Michalsen, A., N. Lehmann, C. Pithan, N. T. Knoblauch, S. Moebus, F. Kannenberg, L. Binder, T. Budde, and G. J. Dobos. 2006. Mediterranean diet has no effect on markers of inflammation and metabolic risk factors in patients with coronary artery disease. *Eur J Clin Nutr* 60: 478–85.

Miettinen, T. A., P. Puska, H. Gylling, H. Vanhanen, and E. Vartiainen. 1995. Reduction of serum cholesterol with sitostanol-ester margarine in a mildly hypercholesterolemic population. *N Engl J Med* 333: 1308–12.

Mitrou, P. N., V. Kipnis, A. C. Thiebaut, J. Reedy, A. F. Subar, E. Wirfalt, A. Flood, T. Mouw, A. R. Hollenbeck, M. F. Leitzmann, and A. Schatzkin. 2007. Mediterranean dietary pattern and prediction of all-cause mortality in a US population: results from the NIH–AARP Diet and Health Study. *Arch Intern Med* 167: 2461–68.

Molyneux, S. L., C. M. Florkowski, P. M. George, A. P. Pilbrow, C. M. Frampton, M. Lever, and A. M. Richards. 2008. Coenzyme Q10: an independent predictor of mortality in chronic heart failure. *J Am Coll Cardiol* 52: 1435–41.

Mudd, J. O., B. A. Borlaug, P. V. Johnston, B. G. Kral, R. Rouf, R. S. Blumenthal, and P. O. Kwiterovich, Jr. 2007. Beyond low-density lipoprotein cholesterol: defining the role of low-density lipoprotein heterogeneity in coronary artery disease. *J Am Coll Cardiol* 50: 1735–41.

Olsson, A. G., J. Pears, J. Mckellar, J. Mizan, and A. Raza. 2001. Effect of rosuvastatin on low-density lipoprotein cholesterol in patients with hypercholesterolemia. *Am J Cardiol* 88: 504–08.

Packard, C. J., and Y. Saito. 2004. Non-HDL cholesterol as a measure of atherosclerotic risk. *J Atheroscler Thromb* 11: 6–14.

Paiva, H., K. M. Thelen, R. Van Coster, J. Smet, B. De Paepe, K. M. Mattila, J. Laakso, T. Lehtimaki, K. Von Bergmann, D. Lutjohann, and R. Laaksonen. 2005. High-dose statins and skeletal muscle metabolism in humans: A randomized, controlled trial. *Clin Pharmacol Ther* 78: 60–68.

Pearson, T. A., S. N. Blair, S. R. Daniels, R. H. Eckel, J. M. Fair, S. P. Fortmann, B. A. Franklin, L. B. Goldstein, P. Greenland, S. M. Grundy, Y. Hong, N. H. Miller, R. M. Lauer, I. S. Ockene, R. L. Sacco, J. F. Sallis, Jr., S. C. Smith, Jr., N. J. Stone, and K. A. Taubert. 2002. AHA Guidelines for primary prevention of cardiovascular disease and stroke: (2002) Update: Consensus panel guide to comprehensive risk reduction for adult patients without coronary or other atherosclerotic vascular diseases. American Heart Association Science Advisory and Coordinating Committee. *Circulation* 106: 388–91.

Pelkman, C. L. 2001. Effects of the glycemic index of foods on serum concentrations of high-density lipoprotein cholesterol and triglycerides. *Curr Atheroscler Rep* 3: 456–61.

Phillips, P. S., R. H. Haas, S. Bannykh, S. Hathaway, N. L. Gray, B. J. Kimura, G. D. Vladutiu, and J. D. England. 2002. Statin-associated myopathy with normal creatine kinase levels. *Ann Intern Med* 137: 581–85.

Pittas, A. G., B. Dawson-Hughes, T., Li, R. M. Van Dam, W. C. Willett, J. E. Manson, and F. B. Hu. 2006. Vitamin D and calcium intake in relation to type 2 diabetes in women. *Diabetes Care* 29: 650–56.

Plat, J., E. N. Van Onselen, M. M. Van Heugten, and R. P. Mensink. 2000. Effects on serum lipids, lipoproteins and fat soluble antioxidant concentrations of consumption frequency of margarines and shortenings enriched with plant stanol esters. *Eur J Clin Nutr* 54: 671–77.

Plourde, M., and S. C. Cunnane. 2007. Extremely limited synthesis of long chain poly-unsaturates in adults: implications for their dietary essentiality and use as supplements. *Appl Physiol Nutr Metab* 32: 619–34.

Poole, K. E., N. Loveridge, P. J. Barker, D. J. Halsall, C. Rose, J. Reeve, and E. A. Warburton. 2006. Reduced vitamin D in acute stroke. *Stroke* 37: 243–45.

Rigby, W. F., S. Denome, and M. W. Fanger. 1987. Regulation of lymphokine production and human T lymphocyte activation by 1,25-dihydroxyvitamin D3. Specific inhibition at the level of messenger RNA. *J Clin Invest* 79: 1659–64.

Roberts, W. C. 1997. The rule of 5 and the rule of 7 in lipid-lowering by statin drugs. *Am J Cardiol* 80: 106–07.

Robins, S. J., D. Collins, J. T. Wittes, V. Papademetriou, P. C. Deedwania, E. J. Schaefer, J. R. Mcnamara, M. L. Kashyap, J. M. Hershman, L. F. Wexler, and H. B. Rubins. 2001. Relation of gemfibrozil treatment and lipid levels with major coronary events: VA-HIT: A randomized controlled trial. *JAMA* 285: 1585–91.

Rosenfeldt, F. L., S. J. Haas, H. Krum, A. Hadj, K. Ng, J. Y. Leong, and G. F. Watts. 2007. Coenzyme Q10 in the treatment of hypertension: a meta-analysis of the clinical trials. *J Hum Hypertens* 21: 297–306.

Ruisinger, J. F., J. M. Backes, C. A. Gibson, and P. M. Moriarty. 2009. Once-a-week rosuvastatin 2.5 to 20 mg in patients with a previous statin intolerance. *Am J Cardiol* 103: 393–94.

Rutter, M. K., J. B. Meigs, L. M. Sullivan, R. B. D'Agostino, Sr., and P. W. Wilson. 2004. C-reactive protein, the metabolic syndrome, and prediction of cardiovascular events in the Framingham Offspring Study. *Circulation* 110: 380–85.

Scarmeas, N., J. A. Luchsinger, N. Schupf, A. M. Brickman, S. Cosentino, M. X. Tang, and Y. Stern. 2009. Physical activity, diet, and risk of Alzheimer disease. *JAMA* 302: 627–37.

Schaefer, E. J., S. Lamon-Fava, J. L. Jenner, J. R. Mcnamara, J. M. Ordovas, C. E. Davis, J. M. Abolafia, K. Lippel, and R. I. Levy. 1994. Lipoproteina levels and risk of coronary heart disease in men. The lipid research clinics coronary primary prevention trial. *JAMA* 271: 999–1003.

Schwab, U., A. Torronen, L. Toppinen, G. Alfthan, M. Saarinen, A. Aro, and M. Uusitupa. 2002. Betaine supplementation decreases plasma homocysteine concentrations but does not affect body weight, body composition, or resting energy expenditure in human subjects. *Am J Clin Nutr* 76: 961–67.

Scragg, R., R. Jackson, I. M. Holdaway, T. Lim, and R. Beaglehole. 1990. Myocardial infarction is inversely associated with plasma 25-hydroxyvitamin D3 levels: A community-based study. *Int J Epidemiol* 19: 559–63.

Selvin, E., N. P. Paynter, and T. P. Erlinger,. 2007. The effect of weight loss on C-reactive protein: a systematic review. *Arch Intern Med* 167: 31–39.

Shai, I., D. Schwarzfuchs, Y. Henkin, D. R. Shahar, S. Witkow, I. Greenberg, R. Golan, D. Fraser, A. Bolotin, H. Vardi, O. Tangi-Rozental, R. Zuk-Ramot, B. Sarusi, D. Brickner, Z. Schwartz, E. Sheiner, R. Marko, E. Katorza, J. Thiery, G. M. Fiedler, M. Bluher, M. Stumvoll, and M. J. Stampfer. 2008. Weight loss with a low-carbohydrate, Mediterranean, or low-fat diet. *N Engl J Med* 359: 229–41.

Simopoulos, A. P., and F. Visioli. 2000. *Mediterranean diets.* Basel and New York: Karger.

Singh, R. B., G. Dubnov, M. A. Niaz, S. Ghosh, R. Singh, S. S. Rastogi, O. Manor, D. Pella, and E. M. Berry. 2002. Effect of an Indo-Mediterranean diet on progression of coronary artery disease in high risk patients Indo-Mediterranean Diet Heart Study: A randomised single-blind trial. *Lancet* 360: 1455–61.

Siscovick, D. S., N. S. Weiss, R. H. Fletcher, and T. Lasky. 1984. The incidence of primary cardiac arrest during vigorous exercise. *N Engl J Med* 311: 874–77.

Sniderman, A. D. 2005. Apolipoprotein B versus non-high-density lipoprotein cholesterol: And the winner is. *Circulation* 112: 3366–67.

Sofi, F., F. Cesari, R. Abbate, G. F. Gensini, and A. Casini. 2008. Adherence to Mediterranean diet and health status: Meta-analysis. *BMJ* 337: a1344.

Suk Danik, J. 2006. Lipoproteina, Measured with an assay independent of apolipoproteina isoform size, and risk of future cardiovascular events among initially healthy women. *JAMA* 296: 1363–70.

Szapary, P. O., M. L. Wolfe, L. T. Bloedon, A. J. Cucchiara, A. H. Dermarderosian, M. D. Cirigliano, and D. J. Rader. 2003. Guggulipid for the treatment of hypercholesterolemia: A randomized controlled trial. *JAMA* 290: 765–72.

Tanasescu, M., M. F. Leitzmann, E. B. Rimm, W. C. Willett, M. J. Stampfer, and F. B. Hu. 2002. Exercise type and intensity in relation to coronary heart disease in men. *JAMA* 288: 1994–2000.

Tangpricha, V., E. N. Pearce, T. C. Chen, and M. F. Holick. 2002. Vitamin D insufficiency among free-living healthy young adults. *Am J Med* 112: 659–62.

Tomasetti, M., R. Alleva, M. D. Solenghi, and G. P. Littarru. 1999. Distribution of antioxidants among blood components and lipoproteins: Significance of lipids/CoQ10 ratio as a possible marker of increased risk for atherosclerosis. *Biofactors* 9: 231–40.

Toole, J. F., M. R. Malinow, L. E. Chambless, J. D. Spence, L. C. Pettigrew, V. J. Howard, E. G. Sides, C. H. Wang, and M. Stampfer. 2004. Lowering homocysteine in patients with ischemic stroke to prevent recurrent stroke, myocardial infarction, and death: The Vitamin Intervention for Stroke Prevention VISP randomized controlled trial. *JAMA* 291: 565–75.

Tribble, D. L., L. G. Holl, P. D. Wood, and R. M. Krauss. 1992. Variations in oxidative susceptibility among six low density lipoprotein subfractions of differing density and particle size. *Atherosclerosis* 93: 189–99.

Wald, D. S., M. Law, and J. K. Morris. 2002. Homocysteine and cardiovascular disease: Evidence on causality from a meta-analysis. *BMJ* 325: 1202.

Wang, T. J., M. J. Pencina, S. L. Booth, P. F. Jacques, E. Ingelsson, K. Lanier, E. J. Benjamin, R. B. D'Agostino, M. Wolf, and R. S. Vasan. 2008. Vitamin D deficiency and risk of cardiovascular disease. *Circulation* 117: 503–11.

Weggemans, R. M., and E. A. Trautwein. 2003. Relation between soy-associated isoflavones and LDL and HDL cholesterol concentrations in humans: A meta-analysis. *Eur J Clin Nutr* 57: 940–46.

Wittstein, I. S., D. R. Thiemann, J. A. Lima, K. L. Baughman, S. P. Schulman, G. Gerstenblith, K. C. Wu, J. J. Rade, T. J. Bivalacqua, and H. C. Champion. 2005. Neurohumoral features of myocardial stunning due to sudden emotional stress. *N Engl J Med* 352: 539–48.

Yeh, E. T., and J. T. Willerson. 2003. Coming of age of C-reactive protein: Using inflammation markers in cardiology. *Circulation* 107: 370–71.

Young, J. M., C. M. Florkowski, S. L. Molyneux, R. G. Mcewan, C. M. Frampton, P. M. George, and R. S. Scott. 2007. Effect of coenzyme Q10 supplementation on simvastatin-induced myalgia. *Am J Cardiol* 100: 1400–03.

Zipitis, C. S., and A. K. Akobeng. 2008. Vitamin D supplementation in early childhood and risk of type 1 diabetes: A systematic review and meta-analysis. *Arch Dis Child* 93: 512–17.

11

The Integrative Approach to Hypertension

STEPHEN T. SINATRA AND MARK C. HOUSTON

KEY CONCEPTS

- Oxidative stress initiates and propagates hypertension and cardiovascular disease.
- Nutrition can prevent, control, and treat hypertension through numerous vascular biology mechanisms.
- There is a role for the selected use of nutritional supplements in the management of hypertension.
- Exercise and weight reduction are integral components of a blood pressure treatment program.
- Mind–body therapies are powerful tools for management of blood pressure, yet they are often ignored by the mainstream medical profession.

■

Introduction

Optimal nutrition, exercise, weight management, nutraceutical supplements, and management of emotional stress, can prevent, delay the onset of, and treat hypertension in many patients. An integrative approach combining these lifestyle suggestions with pharmacologic treatment will best achieve blood pressure goals, and reduce the likelihood of cardiovascular complications.

Epidemiology

Hypertension has become a global public health challenge afflicting approximately one billion individuals worldwide, with the prevalence of hypertension having increased dramatically in developing countries in recent years (Chobanian et al. 2003; Gu et al. 2002; Kearney et al. 2005). The consequence is that hypertension results in a seven-fold increased risk of developing stroke, triple the risk for coronary heart disease, a six-fold risk of developing congestive heart failure, and an alarming increase in end-stage renal disease (Iseki et al. 2000). Fortunately, the treatment of moderate to severe hypertension has resulted in decreased rates of stroke and myocardial infarction (Neaton et al. 1993; Whelton et al. 2002).

THE ROLE OF OXIDATIVE STRESS

Oxidative stress (an imbalance of harmful oxygen species and the antioxidant defense mechanism) may contribute to the etiology of human hypertension (Kitiyakara and Wilco 1998; Nayak et al. 2001; Vaziri, Liang, and Ding 1999). Hypertensive patients have a high level of oxidative stress and a greater than normal response to oxidative stress (Lacy, O'Connor, and Schmid-Schonbein 1998). In addition, hypertensive patients have an impaired endogenous and exogenous antioxidant defense mechanism (Kumar and Das 1993; Russo et al. 1998).

An imbalance of vasodilators (such as nitric oxide), vasoconstrictors (such as angiotension), and radical oxygen species contribute to the initiation and perpetuation of hypertension (McIntyre, Bohr, and Dominiczak 1999).

STAGED THERAPY OF HYPERTENSION

Patients with blood pressure below 140/90 mmHg who have no risk factors, target organ disease, or clinical cardiovascular disease may be initially successfully treated with lifestyle modifications alone. As many as 50 to 60 percent of essential hypertensive patients are included in this classification (Houston 1992). Those with more significant hypertension or with end- organ disease will often require a combination treatment of lifestyle modifications and drugs.

When antihypertensive medication is needed, lifestyle changes potentiate the effects of antihypertensive drugs, often permitting fewer drugs and/or lower doses to be used (Houston 1992; Houston, Meador, and Schipani 2000). In order to obtain optimal results and to keep the patient actively involved in their care, lifestyle modifications should always be continued following initiation of drug therapy (Houston 1992; Houston, Meador, and Schipani 2000).

Role of Prescription Medication

Although a complete discussion of possible pharmacologic therapy for hypertension is beyond the scope of this chapter, a brief overview is provided, to emphasize the importance of balance and integration when treating hypertension.

Lifestyle recommendations are the first-line treatment for high blood pressure, but some patients must take prescription medication, especially those whose hearts or lives are compromised, and those who are resistant to making the lifestyle modifications needed. Blood pressure prescription drugs are strongly recommended:

1. When a patient's blood pressure is more than mildly elevated and immediate action must be taken.
2. When lifestyle modification, weight loss, and exercise have been unsuccessful or have failed to achieve blood pressure goals.
3. When a patient has evidence of end-organ dysfunction, especially kidney disease.

Although antihypertensive drugs are effective, the chronic use of these drugs can cause side effects including impotence, loss of libido, fatigue, drowsiness, dry cough, lightheadedness and depression. For example, diuretics—one of the oldest and most commonly used antihypertensives—can cause muscle cramping, fatigue, weakness, impotence, type 2 diabetes mellitus, and renal insufficiency.

Several years ago, a report in the *Journal of the American Medical Association* noted that properly prescribed medications in a hospital is the fourth leading cause of death in the United States (Lazaron, Pomeranz, and Corey 1998). At that time, over 100,000 inpatient deaths were attributed to adverse reactions to, or drug interactions with, prescription medication.

Even over-the-counter medications can be dangerous. A report from the Harvard School of Medicine's ongoing Nurses' Health Study concluded that women are at increased risk for high blood pressure if they take daily doses of non-aspirin painkillers, including acetaminophen and over-the-counter nonsteroidal antiinflammatory agents (Forman, Stampfer, and Curhan 2005).

The Integrative Approach

Patients diagnosed with hypertension frequently leave their physician's office with prescriptions, and perhaps some advice to lose weight and cut back on consumption of salt and fat. Although this is a good start, a better recommendation incorporates an integrative strategy including nutrition, targeted nutritional supplementation, exercise as well as weight management, and mind–body strategies. Such a structured protocol leads to effective blood pressure lowering and can eventually reduce—and in some cases eliminate—the need for pharmaceutical drugs.

The Role of Nutrition

Humans have evolved away from pre-agricultural, hunter–gatherer traditions toward a commercial agriculture and food industry which produces highly processed foods that impart unnatural and unhealthy nutrition. The human genetic makeup is 99.9 percent that of our Paleolithic ancestors, who date back 35,000 years, yet our nutrition is vastly different (Eaton, Eaton, and Konner 1997). The macronutrient and micronutrient variations contribute to the higher incidence of hypertension and other cardiovascular diseases through a complex nutrient–gene interaction.

The optimal combination of macronutrients and micronutrients significantly impacts on vascular health. The landmark study "Dietary Approaches to Stop Hypertension (DASH)" clearly demonstrated in 1997 that patients who eat more fruits and vegetables and who switch to low-fat dairy foods are able to lower their systolic blood pressure by an average of 11.4 points, and their diastolic pressure by 5.5 points (Appel et al. 1997). This reduction is on par with that observed with many antihypertensive medications. Moreover, the DASH participants achieved these gains without losing weight or cutting back on sodium—two of the most effective non-medical tools for blood pressure lowering.

The average sodium intake in the U.S. is 5,000 mg per day, with people living in some areas of the country consuming 15,000–20,000 mg per day (Warner 2000). However, the necessary amount of sodium is probably only about 500 mg per day (Warner 2000). Epidemiologic, observational, and controlled clinical trials demonstrate that an increased sodium intake is associated with higher blood pressure (Kotchen and McCarron 1998). A reduction in sodium intake in hypertensive patients, especially the salt-sensitive patients, will significantly lower blood pressure by an average of 4–6 mmHg systolic and 2-3 mmHg diastolic (Sacks et al. 2001). The blood pressure reduction is proportional to the severity of sodium restriction (Sacks et al. 2001).

The effect of dietary sodium on blood pressure is modulated by other components of the diet. Sodium chloride-induced hypertension is augmented by diets low in potassium (Hamet et al. 1992), calcium, and magnesium (Hamet et al. 1992; Kotchen and Kotchen 1997) and attenuated by high potassium, magnesium, and calcium (especially Na^+ sensitive). The DASH-II diet is particularly instructive in this regard (Sacks et al. 2001). Gradual reductions in sodium from 150 mmol to 100 mmol to 50 mmol per day in association with a high intake of fruits and vegetables, and intake of low-fat dairy products, with adequate potassium, calcium, magnesium and fiber intake, was the most effective in reducing blood pressure.

The average adult consumes the equivalent of nearly two teaspoons of salt a day—nearly twice the upper limit for good health. The majority of that excess salt is hidden in processed foods such as canned spaghetti sauces, dill pickles, packaged soups, salty nuts, crackers, and sauerkraut as well as fast foods.

MAGNESIUM (MG^{++})

A high dietary intake of magnesium of at least 500–1,000 mg per day reduces blood pressure in most of the reported epidemiologic, observational, and clinical trials, but the results are less consistent than those seen with Na^+ and K^+ (Kotchen and McCarron 1998; Warner 2000). In most epidemiologic studies, there is an inverse relationship between dietary magnesium intake and blood pressure (Kotchen and McCarron 1998).

PROTEIN

Observational and epidemiologic studies demonstrate a consistent association between a high protein intake and a reduction in blood pressure (BP) (Obarzanek, Velletri, and Cutler 1996). The source of that protein is an important factor in the BP effect, animal protein being less effective than non-animal protein for blood pressure lowering (Elliot et al. 2000).

The INTERSALT Study (Stamler et al. 1996) supported the hypothesis that higher dietary protein intake has favorable influences on blood pressure. In 10,020 men and women in 32 countries worldwide, the average systolic blood pressure (SBP) and diastolic blood pressure (DBP) were 3.0 mmHg and 2.5 mmHg lower, respectively, for those whose dietary protein intake was

30 percent above the overall mean than for those 30 percent below the overall mean (81 grams/day versus 44 grams/day).

Soy protein at intakes of 25 to 30 grams/day lowers blood pressure and increases arterial compliance. Soy contains many active compounds that produce these antihypertensive effects, including isoflavones, amino acids, saponins, phytic acid, trypsin inhibitors, fiber, and globulins (Hasler CM, Kundrat S, Wool D 2000).

Sardine muscle protein, which contains Valyl-Tyrosine (VAL-TYR), significantly lowers blood pressure in hypertensive subjects (Kawasaki et al. 2000). Kawasaki et al. (2000) treated 29 hypertensive subjects with 3 mg of Valyl-Tyrosine sardine muscle concentrated extract for four weeks, and lowered BP 9.7 mmHg/5.3 mmHg (p < 0.05). Valyl-Tyrosine is a natural angiotensin converting enzyme inhibitor (ACEI). The antihypertensive effect of sardine may also be due to its high concentration of both calcium and CoQ10.

OMEGA-3 FATTY ACIDS

Alpha-linolenic acid (ALA), eicosapentaenoic acid (EPA), and docosahexanoic acid (DHA) comprise the primary members of the omega-3 PUFA family. Omega-3 fatty acids are found in cold-water fish (herring, haddock, salmon, trout, tuna, cod, and mackerel), fish oils, flax, flax seed, flax oil, and nuts (Warner 2000). Omega-3s stimulate the production of nitric oxide, which relaxes vascular smooth muscle and counteracts the impairment of nitric oxide production caused by atherosclerotic plaques (Braunwald E 1994). Omega-3 fatty acids also attenuate the vasopressor effects of angiotensin 2 and norepinephrine that affect blood pressure (Lorenz et al. 1983). Omega-3 PUFA was found to significantly lower blood pressure in observational, epidemiologic, and in some small prospective clinical trials through a variety of mechanisms (Lorenz et al. 1983; Mori et al. 1999a; Mori et al. 1999b; Warner 2000).

Mori et al. (1999b) studied sixty-three hypertensive, hyperlipidemic subjects treated with omega-3 PUFA, at 3.65 grams/day for sixteen weeks, and found significant reductions in blood pressure (P < 0.01). An average systolic reduction was 5 mmHg. Studies indicate that DHA is more effective in reducing blood pressure and heart rate than EPA supplementation, possibly due to greater improvement of DHA on endothelial function (Mori et al. 1999a; Mori et al. 2000).

Eating cold-water fish three times per week is as effective as high-dose fish oil in reducing blood pressure in hypertensive patients, and the protein in the fish may also have antihypertensive effects (Warner 2000).

Plant sources of omega-3 are metabolized to EPA and DHA, but this conversion is jeopardized in the presence of increased intake of omega-6 fatty acids, saturated and trans fats, alcohol, and aging via inhibitory effects on delta desaturase enzymes.

OMEGA-9 FATTY ACIDS

Olive oil is rich in monounsaturated fats (MUFA) predominantly containing omega 9 fatty acids, which have been associated with blood pressure and lipid reduction in Mediterranean and other diets (Warner 2000). Ferrara and colleagues (2000) studied 23 hypertensive subjects in a double-blind, randomized, crossover study for six months comparing MUFA with PUFA. Extra virgin olive oil (a MUFA) was compared to sunflower oil (a PUFA), abundant in linoleic acid (W-6 FA). The SBP fell 8 mmHg ($p < 0.05$) and the DBP fell 6 mmHg ($p < 0.01$) in the MUFA-treated subjects, compared to the PUFA-treated subjects. In addition, the need for antihypertensive medications was reduced by 48 percent in the MUFA group, versus 4 percent in the PUFA (omega-6 FA) group ($p < 0.005$).

FIBER

The clinical trials with various types of fiber to reduce blood pressure have been generally favorable, but inconsistent. Soluble fiber, guar gum, guava, psyllium, and oat bran lower blood pressure and possibly reduce the need for antihypertensive treatments (Pereira and Pins 2000; Vuksan et al. 1999). Vuskan and colleagues (1999) reduced SBP 9.4 mmHg in hypertensive subjects with the fiber glucomannan. The doses required to achieve these BP reductions are approximately 60 grams of oatmeal (slightly more than one-quarter cup) per day, 40 grams of oat bran (dry weight) per day, or 7 grams a day of psyllium (Stamler et al. 1996).

GARLIC AND ONIONS

Garlic is an outstanding antiinflammatory and antimicrobial agent with a long history of use in traditional folk medicine. A review of eleven studies in which hypertensive patients were randomly given garlic or placebo found that garlic can lower blood pressure as effectively as some pharmaceutical drugs (Ried et al. 2008).

On average, the metaanalysis demonstrated blood pressure reductions of 8 mmHg systolic, and 7 mm diastolic. The higher a patient's blood pressure was at baseline, the more it was reduced with garlic. Dosages taken by the subjects in the studies ranged from 600 to 900 mg over a period of 3 to 6 months. There is a consistent dose-dependent reduction in BP with garlic mediated through the RAAS (renin angiotensin aldosterone system) and the nitric oxide system (Mohamadi et al. 2000)·

Approximately 10,000 mcg of allicin per day (the amount contained in four cloves of garlic, or four grams) is required to achieve a significant blood pressure lowering effect (McMahon and Vargas 1993; Warner 2000). Garlic is probably a natural Angiotensin converting enzyme inhibitor (ACEI) that increases BK and NO-inducing vasodilation, reducing SVR and BP and improving vascular compliance.

Because they are in the same family as garlic, it is no surprise that onions have similar effects. Onions, like garlic, contain sulfur and powerful flavonoids, quercetin being the major health-promoting flavonoid of onions.

NATTO

Natto is a traditional fermented vegetable, a cheese-like food that is a staple in Japan.

Previous studies have shown that consumption of natto enhances the fibrinolytic system while suppressing thrombosis and intimal thickening (Kim et al. 2008; Pais et al. 2006). It also lowers blood pressure by inhibiting plasma renin activity (Kim et al. 2008).

SEAWEED

Another medicinal food in the Asian diet is wakame seaweed. Wakame (undaria pinnatifida) is the most popular edible seaweed in Japan (Suetsuna and Nakano 2000). In humans, 3.3 grams of dried wakame for four weeks significantly reduced both the SBP 14 + 3 mmHg and the DBP 5 + 2 mmHg (p < 0.01) (Nakano et al. 1998). The primary effect of wakame appears to be through its ACEI (Suetsuna and Nakano 2000).

CELERY

Consuming four sticks of celery or eight teaspoons of celery juice three times daily, or the equivalent in the form of extract of celery seed (1,000 mg twice a day) or oil (one-half to one teaspoon three times daily in tincture form) seems to provide an antihypertensive effect in human essential hypertension (Le and Elliot 1991; Duke 2001).

The Role of Nutritional Supplements

While the diet discussed earlier in this chapter can significantly lower blood pressure, it is difficult for most patients to consistently adhere to a prescribed diet. Complementing the diet with targeted nutritional supports may further support blood pressure lowering.

B VITAMINS

Vitamin B-6 is a readily metabolized and excreted water-soluble vitamin. Six different B-6 vitamins exist, but pyridoxal 5' phosphate (PLP) is the primary and most potent active form. A clinical study by Aybak et al. (1995) demonstrated that high-dose vitamin B-6 significantly lowered blood pressure. This study compared nine normotensive men and women with 20 hypertensive subjects, all of whom had significantly higher blood pressure, plasma NE, and HR compared to control normotensive subjects. Subjects received 5 mg/kg/day of vitamin B-6 for four weeks. The SBP fell from 167 ± 13 mmHg to 153 ± 15 mmHg, an 8.4% reduction ($p < 0.01$), and the DBP fell from 108 ± 8.2 mmHg to 98 ± 8.8 mmHg, a 9.3% reduction ($p < 0.005$).

VITAMIN D

Low levels of vitamin D have been linked to the development of high blood pressure. In a 2008 case-controlled study involving 1,484 women between the ages of 32 and 52, plasma levels of vitamin D were found to be lower among women who developed hypertension. The authors concluded that vitamin D levels are inversely and independently associated with the risk of developing hypertension (Forman, Curhan, and Taylor 2008).

In a group of 148 women with low vitamin D levels, the administration of 1,200 mg calcium, plus 800 IU of vitamin D_3 reduced SBP 9.3 percent more ($p < 0.02$), compared to 1,200 mg of calcium alone. The HR fell 5.4 percent ($p = 0.02$), but DBP was not changed (Pfeifer et al. 2001).

VITAMIN C

Vitamin C, a potent water-soluble antioxidant, not only regenerates tocopherol and supports endothelial cell function; it also enhances the body's total antioxidant system by raising levels of glutathione, a polypeptide amino acid and potent free radical scavenger. The dietary intake of vitamin C or plasma ascorbate concentration in humans is inversely correlated to SBP, DBP, and heart rate (Duffy et al. 1999).

Duffy et al. (1999) evaluated 39 hypertensive subjects (DBP 90 mmHg to 110 mmHg) in a placebo-controlled, four-week study. A 2,000-mg loading dose of vitamin C was given initially, followed by 500 mg per day. The SBP was reduced 11 mmHg (p = 0.03), DBP decreased by 6 mmHg (p = 0.24), and MAP fell 10 mmHg (p < 0.02).

COENZYME Q10 (UBIQUINONE)

Coenzyme Q10 is an essential component of the mitochondrial respiratory chain, and has important functions in oxidative phosphorylation and ATP production. It is a potent lipid phase antioxidant, free radical scavenger, cofactor, and coenzyme in mitochondrial energy production that lowers systemic vascular resistance and blood pressure (Cooke 1998; Digiesi et al. 1994; Langsjoen and Langsjoen 1999; Warner 2000).

In its reduced form, coenzyme Q10 protects membrane phospholipids and serum LDL from lipid peroxidation. It safeguards mitochondrial membrane proteins and DNA from free radical-induced oxidative damage (Digiesi et al. 1994; Langsjoen and Langsjoen 1999).

Coenzyme Q10 is commonly found predominantly in animal protein. Sardines, wild Alaskan salmon, mackerel, and organ meats such as beef heart and chicken liver are excellent sources. Serum levels of CoQ10 decrease with age and are lower in patients with diseases characterized by oxidative stress such as hypertension, CHD, hyperlipidemia, diabetes mellitus, and atherosclerosis. Enzymatic assays showed a deficiency of CoQ10 in 39 percent of 59 patients with essential hypertension, versus only 6 percent deficiency in controls (p < 0.01) (Digiesi, Cantini, and Brodbeck 1990).

Studies have also demonstrated significant and consistent reductions in blood pressure in hypertensive subjects following oral administration of 100 mg to 225 mg per day of CoQ10 (Burke, Neustenschwander, and Olson 2001; Digiesi, Cantini, and Brodbeck 1990; Langsjoen and Langsjoen 1999).

Burke, Neustenschwander, and Olson (2001) conducted a 12-week, randomized, double-blind, placebo-controlled trial with 60 mg of oral CoQ10 in 76 subjects with isolated systolic hypertension. The mean reduction in SBP in the treated group was 17.8 ± 7.3 mmHg (p < 0.01), but DBP did not change. Only 55 percent of the subjects were responders achieving a reduction in SBP ≥ 4 mmHg, but in this group the SBP fell 25.9 ± 6.4 mmHg. There was a trend between SBP reduction and increase in CoQ10 levels. Adverse effects were virtually nonexistent.

CoQ10 has consistent and significant antihypertensive effects in patients with essential hypertension. The major conclusions from in vitro, animal, and human clinical trials indicate the following:

1. The bioavailability and delivery of CoQ10 are important considerations when measuring blood levels (Chopra et al. 1998).
2. Compared to normotensive patients, essential hypertensive patients have a high incidence of CoQ10 deficiency documented by serum levels.
3. Doses of 120 to 300 mg per day of CoQ10, depending on the delivery method and concomitant ingestion with a fatty meal, are necessary to achieve a therapeutic level of over 2 ug/ml. This dose is usually 1–2 mg/kg/day of CoQ10. Use of a special delivery system allows better absorption and lower oral doses. Sicker and more compromised patients often require larger doses (2–4 mgs/kg/day of CoQ10).
4. Patients with the lowest CoQ10 serum levels may have the best antihypertensive response to supplementation.
5. The average reduction in SBP is about 15/10 mm Hg based on reported studies.
6. CoQ10's favorable impact on blood pressure may be attributed to its role in reducing oxidative stress in blood vessel tissue, which, in turn, lowers resistance in the blood vessel.
7. The antihypertensive effect takes time to reach its peak level, usually at about four weeks; after that blood pressure remains stable. The antihypertensive effect is gone within two weeks after discontinuation of CoQ10.
8. Some patients with mild hypertension treated with prescription medication who start coenzyme Q10 may be able to lower the dosage of medication, or possibly eliminate the need for its use.
9. Even high doses (>600 mg/daily) of CoQ10 have no acute or chronic adverse effects.

HAWTHORN

Hawthorn, a term encompassing many Crataegus species, is traditionally considered a tonic for the cardiovascular system. Crataegus extract appears to have multiple antioxidant properties that can inhibit the formation of thromboxane A2, a potent inflammatory mediator (Vibes et al. 1994).

Hawthorn exerts a mild hypotensive effect by lowering total peripheral resistance (Schussler, Holzl, and Fricke 1995). Doses of 1000 to 1500 mg per day have been used with success.

The Role of Exercise

Physical activity has many positive attributes, including supporting the maintainance of a healthy weight, as diet alone cannot take and keep weight off in most cases. Only diet and physical activity together can achieve that. Research shows that a minimum amount of some form of activity—a mere 30 minutes a day of walking, for instance—yields major protective benefits. Walking burns approximately 100 calories per mile, and since it is perhaps the safest form of exercise, it must be considered as a key component in any hypertensive management program. Exercise not only helps to lower blood pressure through vasodilatory effects, but it also helps reduce weight and decrease insulin resistance.

A review of the "neurobiology" of exercise (Dishman et al. 2006) demonstrated that regular exercise positively influences brain and nervous system function. Psychological and emotional stress, especially when they cause heightened arousal of the sympathetic nervous system, are major considerations in the hypertensive syndrome.

The Role of Mind–Body Approaches

Mental stress contributes to hypertension through a sustained increase in sympathetic nervous activity. Chronic emotional stress has been linked to psychological and cognitive dysfunction (Rozanski A, Blumenthal JA, Kaplan J 1999) resulting from dysregulation of the hypothalamic-pituitary-adrenal (HPA) network and sympathoadrenal system (Rozanski, Blumenthal, and Kaplan 1999; Tsigos and Chrousos 2002). Undesirable, dysfunctional affective states increase the risk of both hypertension and cardiovascular disease (Todaro et al. 2003).

For example, intense emotional grief and profound sadness can lead to hypertension (Prigerson et al. 1997; Santić et al. 2006). Researchers looked at hypertension in family members of soldiers killed in the 1992–1995 war in Bosnia and Herzegovina. The study involved 1,144 subjects who experienced a loss and compared them to 582 of their close neighbors who did not. Blood pressure was recorded in 1996 and again in 2003. At the time of both readings, the results revealed a significantly higher prevalence of hypertension in the loss group, which the researchers attributed to the psychological stress of mourning—even though more than seven years had passed since their family members had been killed.

Another study related to grief as a predictor of future physical and mental health problems was conducted in 1997 at the University of Pittsburgh School of Medicine. Researchers interviewed 150 women and men with terminally ill spouses. They were first interviewed at the time of their spouses' hospital admission and then again after 6 weeks, 6 months, 13 months, and 25 months. The researchers found that the presence of traumatic grief symptoms at the 6-month mark predicted not only high blood pressure at the 13- and 25-month interviews, but also other negative health outcomes, such as cancer, heart trouble, suicidal thoughts, and unhealthy eating habits. Assessing grief is of critical importance in determining which bereaved individuals will be at higher risk for long-term dysfunction (Prigerson et al. 1997).

Such chronic emotional and psychological stress, or lack of control over one's environment, triggers the pituitary release of ACTH (adrenocorticotropic hormone) (Jezova and Duncko 2002). ACTH catalyzes the release of catecholamines—epinephrine (adrenalin) and norepinephrine (noradrenaline)—into the bloodstream.

The sustained release of these catecholamines, increases cardiac output and systemic vascular resistance, and disrupts the equilibrium between the sympathetic and parasympathetic nervous systems (Goldstein 1995). Hypertension, then, may be viewed as a form of chronic sympathetic overdrive. As people with a compromised autonomic nervous system often exhibit blood pressure problems, it follows that balancing the ANS may be an adjunct to blood pressure and stress management.

Manipulating sympathetic nervous activity through mind–body relaxation techniques helps to assuage emotional stress. Relaxation techniques, such as Transcendental Meditation (TM), Tai Chi, and yoga, help lower sympathetic medullary activity, as well as train the body and mind to adapt to stress (Jacobs 2001). Yoga, TM, and Tai Chi are optimal long-term methods of reducing blood pressure, as they may be regularly practiced anywhere as either group or individual activities.

All relaxation responses involve reduced stress hormones and central nervous system activity, measurable through changes in brain wave activity.

TRANSCENDENTAL MEDITATION (TM)

The Transcendental Meditation program, or TM as it is popularly called, has been the focus of more than 600 scientific studies around the world, including nine randomized controlled trials in patients with hypertension or high blood pressure. Anderson, Liu, and Kryscio (2008) at the University of Kentucky conducted a systematic review and metaanalysis on these randomized trials, which met strict entry criteria for experimental quality. The random-effects metaanalysis model for systolic and diastolic blood pressure, respectively, indicated that TM, compared to control, achieved clinically significant reductions in blood pressure. The results showed the following changes: systolic −4.7 mmHg (−7.4 to −1.9 mm) and diastolic −3.2 mmHg (95% CI −5.4 to −1.3 mmHg). The duration of studies ranged from 8 to 52 weeks, with a median length of 15 weeks.

In 1987, Orme-Johnson reported on a study of health insurance statistics in more than 2,000 individuals practicing the TM program over a 5-year period. He found that those who meditated consistently had less than half the number of hospitalizations and doctor visits than did other groups with comparable age, gender, profession, and insurance terms. There were 87 percent fewer hospitalizations for heart disease (Orme-Johnson 1987).

TM was brought to the West in the late 1950s by Maharishi Mahesh Yogi, a visionary Indian sage trained in physics, who saw meditation as a means of alleviating stress in individuals and society. His emphasis on scientific research proved that the timeless practice of meditation was not just an arcane mystical activity for Himalayan recluses, but rather a mind–body method hugely relevant to and beneficial for modern society.

In 2007, an analysis of 107 studies compared the effects on high blood pressure of multiple stress reduction and relaxation methods. The TM technique was found to produce a statistically significant reduction in high blood pressure not found with relaxation, biofeedback, or stress management training (Rainforth et al. 2007).

Therfore, many studies strongly support the inclusion of TM as a major mind–body tool for blood pressure management, either as the sole or an adjunctive therapy. Side benefits include reductions in related CVD risk factors, such as psychological stress, metabolic syndrome, CVD morbidity, and mortality (Anderson, Liu, and Kryscio 2008; Rainforth et al. 2007).

TAI CHI

Tai Chi, originally a non-competitive form of self-defense, has been referred to as "meditation in motion." Consisting of a series of postures and movements performed slowly and gracefully, Tai Chi focuses on breathing through fluid movements to induce a state of relaxation and tranquility. As *chi* is believed to be the vital force animating the body, Tai Chi aims to circulate chi throughout the body while fostering a calm mind. Practiced regularly, Tai Chi can reduce stress while improving flexibility, strength, and energy (Wang, Collet, and Lau 2004).

Table 11.1. Diet and Lifestyle Recommendations

Nutrition	Daily Intake
1. Dash I, Dash II-Na⁺ and premier diets like Mediterranean and Asian	
2. Sodium restriction	Less than 1.5 grams
3. Potassium	100 mEq
4. Potassium/sodium ratio	>5:1
5. Protein: total intake (30% total calories)	1.0–1.5 gram/kg
A. Non-animal sources preferred but lean or wild free- range animal protein in moderation is acceptable	
B. Soy protein (fermented is best)	30 grams 1–2 x per week
C. Sardine muscle concentrate extract or 2–3 Sardines	1–2 x per week
D. Cold-water wild fish, i.e., Alaskan salmon, no farm-raised fish, fowl, or poultry	4–5 oz, 2–3 x per week
6. Fats: 30% total calories	
A. Omega-3 fatty acids PUFA (DHA, EPA, cold-water fish)	3–4 grams
B. Omega-6 fatty acids PUFA Oatmeal	60 grams=>1/4 cup
C. Omega-9 fatty acids MUFA Extra virgin olive oil, Olives	1–2 tablespoons on steamed veggies or salad or 3–5 olives
D. Saturated FA (lean, wild animal meat) (30%)	<10% total calories
E. P/S ratio (polyunsaturated/saturated_ fats >2.0	
F. Omega-3/Omega-6 PUFA, ratio 1:1 – 1:2	
G. No trans fatty acids (0%) (hydrogenated margarines, vegetable oils)	
H. Nuts: almonds, walnuts, hazelnuts, macadamia.	¼–½ cup one to two times a week
7. Carbohydrates	30–40% calories
A. Reduce or eliminate refined sugars and simple carbohydrates	
B. Increase complex carbohydrates and fiber whole grains (oat, barley, wheat) vegetables, beans, legumes	3–4 times per week for complex carbs
i.e. oatmeal or	60 grams=>1/4 cup
oatbran (dry) or	40 grams, 2–3 times pr/wk
beta-glucan	3 grams
or psyllium	7 grams
8. Garlic	4 cloves/day

(continued)

Table 11.1. (Continued)

Nutrition	Daily Intake
9. Onions	1–2 slices raw/day
10. Wakame seaweed (dried)	3.0–3.5 grams, 2–3 times per week
11. Celery Celery stalks or Celery juice or Celery seed extract Celery Oil (tincture)	 4 stalks/day 8 teaspoons TID 1000 mg BID ½–1 teaspoon TID
12. Natto	100 grams, 2–3 times per week
Exercise • Aerobic • Walk 30–60 minutes daily • 4200 KJ/week • Resistance training	5 days a week 3x/week or daily
Weight Loss • To ideal body weight (IBW) • Lose 1–2 pounds week • BMI <25 • Waist circumference <40 inches for male <35 inches for female • Total body fat <16% in males <22% in females • Increase lean muscle mass	3x/week or daily
Alcohol Restriction • Wine • Beer	<20 grams/day <10 ounces (preferred-red wine)3–4 x per week <12 ounces 3–4 x per week
Caffeine	None
Tobacco and Smoking	None
Avoid drugs and interactions that increase BP	Non-steroidals, acetaminophen
Stress Management	Yoga, TM, Tai Chi

In a study of two groups of 76 healthy subjects with high to normal blood pressure or stage I hypertension, Tai Chi was shown to decrease blood pressure and anxiety. After subjects practiced 50 minutes of Tai Chi three times per week for 12 weeks, the treatment group demonstrated a 15.6 mmHg decrease in systolic blood pressure and a 8.8 mmHg decrease in diastolic blood pressure (Tsai et al. 2003).

YOGA

The practice of yoga can help reduce weight and lower blood pressure as an adjunctive means of treating hypertension, most favorably in conjunction with a healthy diet, exercise, and pharmaceutical treatment (Yang 2007).

In studies of adults with high blood pressure, with and without coronary disease, reductions in medication requirements have been observed among those participants completing a yoga-based intervention, as compared to controlled counterparts receiving usual care (Yang 2007; Yogendra et al. 2004).

For example, in a study of thirteen hypertensive individuals aged 41–60, practicing one hour of yoga per day, six days per week, resulted in a significant drop in blood pressure: systolic dropped from 141.7 to 127.9 mmHg by the third week and then to 120.7 mmHg by the fourth week (Yang 2007). Even 30 minutes of daily yoga has been shown to decrease blood pressure in studies involving hypertensive individuals (Selvamurthy et al. 1998)

Table 11.2 Nutritional Supplements for Hypertension

Supplements	Daily Intake
Coenzyme Q10	120–150 mg 2x a day
Fish Oil	3–4 grams a day
Nattokinase (NSK-SD)	50–100 mg if dietary natto is not consumed
Magnesium	400–800 mg a day
Organic Garlic	1000 mg if not taken in diet
Hawthorn	1000 to 1500 mg per day
Quercetin	500–1000 mg per day 2x a day
Vitamin D3	2000 units per day
Vitamin B6	100 mg 1–2x a day
Vitamin C	250–500 mg 2x a day

In addition to their antihypertensive effects, mind–body interventions provide patients with a proactive process through which they may manage their health, as opposed to passively taking pills. As lack of control over various aspects of life creates stress, empowerment derived from harnessing control over blood pressure and health through such lifestyle modification techniques ultimately improves patients' blood pressure, health, and longevity.

REFERENCES

Anderson J. W., C. X. Liu, and R. J. Kryscio. 2008. Blood pressure response to transcendental meditation: a meta-analysis. *Am J Hypertens* 21: 310–16.

Appel L. J. T. J. Moore, E. Obarzanek, W. M. Vollmer, L. P. Svetkey, F. M. Sacks, G. A. Bray, T. M. Vogt, J. A. Cutler, M. M. Windhauser, P. H. Lin, N. Karanja . 1997. A clinical trial of the effects of dietary patterns on blood pressure. DASH Collaborative Research Group. *N Engl J Med* 336(16): 1117–24.

Aybak, M., A. Sermet, M. O. Ayyildiz, and A. Z. Karakilcik. 1995. Effect of oral pyridoxine hydrochloride supplementation on arterial blood pressure in patients with essential hypertension. *Arzneimittelforschung* 45: 1271–73.

Braunwald, E. 1994. Cellular and molecular biology of cardiovascular disease. In *Harrison's principles of internal medicine*, ed. K. J. Isselbacher, E. Braunwald, J. D. Wilson. 13th ed. New York: McGraw Hill.

Burke, B. E., R. Neustenschwander, and R. D. Olson. 2001. Randomized, double-blind, placebo-controlled trial of coenzyme Q10 in isolated systolic hypertension. *South Med J* 94: 1112–17.

Chobanian, A. V., G. L. Bakris, H. R. Black, W. C. Cushman, L. A. Green, J. L. Izzo Jr., D. W. Jones, B. J. Materson, S. Oparil, J. T. Wright Jr, E. J. Roccella. 2003. National Heart, Lung, and Blood Institute Joint National Committee on Prevention, Detection, Evaluation, and Treatment of High Blood Pressure; National High Blood Pressure Education Program Coordinating Committee: The Seventh Report of the Joint National Committee on Prevention, Detection, Evaluation, and Treatment of High Blood Pressure: the JNC 7 report. *JAMA* 289: 2560–72.

Chopra, R. K., R. Goldman, S. T. Sinatra, and H. N. Bhagavan. 1998. Relative bioavailability of coenzyme Q10 formulations in human subjects. *Int J Vitam Nutr Res* 68(2): 109–13.

Cooke, J. P. 1998. Nutriceuticals for cardiovascular health. *Am J Cardiol* 82(10A): 43S.

DeFronzo, R., and E. Ferrannini. 1991. Insulin resistance: A multifaceted syndrome responsible for NIDDM, obesity, hypertension, and atherosclerotic cardiovascular disease. *Diabetes Care* 14: 173–94.

Digiesi, V., F. Cantini, and B Brodbeck. 1990. Effect of coenzyme Q10 on essential hypertension. *Curr Ther Res* 47: 841–45.

Digiesi, V., F. Cantini, A. Oradei, G. Bisi, G. C. Guarino, A. Brocchi, F. Bellandi, M. Mancini, G. P. Littarru. 1994. Coenzyme Q-10 in essential hypertension. *Mol Aspects Med* 15: S257–S263.

Dishman, R. K, H. R. Berthoud, F. W. Booth, C. W. Cotman, V. R. Edgerton, M. R. Fleshner, S. C. Gandevia, F. Gomez-Pinilla, B.N. Greenwood, C. H. Hillman, A. F. Kramer, B. E. Levin, T. H. Moran, A. A. Russo-Neustadt, J. D. Salamone, J. D. Van Hoomissen, C. E. Wade, D. A. York, M. J. Zigmond. 2006. Neurobiology of exercise. Obesity. I (Silver Spring). 14(3): 345–56.

Duffy, S. J., N. Gokce, M. Holbrook, A. Huang, B. Frei, J. F. Keaney Jr., J. A. Vita. 1999. Treatment of hypertension with ascorbic acid. *Lancet* 354: 2048–49.

Duke, J. A. 2001. The green pharmacy: Herbs, foods and natural formulas to keep you young. Anti-aging prescriptions. Emmaus, PA: Rodale and St. Martin's Press.

Eaton, S. B, S. B. Eaton, III, and M. J. Konner. 1997. Paleolithic nutrition revisited: A twelve-year retrospective on its nature and implications. A review. *Eur J Clin Nutr* 51: 207–216.

Ferrara, L. A., S. Raimondi, and L. d'Episcopa, L. Guida, A. Della Russo, T. Marotta. 2000. Olive oil and reduced need for antihypertensive medications. *Arch Intern Med* 160: 837–42.

Forman, J. P., G. C. Curhan, and E. N. Taylor. 2008. Plasma 25-hydroxy vitamin D levels and risk of incident hypertension among young women. *Hypertension* 52(5): 828–32.

Forman, J. P., Stampfer, M. J., and Curhan, G. C. 2005. Non-narcotic analgesic dose and risk of incident hypertension in U.S. women. *Hypertension* 46: 500.

Goldstein, D. 1995. Stress, catecholamines, and cardiovascular disease. *BMJ* 311: 1580–81.

Gu, D., K. Reynolds, X. Wu, J. Chen, X. Duan, P. Muntner, G. Huang, R. F. Reynolds, S. Su, P. K. Whelton, J. He. 2002. InterASIA Collaborative Group. The International Collaborative Study of Cardiovascular Disease in ASIA. Prevalence, awareness, treatment, and control of hypertension in China. *Hypertension* 40: 920–27.

Hamet, P., M. Daignault-Gelinas, J. Lambert, M. Ledoux, L. Whissell-Cambiotti, F. Bellavance, and E. Mongean. 1992. Epidemiological evidence of an interaction between calcium and sodium intake impacting on blood pressure: A Montreal study. *Am J Hypertens* 5: 378–85.

Hasler, C. M., S. Kundrat, and D. Wool. 2000. Functional foods and cardiovascular disease. *Curr Atheroscler Rep* 2: 467–75.

Houston, M. C. 1992. New insights and approaches to reduce end organ damage in the treatment of hypertension: Subsets of hypertension approach. *Am Heart J* 123: 1337–67.

Houston, M. C., B. P. Meador, and L. M. Schipani. 2000. *Handbook of antihypertensive therapy.* 10th ed. Philadelphia: Hanley and Belfus, Inc.

Iseki, K., Y. Kimura, K. Wakugami, H. Muratani, Y. Ikemiya, K. Fukiyama. 2000. Comparison of the effect of blood pressure on the development of stroke, acute myocardial infraction, and end-stage renal disease. *Hypertens Res* 23: 143–49.

Jacobs, G. 2001. The physiology of mind body interactions: The stress response and the relaxation response. *J Altern Complement Med* 7(1): S83–92.

Jezova, D., and R. Duncko. 2002. Enhancement of stress-induced pituitary hormone release and cardiovascular activation by antidepressant treatment in healthy men. *J psychopharmacol* 16(3): 235–40.

Kawasaki, T., E. Seki, K. Osajima, M. Yoshida, K. Asada, T. Matsui, and Y. Osajima. 2000. Antihypertensive effect of valyl-tyrosine, a short chain peptide derived from sardine muscle hydrolyzate, on mild hypertensive subjects. *J Hum Hypertens* 14: 519–23.

Kearney, P. M., M. Whelton, K. Reynolds, P. Muntner, P. K. Whelton, and J. He. 2005. Global burden of hypertension: Analysis of worldwide data. *Lancet* 365(9455): 217–23.

Kim, J. Y., S. N. Gum, J. K. Paik, H. H. Lim, K. C. Kim, K. Ogasawara, K. Inoue, S. Park, Y. Jang, J. H. Lee. 2008. Effects of nattokinase on blood pressure: a randomized, controlled trial. *Hypertens Res* 31(8): 1583–88.

Kitiyakara, C., and C. S. Wilcox. 1998. Antioxidants for hypertension. *Opin Nephrol Hypertens* 7: 531–38.

Kotchen, T. A., and J. M. Kotchen. 1997. Dietary sodium and blood pressure: Interactions with other nutrients. *Am J Clin Nutr* 65: 708S–711S.

Kotchen, T. A., and D. A. McCarron. 1998. AHA Science Advisory. Dietary electrolytes and blood pressure. *Circ* 98: 613–17.

Kumar, K. V., and U. N. Das. 1993. Are free radicals involved in the pathology of human essential hypertension? *Free Radic Res Commun* 19: 59–66.

Lacy, F., D. T. O'Connor, and G. W. Schmid-Schonbein. 1998. Plasma hydrogen peroxide production in hypertensives and normotensive subjects at genetic risk of hypertension. *J Hypertens* 16: 291–303.

Langsjoen, P. H., and A. M. Langsjoen. 1999. Overview of the use of Co Q 10 in cardiovascular disease. *Biofactors* 9: 273–84.

Lazaron, J., B. Pomeranz, and P. Corey. 1998. Incidence of adverse drug reaction in hospitalized patients. *JAMA* 279: 1200–05.

Le, O. T., and W. J. Elliot. 1991. Dose response relationship of blood pressure and serum cholesterol to 3-N-butyl phthalide, a component of celery oil. *Clinical Research* 139: 750A. Abstract.

Lorenz, R., U. Spengler, S. Fischer, J. Duhm, P. C. Weber. 1983. Platelet function, thromboxane formation and blood pressure control during supplementation of the western diet with cod liver oil. *Circ* 67: 504.

McIntyre, M., D. F. Bohr, and A. F. Dominiczak. 1999. Endothelial function in hypertension: The role of superoxide anion. *Hypertension* 34(4 Pt 1): 539–45.

McMahon, F. G., and R. Vargas. 1993. Can garlic lower blood pressure? A pilot study. *Pharmacotherapy* 13: 406–07.

Mohamadi, A., S. T. Jarrell, S. J. Shi, N. S. Andrawis, A. Myers, D. Clouatre, and H. G. Preuss. 2000. Effects of wild versus cultivated garlic on blood pressure and other parameters in hypertensive rats. *Heart Disease* 2: 3–9.

Mori, T. A., D. Q. Bao, V. Burke, I. B. Puddey, L. J. Beilin. 1999. Docosahexaenoic acid but not eicosapentaenoic acid lowers ambulatory blood pressure and heart rate in humans. *Hypertension* 34: 253–60.

Mori, T. A., D. Q. Bao, V. Burke, I. B. Puddey, G. F. Watts, and L. J. Beilin. 1999. Dietary fish as a major component of a weight-loss diet: effect on serum lipids, glucose and insulin metabolism in overweight hypertensive subjects. *Am J Clin Nutr* 70: 817–25.

Mori, T. A., G. F. Watts, V. Burke, E. Hilme, I. B. Puddey, L. J. Beilin. 2000. Differential effects of eicosapentaenoic acid and docosahexaenoic acid on vascular reactivity of the forearm microcirculation in hyperlipidemic, overweight men. *Circ* 102(11): 1264–69.

Nakano, T., H. Hidaka, J. Uchida, K. Nakajima, and Y. Hata. 1998. Hypotensive effects of wakame. *J Jpn Soc Clin Nutr* 20: 92.

Nayak, D. U., C. Karmen, W. H. Frishman, and B. A. Vakili. 2001. Antioxidant vitamins and enzymatic and synthetic oxygen-derived free radical scavengers in the prevention and treatment of cardiovascular disease. *Heart Disease* 3: 28–45.

Neaton, J. D., R. H. Grimm, Jr., R. J. Prineas, J. Stamler, G. A. Grandits, P. J. Elmer, J. A. Cutler, J. M. Flack, J. A. Schoenberger, R. McDonald. 1993. Treatment of Mild Hypertension Study. Final results. Treatment of Mild Hypertension Study Research Group. *JAMA* 270: 713–24.

Obarzanek, E., P. A. Velletri, and J. A. Cutler. 1996. Dietary protein and blood pressure. *JAMA* 274: 1598–1603.

Orme-Johnson, D. W. 1987. Medical care utilization and the trancendental meditation program. *Psychosom Med* 49: 493–507.

Pais, E., T. Alexy, R. E. Holsworth, Jr., and H. J. Meiselman. 2006. Effects of nattokinase, a pro-fibrinolytic enzyme, on red blood cell aggregation and whole blood viscosity. *Clin Hemorheol Microcirc* 35: 139–42.

Pereira, M. A., and J. J. Pins. 2000. Dietary fiber and cardiovascular disease: Experimental and epidemiologic advances. *Curr Atheroscler Rep* 2: 494–502.

Pfeifer, M., B. Begerow, H. W. Minne, D. Nachtigall, and C. Hansen. 2001. Effects of a short-term vitamin D(3) and calcium supplementation on blood pressure and parathyroid hormone levels in elderly women. *J Clin Endocrinol Metab* 86: 1633–37.

Prigerson, H. G., A. J. Bierhals, S. V. Kasl, C. V. Reynolds, III, M. K. Shear, N. Day, L. C. Beery, J. T. Newsom, S. Jacobs. 1997. Traumatic grief as a risk factor for mental and physical morbidity. *Am J Psychiatry* 154(5): 616–23.

Rainforth, M. V., R. H. Schneider, S. I. Nidich, C. Gaylord-King, J. W. Salerno, J. W. Anderson. 2007. Stress reduction programs in patients with elevated blood pressure: A systematic review and meta-analysis. *Curr Hyperten Reports* 9: 520–28.

Ried, K., O. R. Frank, N. P. Stocks, P. Fakler, T. Sullivan. 2008. Effect of garlic on blood pressure: A systematic review and meta-analysis. *BMC Cardiovasc Disord* 8: 13.

Rozanski, A., J. A. Blumenthal, and J. Kaplan. 1999. Impact of psychological factors on the pathogenesis of cardiovascular disease and implications for therapy. *Circ.* 99(16): 2192–217.

Russo, C., O. Olivieri, D. Girelli, G. Faccini, M. L. Zenari, S. Lombardi, and R. Corrocher. 1998. Antioxidant status and lipid peroxidation in patients with essential hypertension. *J Hypertens* 16: 1267–71.

Sacks, F. M., L. P. Svetkey, W. M. Vollmer, L. J. Appel, G. A. Bray, D. Harsha, E. Obarzanek, P. R. Conlin, E. R. Miller 3rd, D. G. Simons-Morton, N. Karanja,

P. H. Lin. 2001. Effects on blood pressure of reduced dietary sodium and the dietary approaches to stop hypertension (DASH) diet. *N Engl J Med* 344: 3–10.

Santić, Z., A. Lukić, D. Sesar, S. Milicević, and V. Ilakovac. 2006. Long-term follow-up of blood pressure in family members of soldiers killed during the war in Bosnia and Herzegovina. *Croat Med J* 47(3): 416–23.

Schussler, M., J. Holzl, and U. Fricke. 1995. Myocardial effects of flavonoids from Crataegus species. *Arzneim Forsch* 45(8): 842.

Selvamurthy, W., K. Sridharan, U.S. Ray, R. S. Tiwary, K. S. Hegde, U. Radhakrishan, K. C. Sinha. 1998. A new physiological approach to control essential hypertension. *Indian J Physiol Pharmacol* 42(2): 205–13.

Stamler, J., P. Elliott, H. Kesteloot, R. Nichols, G. Claeys, A. R. Dyer, and R. Stamle. 1996. Inverse relation of dietary protein markers with blood pressure. Findings for 10,020 men and women in the Intersalt Study. Intersalt Cooperative Research Group. International study of salt and blood pressure. *Circ* 94: 1629–34.

Suetsuna, K., and T. Nakano. 2000. Identification of an antihypertensive peptide from peptic digest of wakame (undaria pinnatifida). *J Nutr Biochem* 11: 450–54.

Todaro, J. F., B. J. Shen, R. Niaura, A. Spiro, and K. D. Ward. 2003. Effect of negative emotions on frequency of coronary heart disease (The Normative Aging Study*)*. *Am J Cardiol* 92(8): 901–06.

Tsai, J. C., W. H. Wang, P. Chan, L. J. Lin, C. H. Wang, B. Tomlinson, M. H. Hsieh, H. Y. Yang, J. C. Liu. 2003. The beneficial effects of tai chi chuan on blood pressure and lipid profile and anxiety status in a randomized controlled trial. *J Altern Complement Med* 9(5): 747–54.

Tsigos, C., and G. P. Chrousos. 2002. Hypothalamic-pituitary-adrenal axis, neuroendocrine factors and stress. *J Psychosom Res* 53(4): 865–71.

Vaziri, N. D., K. Liang, and Y. Ding. 1999. Increased nitric oxide inactivation by reactive oxygen species in lead-induced hypertension. *Kidney Int.* 56: 1492–98.

Vibes, J., B. Lasserre, J. Gleye, C. Declume. 1994. Inhibition of thromboxane A2 biosynthesis in vitro by the main components of Crataegus oxyacantha (Hawthorn) flower heads. *Prostaglandins Leukot Essent Fatty Acids* 50: 173.

Vuksan, V., D. J. A. Jenkins, P. Spadafora, J. L. Sievenpiper, R. Owen, E. Vidgen, F. Brighenti, R. Josse, L. A. Leiter, C. Bruce-Thompson. 1999. Konjac-Mannan (Glucomannan) improves glycemia and other associated risk factors for coronary heart disease in type 2 diabetes. *Diabetes Care* 22: 913–19.

Wang, C., J. P. Collet, and J. Lau. 2004. The effect of tai chi on health outcomes in patients with chronic conditions: a systematic review. *Arch Intern Med* 164(5): 493:–501.

Warner, M. G. 2000. Complementary and alternative therapies for hypertension. *Comp Health Prac Rev* 6: 11–19.

Whelton, P. K., J. He, L. J. Appel, J. A. Cutler, S. Havas, T. A. Kotchen, E. J. Roccella, R. Stout, C. Vallbona, M. C. Winston, J Karimbakas. 2002. National High Blood Pressure Education Program Coordinating Committee. Primary prevention of hypertension: Clinical and public health advisory from The National High Blood Pressure Education Program. *JAMA* 288(15): 1882–88.

Yang, K. 2007. A review of yoga programs for four leading risk factors of chronic diseases. *Evid Based Complement Alternat Med* 4(4): 487–91.

Yogendra J, H. J. Yogendra, S. Ambardekar, R. D. Lele, S. Shetty, M. Dave, N. Husein. 2004. Beneficial effects of yoga lifestyle on reversibility of ischaemic heart disease: caring heart project of International Board of Yoga. *J Assoc Physicians India.* Apr;52: 283–9.

12

Integrative Approaches to Cardiovascular Disease

MIMI GUARNERI AND CHRISTOPHER SUHAR

KEY CONCEPTS

- The causes of cardiovascular disease are multifactorial, ranging from inflammation and lipid abnormalities to stress, depression, anger, and social isolation.
- An integrative holistic approach to cardiovascular disease entails healing the whole person: mind, body, emotions, and spirit.
- A growing understanding of the science of the human genome, nutraceuticals, and mind–body medicine is paving the way to a multidisciplinary approach to individual risk that is personalized, predictive, proactive, and preventive.

■

Introduction

Cardiovascular disease (CVD) is one of the major progressive lifelong diseases in the modern era, affecting the lives of one out of two men and one out of three women. The disease begins silently in adolescence and slowly progresses in middle age. It results in clinical events starting after 55 years of age in men and after 65 years of age in women. The Interheart Study defined the relative risks for acute myocardial infarction of the various cardiovascular risk factors in a population of 29,972 individuals from fifty-two different countries (Ogden et al. 2006). Nine risk factors were found to account for 90 percent of the populations' attributable risk in men, and 94 percent of the risk in women (see Table 12.1).

Table 12.1. Results of the Interheart Study

Cardiovascular Risk Factor	Relative Risk
Smoking	2.87
Elevated Apo B/Apo A1	3.25
Hypertension	1.91
Diabetes	2.37
Abdominal obesity	1.12
Psychosocial factors	2.67
Daily consumption of fruit and vegetables	0.7
Regular alcohol consumption (≥3/week)	0.91
Regular physical activity	0.86

Although Western allopathic medicine excels in the area of acute care, such as treating heart attacks and providing lifesaving surgeries, it falls short in its treatment of chronic disease management and prevention. It is in the arena of prevention and chronic disease management that integrative cardiology has the opportunity to complete the circle of care, addressing all of the risk factors for cardiovascular disease from a holistic perspective.

Lifestyle Change Intervention

The causes of CVD are multifactorial, and treatment almost always requires lifestyle changes and mind–body interventions. Almost all cardiac risk factors are dependent on lifestyle and environment. Prevention is the best intervention for CVD, yet in a recent survey of primary care physicians and cardiologists, it was found that discussions of lifestyle including nutrition, exercise, and psychosocial stressors continue to be poorly addressed (Mosca et al. 2005; Vogel and Krucoff 2007).

Almost all CVD is closely related to and affected by inflammation, which is a direct result of obesity, poor nutrition, sedentary lifestyle, and maladaptive responses to stress and tension. In fact, poor nutrition and physical inactivity are identified as probably the true leading "actual" causes of death in the U.S. (Mokdad, 2004). Increasing BMI has been linked to an increasing risk of diabetes mellitus, hyperlipidemia, and hypertension. Conversely, as the BMI is lowered, so is the prevalence of all risk factors. Multiple avenues of research have shown that lifestyle intervention alone can alter the course of disease. For example, in the Diabetes Prevention Study, type 2 diabetes was prevented in high-risk individuals who underwent individualized counseling on weight loss and physical activity alone, when compared to appropriately matched controls and patients taking metformin alone (Tuomilehto et al. 2001).

An integrative approach to cardiovascular care broadens the traditional diagnosis and treatment of disease, utilizing both Western-based diagnostic tests and pharmaceuticals along with an aggressive focus on all aspects of health, including nutrition, exercise, and psychosocial stress. In almost all cases, a comprehensive lifestyle change approach is necessary.

From Hippocrates we learned that "food is medicine." In fact, a single high-fat meal transiently impairs endothelial function and blood flow (Vogel, Corretti, and Plotnick 1997). A very large epidemiologic study evaluated the effect of nutrition on disease in rural China and the United States. In this study of over 10,000 individuals, the U.S. fat intake was twice as high, fiber intake was three times lower, animal protein intake was 90 percent higher. The heart disease death rate was 16.7-fold greater for men and 5.6-fold greater for women. The incidence of other diseases were also higher in the U.S. including cancer, osteoporosis, diabetes, and hypertension (Chen et al. 1990). Importantly, Asian immigrants to the U.S. reached the American level of heart disease and cancer deaths within two generations.

In order to fully understand the nutritional status of my patients, a three-day food diary is used to assess the quantity and quality of calories consumed. The Department of Agriculture reported an 8 percent increase in food consumption from 1990 to 2000, and the CDC reports that the doubling of the prevalence of obesity between 1971 and 2000 correlated with a 22 percent increase in calorie consumption for women and a 9 percent increase for men (Ogden et al. 2006). Interestingly, despite indications that the percentage of calories consumed as fat is decreasing, surveys indicate that we are consuming more calories overall (Eckel and Krauss 1998). Reduction in total caloric intake and exercise should be emphasized as a first-line approach to weight loss. Determination of the basal metabolic rate allows a more precise estimate of calories needed, along with exercise and stress management, to achieve an ideal body weight.

Simple handouts to guide patients on nutrition choices can be extremely valuable. It is important to teach patients about the glycemic index; you might consider providing handouts that label food choices as high, moderate, and low on the glycemic index. Patients should be taught to eliminate liquid calories, most notably soda and fruit juice. Our patients are also taught to eliminate high-fructose corn syrup and trans fatty acids. If sweeteners are necessary, organic agave nectar or stevia can be used. A plant-based vegetarian diet is preferred. For those individuals who consume fish, options are suggested that are high in omega-3 fatty acids, low in mercury, and not farm raised, such as wild salmon and sardines. Foods high in antioxidants are strongly recommended. Functional foods, which have bioactive properties as well as nutrient value, are incorporated into the nutrition program. These include almonds, chocolate, tea, soy, and viscous fibers such as eggplant, oats. and psyllium. Tea and chocolate are able to reduce free radicals due to their high concentration of flavonoids. We recommend five cups of green tea daily to reduce cardiovascular mortality and to lower cholesterol (Kuriyama et al. 2006). Flavonoids, especially those found in green tea, have been shown to have antithrombotic effects (Son et al. 2004). Consumption of black tea is associated with a reduction in acute myocardial infarction (Geleijnse 2002), and improved endothelial relaxation (Duffy 2001).Supplements, like nutrition and exercise, play an important role in the prevention of CVD. In my integrative cardiology practice I use omega-3 fish oil, CoQ10, red yeast rice, vitamin D, and niacin on a daily basis. I believe that disorders determine treatment and that a supplement regimen should be tailored to the individual. For example, those individuals with low HDL and/or high triglycerides will be placed on a low glycemic index diet, a daily exercise program, omega-3 fish oil, and niacin. An individual with high LDL may be placed on a low- saturated-fat diet, red yeast rice, plant stanols, soluble fiber, statin therapy (if indicated), and omega-3 fish oil. Green tea, soluble fiber, exercise, low glycemic/antiinflammatory diets, and stress management are universal recommendations for health.

Vitamin E and Antioxidants

The Nurses' Health Study, which was observational in design, concluded a 34 percent reduction in cardiovascular events in subjects taking vitamin E supplementation (Lopez-Garcia et al. 2004). Since that initial observation, multiple studies have attempted to evaluate vitamin E in the primary and secondary prevention of cardiovascular disease. In the primary prevention project, 4,495 patients were followed for 3.6 years on 300 IU of vitamin E supplementation without demonstrating improvement in cardiovascular morbidity (Sacco et al. 2003). Multiple secondary prevention studies, including HOPE (Yusef et al. 2000) and GISSI-P (GISSI-Prevenzione Investigators 1999), failed to demonstrate benefit from vitamin E supplementation. HATS compared treatment regimens of lipid-modifying therapy and antioxidant-vitamin therapy, alone and together (Brown et al. 2001). The three-year, double-blind trial included 160 patients with coronary disease, low levels of HDL-C, and normal levels of LDL-C. Patients were assigned to one of four treatment regimens: simvastatin (10-20 mg/day) plus niacin (2-4 g/day); antioxidants; simvastatin (10-20 mg/day) plus niacin (2-4 g/day) plus antioxidants; or placebo. The primary end points were arteriographic evidence of change in coronary stenosis, and the occurrence of a first cardiovascular event (fatal/nonfatal MI, stroke, or revascularization). The average stenosis progressed with placebo (3.9 percent), antioxidants (1.8 percent), and simvastatin plus niacin plus antioxidants (0.7 percent). There was a 0.4 percent regression with simvastatin plus niacin alone (p<0.001). In conclusion, the combination of simvastatin plus niacin greatly reduced the rate of major coronary events (60–90 percent) and substantially slowed progression of coronary atherosclerosis in patients with low HDL-C. While HATS further supported the use of niacin for raising HDL and reducing plaque formation in combination with statin therapy, no further advantage was seen in the group receiving antioxidants and combination statin–niacin therapy. These studies did not attempt to assess the inflammatory and oxidative state of subjects prior to initiation and following therapy.

In a randomized double-blind placebo control trial, subjects received 1600 IU of RRR-alpha tocopherol versus placebo and followed for six months (Devaraj et al. 2007). Subjects taking the vitamin E had a statistically significant reduction in hs-CRP and urinary F2 isoprostanes and monocyte superoxide anion and tumor necrosis factor release, compared with baseline and placebo. Despite this reduction in oxidative and inflammatory markers, no change was seen in carotid intimal-medial thickness. Multiple trial design concerns have been raised to explain the inconsistency of the observational and randomized study data (Blumberg and Frei 2007). These include:

1. Not using the right type of supplement formulation;
2. Not using the correct dosage;
3. Not using a complex antioxidant mixture;
4. Not choosing the right study population; and
5. Not looking at functional biomarkers.

One of the important variables missing from all of these studies is nutritional status. Until biomarkers and nutritional status are included with these research variables, it is premature to conclude that antioxidants offer no benefit in cardiovascular disease prevention.

Exercise

Exercise is one of the most powerful methods for decreasing cardiac risk and enhancing health. Looking at patients after myocardial infarction, percutaneous coronary intervention (PCI), or coronary artery bypass graft (CABG) surgery, those who participate in a comprehensive exercise rehabilitation program have a six-fold decrease in cardiac death, as compared to those patients not undergoing cardiac rehabilitation (Taylor et al. 2004). Despite these and many other findings showing the benefits of exercise, physicians reported spending an average of eight minutes counseling their patients on lifestyle change at routine annual visits. Furthermore, less than 5 percent of physicians advise patients to engage in physical activity at least six days per week, as recommended by national guidelines.

A provocative study looking at exercise versus angioplasty in patients with coronary artery disease (CAD) determined by >75% stenosis on angiography showed that daily exercise over a 12-month period had a lower cardiovascular event-free survival and equal angina symptom improvement (Hambrecht 2004). Group exercise also provides a valuable social network, which is one of the most powerful interventions available to prevent and treat cardiovascular disease.

Invasive Therapies and Statin Therapy

INVASIVE THERAPIES FOR CAD

Coronary artery bypass grafting is an extremely common procedure, yet the relative gains of its use are limited. The Coronary Artery Surgery Study (CASS) randomized patients with chronic CAD into a bypass group and a medical therapy group. In the long-term follow-up of CASS, only 2.1 percent of bypasses yield improved mortality when compared to medical therapy. Specifically, this was in patients with left main and left main equivalent disease (Caracciolo et al. 1995). It is important to note that the medical therapies available when this study began were nowhere near as comprehensive as currently available medical treatment including a lack of availability of statins. The relative gains of medical therapy, if this study were done today, may be found to be even greater.

STATIN THERAPY

Multiple studies have shown substantial reductions in mortality and procedure rates using statin medications. The Scandinavian Simvastatin Survival Study (4S) was one of the largest of these studies. The trial enrolled 4,444 patients with known CAD and treated them with Simvastatin. This treatment alone decreased revascularization procedures by 37 percent; cardiac death rates and event rates were lowered by 50 percent in the treatment group as well (Pederson et al. 1994).

STATIN THERAPY VS. INVASIVE PROCEDURES

Multiple studies have shown that there is a benefit in using aggressive lipid lowering therapy instead of angioplasty in patients with chronic stable angina (Boden, 2007; Pitt et al. 1999). The AVERT study used 80 mg of Atorvastatin compared to PTCA for chronic stable angina. The Atorvaststin group had fewer ischemic events, including stroke, and a longer time period until a first event (Pitt et al. 1999), thus showing lipid therapy to be preferable in this population. With this and other related studies demonstrating treatment benefit with medication and lifestyle change, the AHA and ACC made the following statement: "Based on the data available from randomized trials comparing medical therapy with PTCA, it seems prudent to consider medical therapy for the initial management of most patients with Canadian Cardiovascular Society Classification Class I and II and reserve PTCA and CABG for those patients with more severe symptoms and ischemia" (Smith et al. 2001).

While statins alone may be preferable to invasive procedures for the patient with chronic stable angina or CAD without ischemia, statin therapy only manages one aspect of coronary disease—the lipids. If you take a truly holistic approach and address diet, exercise, and the patient's emotional health, the gains are far greater.

Coronary Artery Disease Reversal

Multiple studies have been done demonstrating that comprehensive lifestyle change can reverse cardiac atherosclerotic lesions. The majority of this work has been done by Dean Ornish and his colleagues using the Lifestyle Modification Program. This program consists of a very low-fat, (10 percent of total calories consumed) plant-based diet, exercise, yoga, and group support participation. The following abstracts and comments summarize that work.

Effects of stress management training and dietary changes in treating ischemic heart disease

This study evaluated the short-term effects of the Lifestyle Modification Program in patients with coronary heart disease. The study compared the cardiovascular status of 23 patients who received this intervention with a randomized control group of 23 patients who did not. After 24 days, patients in the experimental group demonstrated a 44 percent mean increase in duration of exercise, a 55 percent mean increase in total work performed, significantly improved left ventricular regional wall motion during peak exercise, and a net change in the left ventricular ejection fraction from rest to maximum exercise of +6.4%. Also, there was a 20.5 percent mean decrease in plasma cholesterol levels and a 91 percent mean reduction in frequency of anginal episodes. In this selected sample, short-term improvements in cardiovascular status seem to result from these adjuncts to conventional treatment of coronary heart disease (Ornish et al. 1983).

Can lifestyle changes reverse coronary heart disease? The Lifestyle Heart Trial

In a prospective, randomized, controlled trial to determine whether comprehensive lifestyle changes affect coronary atherosclerosis after one year, patients were assigned to an experimental group asked to follow the Lifestyle Modification Program or to a usual-care control group. One hundred ninety-five coronary artery lesions were analyzed by quantitative coronary angiography. The average percentage diameter stenosis regressed from 40.0 (SD 16.9) percent to 37.8 (16.5) percent in the experimental group, yet progressed from 42.7 (15.5) percent to 46.1 (18.5) percent in the control group. When only lesions greater than 50 percent stenosed were analyzed, the average percentage diameter stenosis regressed from 61.1 (8.8) percent to 55.8 (11) percent in the experimental group, and progressed from 61.7 (9.5) percent to 64.4 (16.3) percent in the control group. Overall, 82 percent of experimental-group patients had an average change toward regression. In summary, comprehensive lifestyle changes may be able to bring about regression of even severe coronary atherosclerosis after only one year, without the use of lipid-lowering drugs (Ornish et al. 1990).

Gould et al. (1995) conducted a study to quantify changes in size and severity of myocardial perfusion abnormalities by PET in patients with coronary artery disease after five years of risk factor modification. The size and severity of perfusion abnormalities on dipyridamole PET images decreased (improved) after risk factor modification in the experimental group compared with an increase (worsening) of size and severity in controls. The percentage of left-ventricle perfusion abnormalities outside 2.5 SDs of those of normal persons (based on 20 disease-free individuals) on the dipyridamole PET image of normalized counts worsened in controls (mean +/- SE, + 10.3% +/- 5.6%) and improved in the experimental group (mean +/- SE, -5.1% +/ 4.8%) (p=0.02); the percentage of left ventricle with activity less than 60 percent of the maximum activity on the dipyridamole PET image of normalized counts worsened in controls (+13.5% +/ 3.8%) and improved in the experimental group (-4.2% +/- 3.8%) (p=0.002); and the myocardial quadrant on the PET image with the lowest average activity expressed as a percentage of maximum activity worsened in controls (-8.8% +/- 2.3%) and improved in the experimental group (+4.9% +/- 3.3%) (p=0.001). The size and severity of perfusion abnormalities on resting PET images were also significantly improved in the experimental group as compared with controls. The relative magnitude of change in size and severity of PET perfusion abnormalities was comparable to or greater than the magnitude of changes in percent diameter stenosis, absolute stenosis lumen area, or stenosis flow reserve documented by quantitative coronary arteriography. These studies, though small in size, provide the most insight into the power of lifestyle change, particularly in coronary artery disease progression.

Additional Cardiovascular Therapies for Consideration

ENHANCED EXTERNAL COUNTERPULSATION (EECP)

EECP uses an inflatable suit that surrounds the lower limbs and expands to compress the extremities during diastole. In doing so, it mimics the effects of intra-aortic balloon counterpulsation. This reduces loading conditions in systole, while increasing coronary perfusion pressures in diastole.

In multiple studies, EECP has been shown to be beneficial in lowering chronic stable angina by one class, while improving quality of life by 50 percent at a two-year follow-up (Michaels et al. 2004). It has also been shown to improve exercise tolerance and decrease anti-anginal medication utilization (Arora et al. 1999; Linnemeier et al. 2003).

An EECP patient registry based on nation-wide data collection demonstrated the following (Bonetti et al. 2003):

- 69 percent of patients improved by at least 1 Canadian Cardiovascular Society (CCS) angina class immediately after EECP
- 72 percent had sustained improvement at one-year follow-up.
- Those with the most severe coronary artery disease and those who had previously undergone a surgical revascularization procedure (89 percent of patients in the registry) seemed to benefit the most.

- In the long-term follow-up:
  - EECP improves coronary perfusion and left ventricular systolic unloading that occurs during a treatment session.
  - EECP increases blood nitric oxide within one week of treatment (nitric oxide has important vasodilatory, antiplatelet, antithrombotic, and antiinflammatory properties).

It is believed that the sheer force induced by EECP may influence atherogenesis and angiogenesis by up-regulating the production of growth factors such as vascular endothelial growth factor and platelet-derived growth factor (Bonetti et al. 2003).

CHELATION FOR CAD

Chelation is an intravenous therapy with ethylenediaminetetra-acetic acid (EDTA). The theory is that components of the plaque can be reabsorbed with treatment. Most practitioners use chelation therapy in combination with lifestyle change and supplements. One randomized controlled trial has been conducted to evaluate chelation therapy in coronary artery disease. In that study, 84 patients, with CAD proven by angiography or a documented MI and stable angina, were randomly assigned to receive infusion with either: weight-adjusted (40 mg/kg) EDTA chelation therapy (n = 41) or placebo (n = 43). The treatments were three hours in length per treatment, twice weekly for 15 weeks and once per month for an additional three months. There was a 27-week follow-up. In this study, there were no differences between chelation and placebo, in time to ischemia on treadmill testing, exercise capacity, or quality of life (Knudtson et al. 2002).

Based on this study and other related studies, the AHA presented the following statement: *The American Heart Association has reviewed the available literature on using chelation to treat arteriosclerotic heart disease. We found no scientific evidence to demonstrate any benefit from this form of therapy.*

A multicenter NHLBI and NCCAM Trial to Assess Chelation Therapy (TACT) was started in 2002. This is a placebo-controlled, double-blind study which will involve 2,372 participants age 50 years and older who have documented coronary artery disease. This larger trial will enhance our understanding of chelation therapy as a treatment for coronary artery disease.

Psychological Risk

Studies by Blumenthal et al. (2005), Dusseldorp et al. (1999), and Schneider et al. (2005) demonstrated the impact of stress reduction on cardiovascular mortality. Blumenthal and colleagues (2005) demonstrated, in a five-year follow-up study, that stress management significantly reduced the risk of cardiovascular events compared to controls. One hundred and thirty-four patients with CVD participated in sixteen 1.5-hour sessions on stress management and exercise. Patients were instructed in biofeedback, a cognitive-social learning model, and progressive muscle relaxation. For patients with stable ischemic heart disease (IHD), exercise and stress management training reduced emotional distress and improved markers of cardiovascular risk more than usual medical care alone.

Randomized controlled trials on stress reduction with the Transcendental Meditation technique show reductions in CVD risk factors, morbidity and mortality (Barnes and Orme-Johnson, 2006; Walton et al. 2004). A systematic review and metaanalysis of 107 well-designed trials on stress reducing methods for high blood pressure found that the Transcendental Meditation program was associated with significant reductions in systolic and diastolic blood pressure (Rainforth et al. 2007). This was confirmed by a later metaanalysis (Anderson et al. 2008) Other meta-analyses have reported reductions in psychosocial stress factors, smoking and alcohol abuse with Transcendental Meditation practice (Orme-Johnson and Walton 1998). A series of NIH-supported RCTs of Transcendental Meditation compared to health education reported improvements in insulin resistance and autonomic tone in CHD patients and reduced atherosclerosis, measured by carotid intima-media thickness [Castillo-Richmond, 2000; Paul-Labrador et al. 2006]. A pooled analysis of long-term trials with an average follow up of 8 years demonstrated 30% reduction in cardiovascular mortality in patients randomized to Transcendental Meditation program compared to controls [Schneider et al. 2005]. The Transcendental Meditation program may be a useful adjunctive therapy in heart failure based on a pilot trial that reported improved functional capacity, reduced depression and enhanced quality of life in the Transcendental Meditation subjects compared to controls [Jayadevappa et al. 2007].

These clinical results are consistent with cost analysis studies that have shown that the practice of Transcendental Meditation lowered health insurance utilization, hospital inpatient days, hospital admissions and hospital outpatient visits, including an 80% reduction in hospitalization rates for cardiovascular disorders (Orme-Johnson 1987; Herron et al. 2000).

I routinely teach my patients two simple stress management techniques. The first technique utilizes a simple five-second-in and five-second-out breath to shift the autonomic nervous system to a more parasympathetic state. Patients are taught to disengage from stress and to not engage in the stress of others. Emphasis is placed on changing one's response to and perception of events. They are also taught to use a mantra on a daily basis to settle their mind. Patients are taught to use their mantra when they need it and when they do not. A list of possible mantras is offered such as "shalom," "Jesus prince of peace," "Om Namo Narayani," depending on the individual's religious and personal preferences. I personally encourage all of my patients to learn to meditate, as I believe meditation is one of the true paths to transformation. The form of meditation varies with the individual.

Guided imagery is a therapeutic technique that allows an individual to use his or her own imagination to achieve desirable outcomes, such as decreased pain perception and reduced anxiety. Imagery has been successfully used as an intervention in patients with pain, cancer, insomnia, post-traumatic stress disorder, and surgery. Guided imagery has been studied as a pre- and post-surgical intervention. A study conducted by the Cleveland Clinic with cardio-thoracic surgery patients demonstrated that both pain and anxiety decreased significantly with guided imagery (Kshettry et al. 2006). In addition, by augmenting pain treatment, guided imagery decreased the length of hospitalization by two days on average.

Qigong and Tai Chi

Qigong is a form of traditional Chinese medicine that implements coordination of different breathing patterns with a variety of physical postures and body motions. It is a very safe, low-impact form of exercise which can be performed by almost anyone, including patients with exercise-limiting diseases or conditions. This practice can be implemented at home on a daily basis. While Qigong is often taught for general health maintenance purposes, it also can be used as a therapeutic intervention where the effectiveness has been studied for disorders such as congestive heart failure, chronic respiratory diseases, hypertension, and generalized stress and anxiety. In an NIH-sponsored pilot trial (Yeh et al. 2004), 30 patients with stable chronic heart failure (ejection fraction <40% and New York heart association class 2) were randomized to receive either 12 weeks of Tai Chi training or usual care. The patients receiving Tai Chi had a statistically significant increase in quality-of-life scores, six-minute walk distances, and a reduction in serum B-type natriuretic peptide levels.

Biofeedback

Biofeedback is a mind–body therapy which involves monitoring and displaying physiological function such as muscle tension, skin temperature, and heart rate. Patients are taught relaxation techniques including deep breathing and muscle relaxation. Biofeedback provides an objective measurement of the impact of these therapies on the autonomic nervous system and is useful to optimize results. Lehrer, Vaschillo, and Vaschillo (2000) demonstrated that training subjects to maximize peak heart rate differences via biofeedback could increase homeostatic reflexes, lower blood pressure, and improve lung function. In cardiovascular patients, biofeedback has been used for stress reduction, blood pressure control and increase in heart rate variability. Biofeedback has been studied in patients with essential hypertension and shown to effectively lower both systolic and diastolic blood pressure (Nakao et al. 1997; Nakao et al. 2000). Where low heart rate variability is an independent risk factor for sudden cardiac death, all-cause death, and cardiac event recurrence, studies support the use of biofeedback and breathing retraining as a treatment to reverse the decrease in heart rate variability that which occurs with heart disease (Bigger et al. 1993; Kleiger et al. 1987). We examined the use of biofeedback in patients with coronary artery disease and found that this technique increases heart rate variability, thus supporting biofeedback as a possible tool for improving cardiac morbidity and mortality (Del Pozo et al. 2004).

Conclusion

Western allopathic medicine excels at treating advanced disease through the use of diagnostic testing, surgery, and pharmaceuticals. Although all of these interventions may be life-saving, they are focused on a diseased care model in which intervention is initiated after the ensuing event. Integrative medicine offers cardiologists the chance to combine the best of Western allopathic medicine with equally strong interventions that focus on lifestyle change. Patients are evaluated from a holistic perspective with all risk factors addressed from a physical, emotional, mental, and spiritual perspective. The ability to motivate patients and empower them with knowledge to take responsibility for their health in partnership with their healthcare provider is at the core of integrative medicine philosophy. As we screen patients for dyslipidemia, inflammation, diabetes, and hypertension we need to add depression, stress, anger, anxiety, and social isolation to the list. Once we identify people at risk we need to have programs and centers of excellence that can guide an individual in proper nutrition counseling, the use of dietary supplements, exercise, and mind–body interventions.

REFERENCES

Anderson, J. W., C. Liu, and R. J. Kryscio 2008. Blood pressure response to transcendental meditation: A meta-analysis. *Am J Hypertens* 21:310–316.

Arora, R. R., T. M. Chou, D. Jain, et al. 1999. The multicenter study of enhanced external counterpulsation (MUST-EECP): Effect of EECP on exercise-induced myocardial ischemia and anginal episodes. *Journal of the American College of Cardiology* 33(7): 1833–40.

Barnes, V. and D. Orme-Johnson 2006. Clinical and Pre-Clinical Applications of the Transcendental Meditation program in the prevention and treatment of essential hypertension and cardiovascular disease in youth and adults. *Current Hypertension Reviews* 2: 207–218.

Bigger, J. T., J. L. Fleiss, L. M. Rolnitzky, and R. C. Steinman. 1993. The ability of several short-term measures of RR variability to predict mortality after myocardial infarction. *Circulation* 88(3): 927–34.

Blumberg, J. B., and Frei, B. 2007. Why clinical trials of vitamin E and cardiovascular diseases may be fatally flawed. Commentary on "The relationship between dose of vitamin E and suppression of oxidative stress in humans". *Free Radical Biology and Medicine* 43(10): 1374–46.

Blumenthal, J. A., A. Sherwood, M. A. Babyak, et al. 2005. Effects of exercise and stress management training on markers of cardiovascular risk in patients with ischemic heart disease: A randomized controlled trial. *Journal of the American Medical Association* 293(13): 1626–34.

Boden, W. E., R. A. O'Rourke, K. K. Teo, et al. 2007. Optimal medical therapy with or without PCI for stable coronary disease. *New England Journal of Medicine* 356(15): 1503–16.

Bonetti, P. O., D. R. Holmes, Jr., A. Lerman, G. W. Barsness. 2003. Enhanced external counterpulsation for ischemic heart disease: What's behind the curtain? *Journal of the American College of Cardiology* 41(11): 1918–25.

Brown, B. G., X. Q. Zhao, A. Chait, et al. 2001. Simvastatin and niacin, antioxidant vitamins, or the combination for the prevention of coronary disease. *New England Journal of Medicine* 345(22): 1583–92.

Caracciolo, E. A., K. B. Davis, G. Sopko, G., et al. 1995. Comparison of surgical and medical group survival in patients with left main equivalent coronary artery disease. Long-term CASS experience. *Circulation* 91(9): 2335–44.

Castillo-Richmond, A., R. Schneider, C. Alexander, R. Cook, H. Myers, S. Nidich, C. Haney, M. Rainforth, J. Salerno 2000. Effects of stress reduction on carotid atherosclerosis in hypertensive African Americans. *Stroke* 31: 568–573.

Chen, J., T. C. Campbell, J. Li, and R. Peto. 1990. *Diet, lifestyle and mortality in China.* Oxford: Oxford University Press.

Del Pozo, J. M., R. N. Gevirtz, B. Scher, and E. Guarneri. 2004. Biofeedback treatment increases heart rate variability in patients with known coronary artery disease. *American Heart Journal* 147(3): E11.

Devaraj, D., R. Tang, B. Adams-Huet, et al. 2007. Effect of high-dose alpha-tocopherol supplementation on biomarkers of oxidative stress and inflammation and carotid atherosclerosis in patients with coronary disease. *American Journal of Clinical Nutrition* 86(5): 1392–98.

Duffy, S. J., J. F. Keaney, Jr, M. Holbrook, et al. 2001. Short- and long-term black tea consumption reverses endothelial dysfunction in patients with coronary artery disease. *Circulation* 104(2): 151–56.

Dusek, J. A., H. H. Out, A. L. Wohlhueter, et al. 2008. Genomic counter-stress changes induced by the relaxation response. *Public Library of Science ONE* 3(7): e25768.

Dusseldorp, E., T. van Elderen, S. Maes, J. Meulman, and V. Kraaij. 1999. A meta-analysis of psychoeduational programs for coronary heart disease patients. *Health Psychology* 18(5): 506–19.

Eckel, R. H., and R. M. Krauss. 1998. American Heart Association call to action: Obesity as a major risk factor for coronary heart disease. AHA Nutrition Committee. *Circulation* 97(21): 2099–100.

Geleijnse, J. M., L. J. Launer, D. A. Van der Kuip, A. Hofman, and J. C. Witteman. 2002. Inverse association of tea and flavonoid intakes with incident myocardial infarction: The Rotterdam Study. *American Journal of Clinical Nutrition* 75(5): 880–86.

GISSI-Prevenzione Investigators. 1999. Dietary supplementation with n-3 polyunsaturated fatty acids and vitamin E after myocardial infarction: Results of the GISSI-Prevenzione trial. *Lancet* 354: 447–55.

Gould, K. L., D. Ornish, L. Scherwitz, et al. 1995. Changes in myocardial perfusion abnormalities by positron emission tomography after long-term, intense risk factor modification. *Journal of the American Medical Association* 274(11):894–901.

Hambrecht, R., C. Walther, S. Mobius-Winkler, et al. 2004. Percutaneous coronary angioplasty compared with exercise training in patients with stable coronary artery disease: A randomized trial. *Circulation* 109(11): 1371–78.

Herron, R. E. and S. L. Hillis 2000. The impact of the Transcendental Meditation program on government payments to physicians in Quebec: An update — accumulative decline of 55% over a 6-year period. *American Journal of Health Promotion* 14:284–293.

Jayadevappa, R., J. Johnson, B. Bloom, S. Nidich, W. Desai, S. Chhatre, D. Raziano, and R. Schneider. 2007. Effectiveness of Transcendental Meditation on Functional Capacity and Quality of Life of African Americans with Congestive Heart Failure: A Randomized Control Study. *Ethnicity and Disease* 17(winter): 72–77.

Kleiger, R. E., J. P. Miller, J. T. Bigger, Jr., and A. J. Moss. 1987. Decreased heart rate variability and its association with increased mortality after acute myocardial infarction. *American Journal of Cardiology* 59(4): 256–62.

Knudtson, M. L., D. G. Wyse, P. D. Galbraith, et al. 2002. Chelation therapy for ischemic heart disease: a randomized controlled trial. *Journal of the American Medical Association* 287(4): 481–86.

Kshettry, V. R., L. F. Carole, S. J. Henly, S. Sendelbach, and B. Kummer. 2006. Complementary alternative medical therapies for heart surgery patients: Feasibility, safety, and impact. *Annals of Thoracic Surgery* 81(1): 201–05.

Kuriyama, S., T. Shimazu, K. Ohmori, et al. 2006. Green tea consumption and mortality due to cardiovascular disease, cancer, and all causes in Japan: The Ohsaki study. *Journal of the American Medical Association* 296(10): 1255–65.

Lehrer, P. M., E. Vaschillo, and B. Vaschillo. 2000. Resonant frequency biofeedback training to increase cardiac variability: Rationale and manual for training. *Applied Psychophysiology and Biofeedback* 25(3): 177–91.

Linnemeier, G., M. K. Rutter, G. Barsness, E. D. Kennard, R. W. Nesto, and IEPR Investigators. 2003. Enhanced external counterpulsation for the relief of angina in patients with diabetes: Safety, efficacy and 1-year clinical outcomes. *American Heart Journal* 146(3): 453–58.

Lopez-Garcia, E., M. B. Schulze, J. E. Manson, et al. 2004. Consumption of (n-3) fatty acids is related to plasma biomarkers of inflammation and endothelial activation in women. *Journal of Nutrition* 134(7): 1806–11.

Michaels, A. D., G. Linnemeier, O. Soran, S. F. Kelsey, and E. D. Kennard. 2004. Two-year outcomes after enhanced external counterpulsation for stable angina pectoris (from the International EECP Patient Registry [IEPR]). *American Journal of Cardiology* 93(4): 461–64.

Mosca, L., A. H. Linfante, E. J. Benjamin, et al. 2005. National study of physician awareness and adherence to cardiovascular disease prevention guidelines. *Circulation* 111(4): 499–510.

Mokdad, A. H., J. S. Marks, D. F. Stroup, and I. L. Gerberding. 2004. Actual causes of death in the United States, 2000. *Journal of the American Medical Association* 291(10): 1238–45.

Nakao, M., S. Nomura, T. Shimosawa, et al. 1997. Clinical effects of blood pressure biofeedback treatment on hypertension by auto-shaping. *Psychosomatic Medicine* 59(3): 331–38.

Nakao, M., S. Nomura, T. Shimosawa, T. Fujita, and T. Kuboki. 2000. Blood pressure biofeedback treatment of white-coat hypertension. *Journal of Psychosomatic Research* 48(2): 161–69.

Ogden, C. L., M. D. Carroll, L. R. Curtin, M. A. McDowell, C. J. Tabak, and K. M. Flegal. 2006. Prevalence of overweight and obesity in the United States, 1999–2004. *Journal of the American Medical Association* 295(13): 1549–55.

Orme-Johnson, D. W. 1987. Medical care utilization and the Transcendental Meditation program. *Psychosomatic Medicine* 49: 493–507.

Orme-Johnson, D. and K. Walton 1998. All approaches to preventing or reversing effects of stress are not the same. *American Journal of Health Promotion* 12(5): 297–299.

Ornish, D., S. E. Brown, L. W. Scherwitz, et al. 1990. Can lifestyle changes reverse coronary heart disease? The Lifestyle Heart Trial. *Lancet* 336(8708): 129–33.

Ornish, D., M. J. Magbanua, G. Weidner, et al. 2008. Changes in prostate gene expression in men undergoing an intensive nutrition and lifestyle intervention. *Proceedings of the National Academy of Sciences U S A* 105(24): 8369–74.

Ornish, D. M., L. W. Scherwitz, R. S. Doody, et al. 1983. Effects of stress management training and dietary changes in treating ischemic heart disease. *Journal of the American Medical Association* 249(1): 54–59.

Paul-Labrador, M., D. Polk, J. H. Dwyer, et al. 2006. Effects of a Randomized Controlled trial of Transcendental Meditation on components of the Metabolic Syndrome in Subjects Coronary Heart Disease. *Archives of Internal Medicine* 166: 1218–1224.

Pedersen, T. R., J. Kjekshus, K. Berg, et al. 1994. Randomised trial of cholesterol lowering in 4444 patients with coronary heart disease: the Scandinavian Simvastatin Survival Study (4S). 1994. *Atherosclerosis Supplement* 5(3): 81–87.

Pitt, B., D. Waters, W. V. Brown, et al. 1999. Aggressive lipid-lowering therapy compared with angioplasty in stable coronary artery disease. Atorvastatin versus revascularization treatment investigators. *New England Journal of Medicine* 341(2): 70–76.

Rainforth, M. V., R. H. Schneider, S. I. Nidich, C. Gaylord-King, J. W. Salerno, and J. W. Anderson. 2007. Stress Reduction Programs in Patients with Elevated Blood Pressure: A Systematic Review and Meta-analysis. *Current Hypertension Reports* 9: 520–528.

Sacco, M., F. Pellegrini, M. C. Roncaglioni, et al. 2003. Primary prevention of cardiovascular events with low-dose aspirin and vitamin E in type 2 diabetic patients: Results of the Primary Prevention Project (PPP) trial. *Diabetes Care* 26(12): 3264–72.

Schneider, R. H., C. N. Alexander, F. Staggers, et al. 2005. Long-term effects of stress reduction on mortality in persons > or = 55 years of age with systemic hypertension. *American Journal of Cardiology* 95(9): 1060–64.

Smith, Jr., S. C., J. T. Dove, A. K. Jacobs, et al. 2001. ACC/AHA guidelines for percutaneous coronary intervention (revision of the (1993) PTCA guidelines)-executive summary: A report of the American College of Cardiology/American Heart Association task force on practice guidelines (Committee to revise the (1993) guidelines for percutaneous transluminal coronary angioplasty) endorsed by the Society for Cardiac Angiography and Interventions. *Circulation* 103(24): 3019–41.

Son, D. J., M. R. Cho, Y .R. Jin, et al. 2004. Antiplatelet effect of green tea catechins: A possible mechanism through arachidonic acid pathway. *Prostaglandins, Leukotrienes and Essential Fatty Acids* 71(1): 25–31.

Taylor, R. S., A. Brown, S. Ebrahim, et al. 2004. Exercise-based rehabilitation for patients with coronary heart disease: Systematic review and meta-analysis of randomized controlled trials. *American Journal of Medicine* 116(10): 682–92.

Tuomilehto, J., J. Lindstrom, J. G. Eriksson, et al. 2001. Prevention of type 2 diabetes mellitus by changes in lifestyle among subjects with impaired glucose tolerance. *New England Journal of Medicine* 344: 1343–50.

Vogel, J. H. K., and M. W. Krucoff. 2007. Integrative Cardiology: Complementary and alternative medicine for the heart. New York: McGraw Hill.

Vogel, R. A., M. C. Corretti, and G. D. Plotnick. 1997. Effect of a single high-fat meal on endothelial function in healthy subjects. *American Journal of Cardiology* 79(3): 350–54.

Walton, K. G., R. H. Schneider, and S. I. Nidich 2004. Review of controlled research on the Transcendental Meditation Program and cardiovascular disease - Risk Factors, Morbidity and Mortality. *Cardiology in Review* 12(5): 262–266.

Yeh, G. Y., M. J. Wood, B. H. Lorell, et al. 2004. Effects of tai chi mind-body movement therapy on functional status and exercise capacity in patients with chronic heart failure: A randomized controlled trial. *American Journal of Medicine* 117(8): 541–48.

Yusuf, S., P. Sleight, J. Pogue, J. Bosch, R. Davies, and G. Dagenais. 2000. Effects of an angiotensin-converting inhibitor, ramipril, on cardiovascular events in high-risk patients. The Heart Outcomes Prevention Evaluation Study Investigators. *New England Journal of Medicine* 342(3): 145–53.

13

Integrative Approaches to Heart Failure

ELIZABETH KABACK, LEE LIPSENTHAL
AND MIMI GUARNERI

KEY CONCEPTS

■ Coronary artery disease is the number-one cause of congestive heart failure. The development of coronary artery disease and, therefore, congestive heart failure is preventable through lifestyle change.

■ Nutrition, nutraceuticals, exercise, and changing one's response to stress and tension are key components in coronary disease prevention.

■ Psychosocial factors such as anger, stress, and social isolation are important determinants of cardiovascular events.

■

Introduction

An estimated 550,000 individuals are diagnosed with heart failure each year. More than 5 million Americans suffer from heart failure, which is the leading cause of hospitalizations in the United States. In the year 2007, it was estimated by the American Heart Association that approximately 432 billion dollars was spent on cardiovascular disease. An estimated 33 billion dollars was spent on heart failure alone. While the mortality rate for acute myocardial infarction has decreased, it has increased for heart failure, because more people are living with chronic heart problems that result in heart failure. The mortality statistics for heart failure are frightening. An astounding percentage (80 percent of men and 70 percent of women under the age of 65) diagnosed with heart failure will die within eight years (Rosamond et al. 2007).

It is therefore not surprising that a diagnosis of heart failure has a detrimental impact on a patient. Just the term—*heart failure*—is terrifying for patients and their families. We try to avoid this term whenever possible, choosing instead words like *heart recovery* and *heart health*. We have changed the name of the Scripps Heart Failure Clinic to the Heart Recovery Clinic. The latter confers a sense of hope, which is crucial to the healing process.

Heart failure is the final common pathway of varying etiologies, including coronary artery disease, hypertension, obesity, diabetes, congenital cardiomyopathies, idiopathic dilated cardiomyopathies, valvular heart disease, pregnancy, viral or bacterial infections, inborn errors of metabolism, and drug and alcohol abuse. In simple terms, it is a condition whereby the heart is unable to pump enough oxygenated blood to meet the body's demand. In technical terms this is described as an oxygen/demand mismatch. This leads to a constellation of symptoms including fatigue, shortness of breath, fluid retention, and in many instances, kidney dysfunction.

Given the number of patients diagnosed with heart failure each year, there is a need to address both secondary as well as primary prevention. Risk factors contributing to disease development include hypertension, diabetes, dyslipidemia, obesity, smoking, aging, stress, genes, valvular abnormalities, and toxins. If addressed early, the development of disease may be slowed or entirely avoided by simple lifestyle change recommendations, in most cases.

Fortunately, there are many treatments for heart failure that have been shown to improve quality of life. Conventional treatments include renin-angiotensin-aldosterone system antagonists, adrenergic blockers (commonly referred to as beta blockers), diuretics, nitrates, ionotropes, as well as sodium and volume restriction. Complementary approaches include herbal or botanical supplementation, minerals, vitamins, amino acids, fish oil, meditation or guided imagery, and Tai Chi. Goals common to both integrative and conventional therapies include nutritional counseling, weight management, and exercise.

The patient–physician relationship is crucial and can have a tremendous impact on the health and well-being of the patient. Patients who are cared for, feel supported by, and trust the medical judgment of their physician will almost always have better outcomes. Setting short-, medium- and long-term goals is also very helpful. They can aid in the setting or resetting of expectations of a patient, the patient's family, and the physician. These goals should be individualized depending on the patient's functional status and willingness to change. The medical management of the patient who is acutely sick is different than the management of one who is chronically well compensated. The acutely ill patient requires conservative traditional therapies. Short-term goals are clearly defined and may include aggressive diuresis and intravenous ionotropic support.

Once beyond the acute care period, a shift in focus to other issues harnessing mind–body interactions is helpful, including Healing Touch. Healing touch treatments are ideal for patients with heart failure because they promote a state of deep relaxation, which decreases stress hormones. The Healing Touch treatments allow for healing on all levels: emotional, mental, spiritual, and physical, providing a great complement to Western allopathic methods. Once discharged from the hospital, an integrative approach to heart failure like coronary artery disease gives a person the greatest opportunity to achieve optimum health, well-being and healing. Long-term goal setting might include conventional medications, herbs, and supplements, as well as dietary and lifestyle changes including exercise, Tai Chi or guided imagery and meditation.

Pathophysiology

The pathophysiology of heart failure is multifactorial, including coronary artery disease, hypertension, genetic factors, idiopathic, and post-viral syndromes just to mention a few causes. Overlaying all of these cardiac insults is prolonged exposure of the heart to stress hormones. Calcium influx into myocytes is triggered, the cells of the heart hypertrophy, and interstitial fibrosis ensues. In ischemic heart disease, scar tissue and fibrosis result in left ventricular remodeling and dysfunction. Myocardial energy demands increase, cardiac output decreases, and sodium and water retention occurs due to the kidneys' response to perceived hypovolemia. The kidneys activate the renin-angiotensin-aldosterone system (RAAS); catecholamines and inflammatory cytokines such as tumor necrosis factor-alpha (TNF-a) increase. This leads to additional salt and water retention, resulting in congestion of the capillaries of the lung, in turn causing leakage of fluid into the alveolar spaces and poor gas exchange, otherwise known as pulmonary edema or congestive heart failure.

Classification of Heart Failure

There are two classification systems of heart failure. The first is the New York Heart Association (NYHA) system which classifies patients based on functional capacity (Table 13.1). Many patients do not come to medical attention until they are Class II, and often times Class III. This is easily understood, as a person with Class I heart failure is asymptomatic, having no physical limitations. In Class II, a person has slight limitation of physical activity. They are comfortable with normal daily physical activity, but moderate exercise such as walking long distances or inclines or climbing two flights of stairs is limited by

Table 13.1. New York Heart Association Functional Classification (ACC/AHA, 2005)

Class	Patient Symptoms
Class I (Mild)	No limitation of physical activity. Ordinary physical activity does not cause undue fatigue, palpitation, or dyspnea (shortness of breath).
Class II (Mild)	Slight limitation of physical activity. Comfortable at rest, but ordinary physical activity results in fatigue, palpitation, or dyspnea.
Class III (Moderate)	Marked limitation of physical activity. Comfortable at rest, but less than ordinary activity causes fatigue, palpitation, or dyspnea.
Class IV (Severe)	Unable to carry out any physical activity without discomfort. Symptoms of cardiac insufficiency at rest. If any physical activity is undertaken, discomfort is increased.

shortness of breath (or dyspnea), resulting in fatigue. Marked limitation of normal daily physical activity—such as walking short distances on level ground, walking a short flight of stairs, or grocery shopping—by fatigue and dyspnea places a patient in Class III. Lastly, symptoms of shortness of breath with minimal activity such as simply getting dressed or bathing is considered Class IV. This classification system falls short in the detection of early disease; it does not allow for primary prevention as it identifies those who already have significant secondary symptoms.

In an attempt to better define the progression of disease, the American Heart Association (AHA) and American College of Cardiology (ACC) developed a new classification system (Table 13.2). This classification enables the physician to identify patients who are at risk of disease development, allowing for earlier intervention and primary prevention in the hope of intervening before disease has occurred. For example, a Stage A patient may have a history of hypertension, diabetes mellitus, coronary artery disease, and\or family history of cardiomyopathy with no symptoms of heart failure. Stage B would be an individual who has structural heart disease (myocardial infarction, left ventricular dysfunction, or valvular heart disease) and no symptoms of heart failure. Those with structural heart disease and symptoms of heart failure including shortness of breath, dyspnea on exertion, fatigue, and exercise intolerance would be included in Stage C. Lastly, those who have significant symptoms at rest or with activity despite maximal medical therapy fall into Stage D. The two different classification systems are often used together to provide insight into functional capacity as well as diagnostic and therapeutic intervention.

An integrative approach to heart failure should be primarily directed at prevention. There are many forms of heart failure including systolic, diastolic,

Table 13.2. American College of Cardiology/American Heart Association
Classification of Chronic Heart Failure (ACC/AHA, 2005)

Stage	Description
A—high risk for developing heart failure	At risk of HF but without structural heart disease or HF symptoms
B—asymptomatic heart failure	Structural heart disease but without signs or symptoms of HF
C—symptomatic heart failure	Structural heart disease with prior or current symptoms of HF
D—refractory end-stage heart failure	Refractory HF requiring specialized intervention

HF = Heart Failure

a combination of systolic and diastolic, acute, chronic, and left- or right-sided. This chapter is written specifically with systolic heart failure in mind, where the left ventricular ejection fraction (the volume of blood ejected from the heart with each beat) is ≤45%.

Conventional Medicines

DIGITALIS

Digoxin is a botanical isolated from the foxglove plant (Digitalis purpurea), which is typically used in the conventional setting to treat heart failure. Many studies demonstrate that digoxin decreases hospital readmission rates and, if discontinued, is associated with worsening heart failure symptoms (Adams et al. 1997; Packer et al. 1993; Uretsky et al. 1993). Fewer studies have demonstrated the effects of digoxin discontinuation on mortality and morbidity. Ahmed et al. (2007) retrospectively used multivariable Cox-regression analysis to determine the effect of discontinuation of digoxin versus various serum digoxin levels on all-cause mortality and hospitalization within the first 40 months in the original DIG study (Digitalis Investigation Group 1997). Thirty-eight percent of patients whose long-term digoxin therapy was discontinued, 32 percent of patients in the low-serum digoxin concentration group, and 45 percent of patients in the high-serum digoxin concentration group died of all-cause mortality. All-cause hospitalization occurred in 70 percent of patients in the digoxin discontinuation group, in 66 percent of patients in the low-serum digoxin concentration group, and 69 percent of those in the high serum digoxin concentration group (Ahmed et al. 2007).

ANGIOTENSIN CONVERTING ENZYME (ACE) INHIBITORS

ACE inhibitors suppress the renin-angiontensin-aldosterone system by inhibiting the conversion of angiotensin I to angiotensin II. Numerous studies have shown that ACE inhibitors slow progression of heart disease, favorably affect left-ventricular remodeling, and improve overall prognosis, including morbidity and mortality (CONSENSUS Trial Study Group 1987; Pfeffer MA, et al. 1992; Garg and Yusuf 1995; SOLVD Investigators 1991). Typically used agents include captopril, enalapril, fosinopril, lisinopril, ramipril, trandolapril, and quinapril. Side effects are many and include, but are not limited to, worsening kidney function (increase in creatinine), electrolyte disturbances (hyperkalemia), hypotension, angioedema, and ACE-induced cough (secondary to increased bradykinin levels). Cough, however, should be evaluated to rule out congestive heart failure exacerbation. ACE inhibitors are considered a mainstay in conventional practice and should be used in all cases of heart failure except when contraindicated, as described above.

ANGIOTENSIN RECEPTOR BLOCKERS (ARB)

ARBs provide additional inhibition of the renin-angiontensin-aldosterone system through the binding of the angiotensin II receptor. Similar to ACE inhibition, ARBs improve morbidity and mortality, favorably affect left ventricular remodeling, and have been shown to increase cardiac output. Importantly, they do not cause the cough sometimes associated with ACE inhibition. Side effects are similar to those for ACE inhibitors, and include renal dysfunction (increase in creatinine), electrolyte disturbance (hyperkalemia), hypotension, angioedema, and a drop in white blood cell counts (Cohn and Tognoni 2001; McKelvie et al. 1999; Pitt et al. 2000; Young et al. 2004). In general ARBs are well tolerated; examples include candesartan, eprosartan, irbesartan, losartan, olmesartan, telmisartan, and valsartan.

ALDOSTERONE ANTAGONISTS

Spironolactone (nonselective) and eplerenone (selective) are aldosterone antagonists. Both have been shown to reduce the readmission rates and risk of sudden death when added to other conventional heart failure medications. Although usage has been demonstrated to be safe, due to potential electrolyte abnormalities, caution is advised when starting these drugs. Renal function should be evaluated prior to the initiation, and all potassium supplementation discontinued, as both can promote hyperkalemia (Ezekowitz and McAlister 2009; Pitt et al. 1999; Pitt et al. 2003; Pitt et al. 2006; Pitt et al. 2008; RALES Investigators 1996).

BETA-BLOCKADE

In the past, treatment of heart failure with beta-blockade was contraindicated. However, in the mid- to late 1990s, beta-blockade alone, or when added to ACE or ARB, was shown to be beneficial and is now considered standard of care in the treatment of heart failure. Beta-blockers favorably affect morbidity and mortality (decreasing the incidence of sudden death), decrease hospital readmission rates, and improve cardiac output and quality of life. They reestablish neurohormonal balance, blunting the ill effects (improving left-ventricular function) of catecholamine bombardment on the heart. Beta-blockage usage in Class IV/Stage D, or decompensated chronic heart failure, is contraindicated due to the possibility of further worsening heart failure. However, once an acute CHF exacerbation has resolved, one can consider introducing beta-blockade. Beta-blockers that have been shown to be beneficial include metoprolol succinate extended release, carvedilol, and bisoprolol. Some more common side effects include worsening heart failure, bradycardia, hypotension, and fatigue (CAPRICORN Investigators 2001; MERIT-HF Study Group 1999; Packer et al. 1996; Packer et al. 2001; Packer et al. 2002; Poole-Wilson et al. 2003; Shibata, Flather, and Wang 2001).

Supplements in CHF

HAWTHORN

Hawthorn (Crataegus monogyna or Crataegus laevigata) is a popular herb used as an adjuvant treatment in mild heart failure. The flower and leaf are considered to be the most therapeutic parts of the plant and recommended for use by the German Commission E. Active constituents are considered to be flavonoids and oligomeric proanthocyanidins. Cardiovascular effects include positive inotropic effects, negative chronotropic effects, vasodilatory properties (both increasing coronary artery blood flow and decreasing peripheral vascular resistance), antioxidant properties, angiotensin converting enzyme inhibition, and antiarrhythmic activity (Chang et al. 2002; Loew 1997). Lastly, immunomodulatory effects have also been implicated, but not clearly established (Bleske et al. 2007).

Two metanalyses suggest that hawthorn is superior to placebo as adjuvant treatment in NYHF class I-III heart failure. The first of the two studies included eight (totaling 632 patients) and the second 14 (totaling 855 patients) small randomized, double-blind, placebo-controlled trials. In both metanalyses, all included studies were required to use a monopreparation of hawthorn, although the dosage used varied between 600–1800 mg/day. Primary end points were not the same in all studies. Some used maximum workload as a primary end point, while others used the six-minute walk test or a combination. The authors concluded in both metanalyses that there was a trend toward significance in favor of hawthorn (Pittler, Schmidt, and Ernst 2003; Tauchert, 2002). While Pittler et al. in their metaanalysis concluded that there was a favorable trend toward significance in heart failure symptoms and left-ventricular ejection fraction (LVEF), authors of the primary studies felt hawthorn did not have a measurable substantial benefit on submaximal exercise capacity, LV function, or quality of life in patients with heart failure (Liu, Konstam, and Force 2005). Still, in a second original trial called SPICE (Survival and Prognosis: Investigation of Crataegus Extract WS 1442 in CHF), the authors concluded a neutral effect on heart failure outcome. The primary end point was defined as a composite of sudden cardiac death, death due to progressive heart failure, fatal MI, nonfatal MI, or hospitalization due to HF progression. The primary end point was measured at 24 months in patients treated with conventional heart failure medications plus hawthorn, versus conventional medications and no hawthorn. The results were not found to be significant, revealing rates of 28 percent for actively treated patients versus 29 percent for controls. It was concluded, however, that hawthorn could safely be added to standard heart failure medications without negative effect (Holubarsch et al. 2000).

Hawthorn was reasonably well tolerated, with the most commonly reported side effects being dizziness, vertigo, and nausea. However, gastrointestinal complaints, fatigue, sweating, rash, palpitations, headache, sleeplessness, agitation, and circulatory disturbances have been reported as well (Pittler, Schmidt, and Ernst 2003; Tauchert, 2002). Hawthorn has the potential to cause hypotension and should be used with caution with conventional medications that lower blood pressure. Potential adverse drug–herb interactions may exist between hawthorn and conventionally used pharmaceuticals including anticoagulants, cardiac glycosides, and antihypertensives (Chang et al. 2002). Until further double-blind prospective randomized controlled trials have been completed, the usage of hawthorn with conventional heart failure medications should be undertaken with care.

L-CARNITINE

L-Carnitine (or Propionyl L-Carnitine [PLC]) is a key player in cellular energy production. It functions to shuttle free fatty acids from the cytoplasm to the mitochondria, where beta oxidation to adenosine tri-phosphate (ATP) occurs (Arseian M.A.,1997), and cellular energy. L-carnitine is most highly concentrated in the heart and skeletal muscle—organs with high fatty acid metabolism and energy requirements. It has been suggested that chronic administration of PLC improves left-ventricular function, improves exercise time and lowers peripheral vascular resistance (Mancini M., 1992; The Investigators of the Study on Propionyl-L-Carnitine in Chronic Heart Failure., 1999; Soukoulis et al. 2009). In the acute setting it has been shown to decrease pulmonary artery and pulmonary wedge pressures (Anand I., et al. 1998). PLC is a reasonable adjunct to other therapies with no known side effects. The recommended dose is 1–3 gm/day.

D-RIBOSE

D-Ribose is a pentose sugar. It is a substrate involved in the salvage and de novo biochemical pathways that are involved in the synthesis of ATP. It has been shown that the infusion of D-ribose following an ischemic event improves recovery of heart function in a rat model (Pasque et al. 1982). A prospective feasibility study examined quality of life, functional capacity, and echocardiographic parameters that assessed myocardial function of D-ribose in heart failure patients. Quality of life and myocardial function were statistically shown to be improved. In particular, diastolic dysfunction (the relaxation phase or filling phase of the heart) was improved (Omran et al. 2003). Larger studies are warranted.

COENZYME Q10

Coenzyme Q10 (CoQ10), a ubiquinone, is a constituent of the respiratory chain in the mitochondrial cell membrane. It plays a key role in oxidative phosphorylation, assisting in the mitochondrial synthesis of adenosine triphosphate, or cellular energy. It is also a potent antioxidant, acting at both the cellular and subcellular levels. Lastly, it has been shown to stabilize cell membranes. On the basis of its antioxidant properties and its role in energy production, CoQ10 has been used to treat a wide variety of cardiovascular disorders.

There is conflicting evidence for the benefits of CoQ10 in the treatment of heart failure, hypertension, and ischemic heart disease. The mechanism of these effects is multifaceted, with increased energy production, protection against lipid peroxidation, and attenuation of ischemic injury all contributing to potential improvements following CoQ10 therapy. CoQ10 is decreased in the myocardial cells of patients with heart failure. The extent of cellular deficiency has been correlated with the clinical severity of heart failure (Folkers et al. 1985; Mortensen 1993). Plasma CoQ10 concentrations have been shown to be an independent predictor of survival in patients with acute congestive heart failure exacerbation. The implication that CoQ10 deficiency may be detrimental to the outcome of patients with CHF suggests that there is reason to examine the possible benefits of supplementation with intervention trials (Molyneux et al. 2008). A small randomized, double-blind, placebo-controlled trial compared the effects of oral CoQ10 (200 mg/d) versus placebo over six months. Parameters examined included left-ventricular ejection fraction, peak oxygen consumption, and exercise duration in patients with New York Heart functional class (NYHF class) III-IV symptoms. No benefit was observed in the CoQ10-treated group (Khatta et al. 2000). In direct contrast, a second study with a similar patient population reported an improvement in ejection fraction following the administration of 100 mg CoQ10 (Langsjoen, Vadhanavikit, and Folkers 1985). A third study involving NYHF class II-III patients in a double-blind, placebo-controlled cross-over design used oral CoQ10 at 100 mg three times daily. Exercise training, peak oxygen consumption, left-ventricular contractility as measured by systolic wall thickening score (SWTI), and endothelial dependent relaxation were examined. Exercise capacity, LV contractility, and endothelial function were shown to improve (Belardinelli et al. 2006). Still other studies have noted improvement in pulmonary capillary wedge pressure (Munkholm et al. 1999), improvement in NYHA functional class (Keogh et al. 2003) and decreased hospitalization as well as decrease in life threatening pulmonary edema (Morisco et al. 1993) Of note, ejection fraction and outcome measures examined were different in each study. These inconsistencies may explain the controversial results noted in the literature, and support the need for large standardized double-blind randomized control trials to further elucidate the true efficacy of CoQ10 in heart failure. Trials involving CoQ10 supplementation use doses ranging from 60-300mg/day (Soukoulis et al. 2009).

In general, CoQ10 is well tolerated. Its side effect profile is relatively benign. No major adverse side effects have been reported in the literature. Minor side effects reported include: gastric upset (including diarrhea, nausea, vomiting, appetite suppression, and epigastric discomfort in < 1 percent of cases) and rash. Side effects appear to occur at larger doses (Pittler, Schmidt, and Ernst 2003; Tauchert, 2002; see also www.naturaldatabase.com). Based on available data, the cost–benefit ratio appears reasonably in favor of its use in patients with congestive heart failure.

MAGNESIUM

Magnesium is used to treat and prevent hypomagnesemia. It is used to treat heart failure for a number of reasons, the first of which is simply poor dietary intake. Loop diuretics used in the treatment of heart failure increase the urinary excretion of magnesium, resulting in low blood levels. Magnesium is effective in the treatment of arrhythmias that are often seen in heart failure, including ventricular tachycardia. One study demonstrated that replacing magnesium alleviated these arrhythmias (Ceremuzyński et al. 2000). Aldosterone antagonist diuretics, such as spironolactone, have been shown to increase plasma and erythrocyte magnesium concentrations and decrease magnesium transport out of the cell. This was shown to decrease heart rate and premature ventricular contractions, and lower the risk of atrial fibrillation and atrial flutter (Gao et al. 2007). Without sufficient magnesium levels the heart cannot pump adequately, as magnesium is intimately involved in the production of ATP, or cellular energy. One small study examined the influence of micronutrients (including magnesium) on left ventricular function, proinflammatory cytokine levels (TNF-alpha and its soluble receptors), and quality of life. In a double-blind, randomized fashion, patients received either placebo or micronutrient for nine months. Left ventricular function and quality of life was shown to improve, while inflammatory cytokine levels were not significantly changed (Witte et al. 2005). Although further research is necessary to fully understand the effects of magnesium, in our clinical practice it is a key micronutrient supplement in patients with normal renal function.

THIAMINE

Thiamine is a water-soluble vitamin. It is also known as vitamin B1. Dietary sources include nuts, citrus fruits, rice, seeds, beef, pork, legumes, brewer's yeast, and whole grains. Very little thiamine is stored in the body, and therefore it can be depleted within a couple of weeks. Chronic severe thiamine deficiency can result in cardiovascular, skeletal muscle, gastrointestinal, brain, and nervous system pathology. "Wet" beriberi affects the cardiovascular system, causing heart failure through peripheral vasodilation and activation of the rennin-angiotensin-aldoserone system. Studies have shown that loop diuretics (such as furosemide) lead to the depletion of thiamine (Seligmann et al. 1991; Zenuk, 2003). In fact patients with NYHF functional class III/IV heart failure have significantly higher thiamine deficiencies than those with NYHF functional class I/II heart failure (Soukoulis et al. 2009). Ironically, the very treatment used to treat heart failure (diuretic therapy) is possibly contributing to left ventricular dysfunction. Heart failure patients tend to have poor nutrition, and it would logically follow that supplementation with thiamine would improve function (Wooley 2008). Additional large studies are needed to examine the potential beneficial effects of thiamine replacement in patients with heart failure.

POLYUNSATURATED FREE FATTY ACIDS (PUFA)

Omega-3 Fatty Acids

Several studies have demonstrated the favorable effects of omega-3 fatty acids in treating cardiovascular disease, including dyslipidemia, coronary artery disease, sudden death due to arrhythmia, and most recently heart failure. Consuming two servings of fatty fish per week seems to reduce the risk of developing cardiovascular disease in primary prevention (Ascherio et al. 1995). Cold-water fish such as salmon, sardine, trout, herring, kipper, mackerel, and to a lesser extent shellfish including scallops, oysters, and shrimp contain omega-3 fatty acid or n-3 polyunsaturated fatty acids (PUFA). Specifically, these fatty acids include eicosapentaenoic acid (EPA) and docosahexaenoic acid (DHA). Consuming 1gm/day of omega-3 fatty acids (three ounces of fatty fish) seems to decrease the risk of recurrent myocardial infarction, sudden death, stroke, and progression of atherosclerotic disease (secondary prevention) (Burr et al. 1989; GISSI-Prevenzione Investigators 1999). A recent large-scale, double-blind, placebo-controlled multicenter trial (the GISSI-HF trial) showed mortality benefit in heart failure—specifically with NYHF class II-IV patients who took 1gm of omega-3 fatty acids daily. It was demonstrated that 56 patients needed to be treated for a median of 3.9 years to avoid one death, or 44 patients required treatment to avoid one major cardiovascular event such as death or a cardiac-induced hospital admission (GISSI-HF Investigators et al. 2008).

Omega-3 fatty acids inhibit platelet activity (but to a 'esser degree than aspirin) by inhibiting platelet aggregation, and cause modest vasodilation by inhibiting the synthesis of thromboxane A2 and increasing the production of prostacyclin. Omega-3s are well known for their potent antiinflammatory effects, as they suppress the expression of proinflammatory cytokines and leukotrienes and are used in many inflammatory states, including cardiovascular disease. They have additional immuno-modulating effects by inhibiting cell adhesion molecules, resulting in decreased endothelial cell activation. The vasodilatory and positive endothelial cell effects may contribute to the increased survival noted in heart failure. However, stabilization of the myocardial cell membrane by the incorporation of omega-3s is likely to have reduced electrical excitability of the myocyte. This in turn decreases the incidence of arrhythmic death.

Fish oil by oral administration is in general well tolerated. The most common side effects include belching, halitosis, heartburn, nausea, loose stool and rash. Taking supplements that are frozen or with meals has been reported to decrease the incidence of belching (Harris, 2004). There is potential for increased bleeding, bruising, and possible hemorrhagic stroke with 3 gm/day or more of omega-3 due to platelet inhibition (Pedersen et al. 1999). The potential for platelet inhibition is greatly affected by conventional medications such as aspirin and Plavix. We routinely use fish oil as an antiinflammatory/antiarrhythmic agent and for hypertriglyceridemia. Fish oil is also added to statin therapy at 1800 mg EPA following the results of the JELIS trial, which demonstrated a 19% reduction in cardiovascular events (Yokoyama, 2003).

L-ARGININE

Studies examining the effects of the amino acid L-arginine on heart failure are small but the results are promising, and certainly suggest the need for further research. Given the activation of the renin-angiotensin-aldosterone axis in heart failure and resultant endothelial cell dysfunction, it is not surprising that l-arginine would be effective. L-arginine is the substrate for nitric oxide synthetase, whose end product nitric oxide—otherwise known as endothelium-derived relaxation factor (EDRF)—is a potent vasodilator. Studies have demonstrated that positive vasodilatory effects may increase coronary artery blood flow and decrease peripheral vascular resistance, resulting in increased cardiac output and improved organ perfusion. The exact cellular mechanism by which this occurs is unknown, but may be secondary to increased production of nitric oxide (EDRF), resulting in vasodilation or reducing the concentration of circulating endothelin, a potent vasoconstrictor (Rector et al. 1996). It has been shown that the production of EDRF is impaired in patients with heart failure (Katz et al. 1999). Presumably because of the positive effects of l-arginine on EDRF production, the following clinical effects have been shown:

1. Improved kidney function (Watanabe, Tomiyama, and Doba 2000).
2. Improved exercise capacity (Bednarz et al. 2004; Rector et al. 1996).
3. Increased cardiac output and stroke volume.
4. Decreased heart rate and systemic vascular resistance (Bocchi et al. 2000; Koifman et al. 1995).

L-arginine doses of 3–8 gm/day in general do not cause significant gastrointestinal side effects. However, at higher doses side effects include abdominal pain, bloating, and diarrhea (Grimble 2007). L-arginine can also exacerbate gout and asthma and cause other allergic reactions resulting in airway inflammation (King et al. 2004; Resnick et al. 2002; Sapienza et al. 1998). Bioavailability may vary between preparations.

DIURETICS

Dandelion (Taraxacum Officinale) has been used in heart failure for its diuretic effect. It has been studied in animal models with mixed results, and further evaluation in humans is needed. It has been traditionally used for gastrointestinal maladies as well as for its antiinflammatory properties. Other natural medicines used in heart failure but not yet proven to be effective or safe include corn silk and stinging nettle (see www.naturaldatabase.com; www.nlm.nih.gov).

Nutrition

Multiple diets have been tested in patients with coronary artery disease (CAD) to evaluate the relative benefits in risk factor reduction and cardiovascular adverse events. Preventing CAD is the best way to prevent congestive heart failure.

The relationship between incident heart failure (death or hospitalization) and intake of seven food categories (whole grains, fruits and vegetables, fish, nuts, high-fat dairy, eggs, and red meat) were investigated in the Atherosclerosis Risk in Communities (ARIC) Study, an observational cohort of 14,153 African-American and Caucasian adults, age 45 to 64 years, sampled from four American communities. Between baseline (1987–1989) and Exam 3 (1993–1995), dietary intake was based on responses to a 66-item food frequency questionnaire. During a mean of 13 years, 1,140 heart failure hospitalizations were identified. After multivariable adjustment (energy intake, demographics, lifestyle factors, prevalent cardiovascular disease, diabetes, hypertension), heart failure risk was lower with greater whole-grain intake (0.93 [0.87, 0.99]), but heart failure risk was higher with greater intake of eggs (1.23 [1.08, 1.41]) and high-fat dairy (1.08 [1.01, 1.16]). These associations remained significant independent of intakes of the five other food categories, which were not associated with heart failure. The authors concluded that whole-grain intake was associated with lower heart failure risk, whereas intake of eggs and high-fat dairy were associated with greater heart failure risk, after adjustment for several confounders (Nettleton 2008).

Decreasing salt intake, often in the range of 2 grams of sodium per day, is felt to be beneficial (Hunt S. A., et al. 2001). In addition, the patient with ischemic cardiomyopathy and resultant heart failure should follow a low-saturated-fat, antiinflammatory diet. Of note, when a person is on a low-fat diet, a natriuresis typically occurs, which may decrease the intensive need for salt restriction in some patients.

Exercise

In counseling a patient with coronary artery disease (CAD) and congestive heart failure (CHF) who is seeking to decrease their body weight, it is important to remember that weight loss without physical activity can lead to "yo-yo" dieting. This is due to the loss of muscle mass early in the dieting process. As muscle mass contributes significantly to the body's metabolism, its loss decreases metabolism, and thus the ability to lose weight. This is one of the main causes for plateaus in weight reduction after three to four weeks on any diet. Yo-yo dieting actually increases cardiovascular risk over time (Klein et al. 2004).

A study of the relative benefits of exercise and lean weight in 22,000 participants, who were followed for eight years, showed that physical activity was a better predictor of cardiovascular outcomes than percentage body fat. Lean, unfit individuals had a higher morbidity and mortality than obese fit people (Lee, Blair, and Jackson 1999). Exercise also has particular value for the patient with CHF. Exercise training improves autonomic balance and decreases ventricular remodeling in CHF patients. Exercise attenuates the rate of progression of CHF, while reducing the risk of hospitalization and death (Belardinelli et al. 1999; Orenstein, Parker, and Butany 1995).

How much exercise is the right amount? General recommendations have been increasing over time. The recommendations vary from a minimum of 40 minutes of aerobic exercise daily to one hour daily. This should be combined with muscle building activity at least three times per week (Thompson 2003). However, many patients may not be physically able to start at this level. Blair and colleagues (1998) showed that modest exercise, such as walking daily, decreased heart disease deaths by 50 percent in both men and women. Certified cardiac rehabilitation programs are an excellent way to conduct safe graded exercise.

Mind–Body Interactions

Stress remains one of the most important triggers for a CHF exacerbation and decompensation. Most notably, the stress hormones aldosterone, epinephrine, and cortisol set up a cascade of events that lead to salt and water retention, coronary vasoconstriction, platelet adhesion, and arrhythmia. All of these events, plus the activation of inflammatory cytokines and the renin- angiotensin-aldosterone system, can rapidly lead to clinical decompensation. Many of the medications prescribed for the treatment of CHF target the stress hormones (beta-blockers block adrenaline, aldactone blocks salt and water retention, ACE inhibitors and ARBs block the renin-angiotensin-aldosterone axis).

To further combat the effects of stress, harnessing mind–body interactions such as meditation, yoga, Tai Chi and biofeedback maybe helpful. Tai Chi has been shown to enhance the quality of life, exercise capacity, and sleep stability in patients with New York Heart Functional Class I-IV heart failure (Yeh et al. 2004; Yeh, Wayne, and Phillips 2008). An 18-week study of biofeedback in 29 patients with New York Heart Functional Class I-III heart failure showed an increase in exercise tolerance ($p = 0.05$) in patients with left-ventricular ejection fraction >31% (Swanson et al. 2009).

These techniques have the potential to modulate the effects of stress on the sympathetic nervous system and neurohormonal bombardment of the cardiovascular system by stimulating the autonomic nervous system.

Enhanced External Counterpulsation (EECP) and CHF

Enhanced External Counterpulsation (EECP) may be a useful adjunct in patients with CHF. EECP improved exercise tolerance and quality of life for patients with New York Heart Functional class II-III heart failure (average ejection fraction of 23 percent), secondary to ischemic or dilated cardiomyopathy without significant adverse events (Soran et al. 2002). The use of EECP in heart failure is suggestive. A study using EECP for seven weeks demonstrated modest improvements in heart failure symptoms and exercise duration, but no changes in peak oxygen consumption, suggesting a possible placebo effect (Feldman et al. 2006).

Mechanical Devices and Percutaneous and Surgical Approaches

The treatment of heart failure with biventricular pacemakers for cardiac resynchronization therapy has been shown to improve quality of life, decrease the combined risk of death of any cause or first hospitalization, and when combined with an AICD, decrease mortality (Bristow, Saxon, and Boehmer 2004; Young et al. 2003). In addition, automatic implantable cardiac defibrillators, in comparison to medications alone, are now well-established to improve mortality in all patients with heart failure and ejection fractions $\leq$ 35–40% (Bardy et al. 2005; Buxton et al. 1999; Moss et al. 1996; 2002). In end-stage heart failure, where life expectancy is limited, left ventricular assist devices (external mechanical circulatory-support devices) have been shown to prolong survival, improve quality of life, functional capacity and have been used as bridges to cardiac transplantation. (Rose E.A., et al. 2001; Rogers J.G., et al. 2007; Slaughter M.S., et al. 2009). Percutaneous coronary artery intervention and surgical revascularization may improve heart failure due to coronary artery disease. Similarly, left-ventricular dysfunction caused by underlying valvular pathology, as in aortic stenosis, can be significantly improved by valve replacement. Following percutaneous intervention or surgery, left-ventricular function often returns to normal and symptoms of heart failure resolve.

Conclusion

It is important to explain the causes of congestive heart failure and to develop an individualized, personalized plan to decrease risk and recurrent events. Frequently this plan includes conventional pharmaceuticals combined with nutraceuticals, nutritional guidance, and mind–body interventions. The role of stress, anger, social isolation, and depression must be considered with the same level of importance as blood pressure control and food choices. Conventional treatments shown to improve quality of life and mortality are in general well-studied, with evidence from double-blind randomized control trials to prove efficacy. However, in the outpatient setting, conventional treatments often fall short, as they only address symptoms related to the physical body in what we feel is a myopic manner. Eliminating the term *heart failure* and replacing it with *heart recovery* or *heart health* offers the opportunity to shift the underlying message we give our patients from one of defeat to hope.

REFERENCES

American College of Cardiology and American Heart Association. 2005. Guideline update for the diagnosis and management of chronic heart failure in the adult— Summary article: A report of the American College of Cardiology/American Heart Association task force on practice guidelines (writing committee to update the (2001) guidelines for the evaluation and management of heart failure). *Journal of the American College of Cardiology* 46: 1116–43.

Adams, Jr., K. F., M. Gheorghiade, B. F. Uretsky, et al. 1997. Patients with mild heart failure worsen during withdrawal from digoxin therapy. *Journal of the American College of Cardiology* 30(1): 42–48.

Ahmed, A., G. Gambassi, M. T. Weaver, J. B. Young, W. H. Wehrmacher, and M. W. Rich. 2007. Effects of discontinuation of digoxin versus continuation at low serum digoxin concentrations in chronic heart failure. *American Journal of Cardiology* 100(2): 280–84.

Anand I., Chandrashekhan Y., De Giuli F., et al. 1998. Acute and chronic effects of propionyl-L-carnitine on the hemodynamics, exercise capacity and and hormones in patients with congestive heart failure. *Cardiovasc Drugs Ther* 12: 291–9.

Arsenian, M. A., 1997. Carnitine and its derivatives in cardiovascular disease. *Prog Cardiovasc Dis* 40: 265–86.

Ascherio, A., E. B. Rimm, M. J. Stampfer, E. L. Giovannucci, and W. C. Willett. 1995. Dietary intake of marine n-3 fatty acids, fish intake, and the risk of coronary disease among men. *New England Journal of Medicine* 332(15): 977–82.

Bardy, G. H., K. L. Lee, D. B. Mark, J. E. Poole, D. L. Packer, R. Boineau, M. Domanski, C. Troutman, J. Anderson, G. Johnson, S. E. McNulty, N. Clapp-Channing, L. D. Davidson-Ray, E. S. Fraulo, D. P. Fishbein, R. M. Luceri, and J. H. Ip, for the Sudden Cardiac Death in Heart Failure Trial (SCD-HeFT) Investigators*. 2005. *New England Journal of Medicine* 352(3): 225–37.

Bednarz, B., T. Jaxa-Chamiec, J. Gebalska, K. Herbaczyńska-Cedro, and L. Ceremuzyński. 2004. L-arginine supplementation prolongs exercise capacity in congestive heart failure. *Kardiologia Polska* 60(4): 348–53.

Belardinelli, R., D. Georgiou, G. Cianci, and A. Purcaro. 1999. Randomized, controlled trial of long-term moderate exercise training in chronic heart failure: Effects on functional capacity, quality of life, and clinical outcome. *Circulation* 99(9): 1173–82.

Belardinelli, R., A. Muçaj, F. Lacalaprice, et al. 2006. Coenzyme Q10 and exercise training in chronic heart failure. *European Heart Journal* 27(22): 2675–81.

Blair, S. N., H. W. Kohl, III, R.S. Paffenbarger, Jr., D. G. Clark, K. H. Cooper, and L. W. Gibbons. 1989. Physical fitness and all-cause mortality. A prospective study of healthy men and women. *Journal of the American Medical Association* 262(17): 2395–401.

Bleske, B. E., I. Zineh, H. S. Hwang, G. J. Welder, M. M. J. Ghannam, and M. O. Boluyt. 2007. Evaluation of hawthorn extract on immunomodulatory biomarkers in a pressure overload model of heart failure. *Medical Science Monitor* 13(12): BR255–58.

Bocchi, E. A., A. V. Vilella de Moraes, A. Esteves-Filho, et al. 2000. L-arginine reduces heart rate and improves hemodynamics in severe congestive heart failure. *Clinical Cardiology* 23(3): 205–10.

Bristow, M. R., L. A. Saxon, and J. Boehmer. 2004. Cardiac-resynchronization therapy with or without an implantable defibrillator in advanced chronic heart failure. *New England Journal of Medicine* 350(21): 2140–50.

Burr, M. L., A. M. Fehily, J. F. Gilbert, et al. 1989. Effects of changes in fat, fish, and fibre intakes on death and myocardial reinfarction: diet and reinfarction trial (DART). *Lancet* 2(8666): 757–61.

Buxton, A. E., et al. 1999. A randomized study of the prevention of sudden death in patients with coronary artery disease. *New England Journal of Medicine* 341(25): 1882–90.

CAPRICORN Investigators. 2001. Effect of carvedilol on outcome after myocardial infarction in patients with left ventricular dysfunction: The CAPRICORN randomised trial. *Lancet* 357: 1385–90.

Ceremuzyński, L., J. Gebalska, R. Wolk, and E. Makowska. 2000. Hypomagnesemia in heart failure with ventricular arrhythmias. Beneficial effects of magnesium supplementation. *Journal of Internal Medicine* 247(1): 78–86.

Chang, Q., Z. Zuo, F. Harrison, and M. S. Chow. 2002. Hawthorn. *Journal of Clinical Pharmacology* 42(6): 605–12.

Cohn, J. N., and G. Tognoni. 2001. Valsartan Heart Failure Trial Investigators. A randomized trial of the angiotensin-receptor blocker valsartan in chronic heart failure. *New England Journal of Medicine* 345(23): 1667–75.

CONSENSUS Trial Study Group. 1987. Effects of enalapril on mortality in severe congestive heart failure. Results of the Cooperative North Scandinavian Enalapril Survival Study (CONSENSUS). The CONSENSUS Trial Study Group. *New England Journal of Medicine* 316(23): 1429–35.

Digitalis Investigation Group. 1997. The effect of digoxin on mortality and morbidity in patients with heart failure. *New England Journal of Medicine* 336(8): 525–33.

Ezekowitz, J. A., F. A. McAlister. 2009. Aldosterone blockade and left ventricular dysfunction: A systematic review of randomized clinical trials. *European Heart Journal* 30(4): 469–77.

Feldman, A. M., M. A. Silver, G. S. Francis, et al. 2006. Enhanced external counterpulsation improves exercise tolerance in patients with chronic heart failure. *Journal of the American College of Cardiology* 48(6): 1198–205.

Folkers, K., S. Vadhanavikit, and S. A. Mortensen. 1985. Biochemical rationale and myocardial tissue data on the effective therapy of cardiomyopathy with coenzyme Q10. *Proceedings of the National Academy of Sciences USA* 82(3): 901–04.

Gao, X., L. Peng, C. M. Adhikari, J. Lin, and Z. Zuo. 2007. Spironolactone reduced arrhythmia and maintained magnesium homeostasis in patients with congestive heart failure. *Journal of Cardiac Failure* 13(3): 170–77.

Garg, R., and S. Yusuf. Overview of randomized trials of angiotensin-converting enzyme inhibitors on mortality and morbidity in patients with heart failure. Collaborative Group on ACE Inhibitor Trials. *Journal of the American Medical Association* 273(18): 1450–56.

Gissi-HF Investigators, L. Tavazzi, A. P. Maggioni, et al. 2008. Effect of n-3 polyunsaturated fatty acids in patients with chronic heart failure (the GISSI-HF trial): A randomised, double-blind, placebo-controlled trial. *Lancet* 372(9645): 1223–30.

Grimble, G. K. 2007. Adverse gastrointestinal effects of arginine and related amino acids. *Journal of Nutrition* 137(6 Suppl 2): 1693S–1701S.

Harris, W.S. 2004. Fish oil supplementation: evidence for health benefits. *Cleveland Clinic Journal of Medicine* 71(3): 208–10, 212, 215–18.

Holubarsch, C. J., W. S. Colucci, T. Meinertz, W. Gaus, and M. Tendera. 2000. Survival and prognosis: Investigation of Crataegus extract WS 1442 in congestive heart failure (SPICE) rationale, study design and study protocol. *European Journal of Heart Failure* 2(4): 431–37.

Hunt S. A., Baker D.W., Chin M.H., et al. 2001. ACC/AHA guidelines for the evaluation and management of chronic heart failure in the adult: executive summary: A report of the American college of cardiology/American heart association task force on practice guidelines (committee to revise the (1995) guidelines for the evaluation and management of heart failure) developed in collaboration with the international society for heart and lung transplantation endorsed by the heart failure society of America. *J. Am. Coll. Cardiol*; 38: 2101–2113.

Katz, S. D., T. Khan, G. A. Zeballos, et al. 1999. Decreased activity of the L-arginine-nitric oxide metabolic pathway in patients with congestive heart failure. *Circulation* 99(16): 2113–37.

Keogh A., Fenton S., Leslie C., et al. 2003. Randomised double-blind, placebo-controlled trial of coenzyme Q therapy in class II and III systolic heart failure. *Heart Lung Circ* 12: 135–41.

Khatta, M., B. S. Alexander, C. M. Krichten, et al. 2000. The effect of coenzyme Q10 in patients with congestive heart failure. *Annals of Internal Medicine* 132(8): 636–40.

King, N. E., M. E. Rothenberg, and N. Zimmermann. 2004. Arginine in asthma and lung inflammation. *Journal of Nutrition* 134(10 Suppl): 2830S–2836S.

Klein, S., L. E. Burke, G. A. Bray, et al. 2004. Clinical implications of obesity with specific focus on cardiovascular disease: A statement for professionals from the American Heart Association Council on Nutrition, Physical Activity, and Metabolism: Endorsed by the American College of Cardiology Foundation. *Circulation* 110(18): 2952–67.

Koifman, B., Y. Wollman, N. Bogomolny, et al. 1995. Improvement of cardiac performance by intravenous infusion of L-arginine in patients with moderate congestive heart failure. *Journal of the American College of Cardiology* 26(5): 1251–56.

Langsjoen, P. H., S. Vadhanavikit, and K. Folkers. 1985. Response of patients in classes III and IV of cardiomyopathy to therapy in a blind and crossover trial with coenzyme Q10. *Proceedings of the National Academy of Sciences USA* 82(12): 4240–44.

Lee, C. D., S. N. Blair, and A. S. Jackson. 1999. Cardiorespiratory fitness, body composition, and all-cause and cardiovascular disease mortality in men. *American Journal of Clinical Nutrition* 69(3): 373–80.

Liu, P., M. A. Konstam, and T. Force. 2005. Highlights of the (2004) scientific sessions of the Heart Failure Society of America, Toronto, Canada, September 12–15, (2004). *Journal of the American College of Cardiology* 45(4): 617–25.

Loew, D. 1997. Phytotherapy in heart failure. *Phytomedicine* 4: 267–71.

Mancini M., Rengo F., Lingetti M., Sorrentino G. P., Nolfe G. 1992. Controlled study on the therapeutic efficacy of propionyl-L-carnitine in patients with congestive heart failure. *Arzneimittelforschung* 42: 1101–4.

McKelvie, R. S., S. Yusuf, D. Pericak, D. 1999. Comparison of candesartan, enalapril, and their combination in congestive heart failure: Randomized evaluation of strategies for left ventricular dysfunction (RESOLVD) pilot study. The RESOLVD Pilot Study Investigators. *Circulation* 100(10): 1056–64.

MERIT-HF Study Group. 1999. Effect of metoprolol CR/XL in chronic heart failure: Metoprolol CR/XL randomised intervention trial in congestive heart failure (MERIT-HF). *Lancet* 353(9169): 2001–07.

Molyneux, S. L., C. M. Florkowski, P. M. George, et al. 2008. Coenzyme Q10: An independent predictor of mortality in chronic heart failure. *Journal of the American College of Cardiology* 52(18): 1435–41.

Morisco C., Trimarco B., Condorelli M. 1993. Effect of coenzyme Q10 therapy in patients with congestive heart failure: a long-term multicenter randomized study. *Clin Investig* 71: S134–6.

Mortensen, S. A. 1993. Perspectives on therapy of cardiovascular diseases with coenzyme Q10 (ubiquinone). *Clinical Investigations* 71(8 Suppl): S116–23.

Moss, A. J., W. Zareba, W. J. Hall, H. Klein, D. J. Wilber, D. S. Cannom, J. P. Daubert, S. L. Higgins, M. W. Brown, and M. L. Andrews. 2002. Prophylactic implantation of a defibrillator in patients with myocardial infarction and reduced ejection fraction. *New England Journal Medicine* 346(12): 877–83.

Moss, A. J., et al. 1996. Improved survival with an implanted defibrillator in patients with coronary disease at high risk for ventricular arrhythmia. Multicenter Automatic Defibrillator Implantation Trial Investigators. *New England Journal of Medicine* 335: 1933–40.

Munkholm H., Hansen H. H., Rasmussen K. 1999. Coenzyme Q10 treatment in serious heart failure. *Biofactors* 9: 285–9.

Nettleton, J. A., L. M. Steffen, L. R. Loehr, W. D. Rosamond, and A. R. Folsom. 2008. Incident heart failure is associated with lower whole-grain intake and greater high-fat dairy and egg intake in the Atherosclerosis Risk in Communities (ARIC) study. *Journal of the American Dietetic Association* 108(11): 1881–87.

Omran, H., S. Illien, D. MacCarter, J. St. Cyr, and B. Lüderitz. 2003. D-Ribose improves diastolic function and quality of life in congestive heart failure patients: a prospective feasibility study. *European Journal of Heart Failure* 5(5): 615–19.

Orenstein, T. L., T. G. Parker, and J. W. Butany. 1995. Favorable left ventricular remodeling following large myocardial infarction by exercise training. Effect on ventricular morphology and gene expression. *Journal of Clinical Investigation* 96(2): 858–66.

Packer, M. 1992. The neurohormonal hypothesis: A theory to explain the mechanism of disease progression in heart failure. *Journal of the American College of Cardiology* 20(1): 248–54.

Packer, M. 1993. How should physicians view heart failure? The philosophical and physiological evolution of three conceptual models of the disease. *American Journal of Cardiology* 71(9): 3C–11C.

Packer, M., M. R. Bristow, J. N. Cohn, et al. 1996. U.S Carvedilol Heart Failure Study Group. The effect of carvedilol on morbidity and mortality in patients with chronic heart failure. *N Engl J Med* 334: 1349–55.

Packer, M., A. J. Coats, M. B. Fowler, et al. 2001. Effect of carvedilol on survival in severe chronic heart failure. *New England Journal of Medicine* 344(22): 1651–58.

Packer, M., M. B. Fowler, E. B. Roecker, et al. 2002. Carvedilol Prospective Randomized Cumulative Survival (COPERNICUS) Study Group. Effect of carvedilol on the morbidity of patients with severe chronic heart failure: Results of the Carvedilol Prospective Randomized Cumulative Survival (COPERNICUS) study. *Circulation* 106: 2194–99.

Packer, M., M. Gheorghiade, J. B. Young, et al. 1993. Withdrawal of digoxin from patients with chronic heart failure treated with angiotensin-converting-enzyme inhibitors. RADIANCE Study. *New England Journal of Medicine* 329(1): 1–7.

Pasque, M. K., T. L. Spray, G. L. Pellom, et al. 1982. Ribose-enhanced myocardial recovery following ischemia in the isolated working rat heart. *J Thorac Cardiovasc Surg* 83(3): 390–98.

Pedersen, H. S., G. Mulvad, K. N. Seidelin, G. T. Malcom, and D. A. Boudreau. 1999. N-3 fatty acids as a risk factor for haemorrhagic stroke. *Lancet* 353(9155): 812–13.

Pfeffer, M.A., Braunwald E., Moye L.A., Basta L., Brown E.J., Jr., Cuddy T.E., Davis B.R., Geltman E.M., Goldman S., Flaker G.C., et al. 1992. Effect of captopril on mortality and morbidity in patients with left ventricular dysfunction after myocardial infarction. Results of the survival and ventricular enlargemetn trial. The SAVE Investigators. *N Engl J Med 3*; 327(10): 669–77.

Pitt, B., G. Bakris, L. M. Ruilope, L. DiCarlo, R. Mukherjee, and EPHESUS Investigators. 2008. Serum potassium and clinical outcomes in the Eplerenone Post-Acute Myocardial Infarction Heart Failure Efficacy and Survival Study (EPHESUS). *Circulation* 118(16): 1643–50.

Pitt, B., M. Gheorghiade, F. Zannad, et al. 2006. Evaluation of eplerenone in the subgroup of EPHESUS patients with baseline left ventricular ejection fraction <or= 30%. *European Journal of Heart Failure* 8(3): 295–301.

Pitt, B., P. A. Poole-Wilson, R. Segal, et al. 2000. Effect of losartan compared with captopril on mortality in patients with symptomatic heart failure: Randomised trial— the Losartan Heart Failure Survival Study ELITE II. *Lancet* 355(9215): 1582–87.

Pitt, B., W, Remme, F. Zannad, et al. 2003. Eplerenone, a selective aldosterone blocker, in patients with left ventricular dysfunction after myocardial infarction. *New England Journal of Medicine* 348(14): 1309–21.

Pitt, B., F. Zannad, W. J. Remme, et al. 1999. The effect of spironolactone on morbidity and mortality in patients with severe heart failure. Randomized Aldactone Evaluation Study Investigators. *New England Journal of Medicine* 341(10): 709–17.

Pittler, M. H., K. Schmidt, and E. Ernst. 2003. Hawthorn extract for treating chronic heart failure: meta-analysis of randomized trials. *American Journal of Medicine* 114(8): 665–74.

Poole-Wilson, P. A., K. Swedberg, J. G. Cleland, et al. 2003. Comparison of carvedilol and metoprolol on clinical outcomes in patients with chronic heart failure in the Carvedilol Or Metoprolol European Trial (COMET): Randomised controlled trial. *Lancet* 362(9377): 7–13.

RALES Investigators. 1996. Effectiveness of spironolactone added to an angiotensin-converting enzyme inhibitor and a loop diuretic for severe chronic congestive heart failure (the Randomized Aldactone Evaluation Study [RALES]). *American Journal of Cardiology* 78: 902–07.

Rector, T. S., A. J. Bank, K. A. Mullen, et al. 1996. Randomized, double-blind, placebo-controlled study of supplemental oral L-arginine in patients with heart failure. *Circulation* 93(12): 2135–41.

Resnick, D. J., B. Softness, A. R. Murphy, G. S. Aranoff, and L. S. Levine. 2002. Case report of an anaphylactoid reaction to arginine. *Annals of Allergy, Asthma and Immunology* 88(1): 67–68.

Rogers, J.G., Butler, J., Lansman, S.L., et al. 2007. Chronic Mechanical Circulatory Support for Inotrope-Dependent Heart Failure Patients who are not Transplant Candidates. *J AM Coll Cardiol* 50: 741–7.

Rosamond, W., K. Flegal, G. Friday, et al. 2007. Heart disease and stroke statistics—2007 update: A report from the American Heart Association Statistics Committee and Stroke Statistics Subcommittee. *Circulation* 115(5): e69–171.

Rose, E.A., Gelijns A.C., Moskowitz A.J., et al. 2001. Longterm Use of Left Ventricular Assist Device for End-stage Heart Failure. *N Engl J Med* 345(20): 1435–43.

Sapienza, M. A., S. A. Kharitonov, I. Horvath, K. F. Chung, and P. J. Barnes. 1998. Effect of inhaled L-arginine on exhaled nitric oxide in normal and asthmatic subjects. *Thorax* 53(3): 172–25.

Seligmann, H., H. Halkin, S. Rauchfleisch, et al. 1991. Thiamine deficiency in patients with congestive heart failure receiving long-term furosemide therapy: A pilot study. *American Journal of Medicine* 91(2): 151–55.

Shibata, M. C., M. D. Flather, and D. Wang. 2001. Systematic review of the impact of beta blockers on mortality and hospital admissions in heart failure. *European Journal of Heart Failure* 3(3): 351–57.

Slaughter, M.S., Rogers, J.G., Milano, C.A., et al. 2009. Advanced Heart Failure Treated with Continuous-Flow Left Ventricular Assist Device. *N Engl J Med* 361: 2241–51.

SOLVD Investigators. 1991. Effect of enalapril on survival in patients with reduced left ventricular ejection fractions and congestive heart failure. The SOLVD Investigators. *New England Journal of Medicine* 325(5): 293–302.

Soran, O., B. Fleishman, T. Demarco, et al. 2002. Enhanced external counterpulsation in patients with heart failure: A multicenter feasibility study. *Congestive Heart Failure* 8(4): 204–08, 227.

Soukoulis V., Dihu J. B., Sole M., Anker S. D., et al. 2009. Micronutrient Deficiences An Unmet Need in Heart Failure. *J Am Coll Cardiol* 54(18): 1660–73.

Swanson, K. S., R. N. Gevirtz, M. Brown, J. Spira, E. Guarneri, and L. Stoletniy. 2009. The effect of biofeedback on function in patients with heart failure. *Applied Psychophysiology and Biofeedback* Feb 10, 2009 [Epub ahead of print].

Tauchert, M. 2002. Efficacy and safety of crataegus extract WS 1442 in comparison with placebo in patients with chro nic stable New York Heart Association class-III heart failure. *American Heart Journal* 143(5): 910–15.

The Investigators of the Study on Propionyl-L-Carnitine in Chronic Heart Failure. 1999. Study on propionyl-L-carnitine in chronic heart failure. *Eur Heart Journal* 20: 70–76.

Thompson, P. D., D. Buchner, I. L. Pina, et al. 2003. Exercise and physical activity in the prevention and treatment of atherosclerotic cardiovascular disease: A statement from the Council on Clinical Cardiology (Subcommittee on Exercise, Rehabilitation, and Prevention) and the Council on Nutrition, Physical Activity, and Metabolism (Subcommittee on Physical Activity). *Circulation* 107(24): 3109–16.

Uretsky, B. F., J. B. Young, F. E. Shahidi, L. G. Yellen, M. C. Harrison, and M. K. Jolly. 1993. Randomized study assessing the effect of digoxin withdrawal in patients with mild to moderate chronic congestive heart failure: Results of the PROVED trial. PROVED Investigative Group. *Journal of the American College of Cardiology* 22(4): 955–62.

Watanabe, G., H. Tomiyama, and N. Doba. 2000. Effects of oral administration of L-arginine on renal function in patients with heart failure. *Journal of Hypertension* 18(2): 229–34.

Witte, K. K., N. P. Nikitin, A. C. Parker, et al. 2005. The effect of micronutrient supplementation on quality-of-life and left ventricular function in elderly patients with chronic heart failure. *European Heart Journal* 26(21): 2238–44.

Wooley, J. A. 2008. Characteristics of thiamin and its relevance to the management of heart failure. *Nutrition in Clinical Practice* 23(5): 487–93.

Yeh, G. Y., M. J. Wood, B. H. Lorell, et al. 2004. Effects of tai chi mind–body movement therapy on functional status and exercise capacity in patients with chronic heart failure: A randomized controlled trial. *American Journal of Medicine* 117(8): 541–48.

Yeh, G. Y., P. M. Wayne, and R. S. Phillips. 2008. T'ai Chi exercise in patients with chronic heart failure. *Medicine and Sport Science* 52: 195–208.

Young, J. B., W. T. Abraham, A. L. Smith, et al. 2003. Combined cardiac resynchronization and implantable cardioversion defibrillation in advanced chronic heart failure: The MIRACLE ICD Trial. *Journal of the American Medical Association* 289(20): 2685–94.

Young, J. B., M. E. Dunlap, M. A. Pfeffer, et al. 2004. Mortality and morbidity reduction with Candesartan in patients with chronic heart failure and left ventricular systolic dysfunction: Results of the CHARM low-left ventricular ejection fraction trials. *Circulation* 110(17): 2618–26.

Zenuk, C., J. Healey, J. Donnelly, R. Vaillancourt, Y. Almalki, and S. Smith. 2003. Thiamine deficiency in congestive heart failure patients receiving long term furosemide therapy. *Canadian Journal of Clinical Pharmacology* 10(4): 184–88.

14

A Brief Note About Arrhythmias

THOMAS B. GRABOYS

Editors' Note

The treatment of cardiac arrhythmias has become extraordinarily complex. Practitioners are faced with a rapidly expanding—and often bewildering—set of options, including a growing armamentarium of medications, as well as invasive therapies, including catheter-based procedures and surgery.

A detailed examination of specific treatments for these conditions is not the subject of this chapter. Instead, we chose to step back and explore some basic concepts that underlie an integrative approach to arrhythmia management. We asked Dr. Thomas B. Graboys, a distinguished Harvard cardiologist and president emeritus of the Lown Cardiovascular Research Foundation in Brookline, Massachusetts, to distill this complex field down to a few clinical pearls. Dr. Graboys, while battling a chronic decline in his own health, has graciously responded to our request and shares his clinical wisdom in the following insightful axioms, which speak to the core of integrative practice.

KEY CONCEPTS:

- Overriding principle of arrhythmia management: try simple measures first before considering drug therapy.
- Be the patient's advocate.
- Minimize tests, especially invasive tests in the elderly.
- Maintain a sense of humor and optimism.

■

Key Factors in Treating Arrhythmias

1. **Diet**: Changes in diet may play a role in the development of arrthythmias. Food allergies have been reported as a trigger of arrhythmia. Comorbid eating disorders may also be a factor.
2. **Hydration**: Check the patient's level of hydration. Many patients are chronically dehydrated. I have seen a number of patients whose arrhythmia "disappeared" after adequate hydration was restored.
3. **Stress**: Assess whether the patient is experiencing psychosocial stressors. As William Harvey wrote in 1628, "Every affection of the mind that is attended with either pain or pleasure, hope or fear, is the cause of an agitation whose influence extends to the heart" (pp. 73). I frequently ask the patient precisely when his or her symptoms began, which may allow us to identify a "trigger" which defines and unlocks the problem without the use of medication (Graboys 1984). Since stress has a direct bearing on sympathetic tone, which raises blood pressure and pulse, these simple vital signs may offer some insight into your patient's level of stress.
4. **Medication-Induced Nutritient Depletion**: Determine if the patient is currently taking any medications (including vitamins and supplements) that could impact on arrhythmias. Many medications and supplements lead to nutrient depletion, which can trigger arrhythmias. Polypharmacy is an essential risk factor to be considered.

Principles to Guide Treatment

1. **Are we treating the patient—or ourselves?** When in doubt, do not treat the patient with any medication unless there is compelling evidence to do so. It is not uncommon for a patient to be prescribed medications simply due to the physician's own anxiety.
2. **Is the problem frequent or severe enough to treat?** Renowned cardiologist Samuel A. Levine chastised us: "It hardly seems wise to institute a course of drug therapy for rare spells" (Graboys 1985, pp. 64).
3. **What is the impact of treatment on the patient's quality of life?** The physician should take care not to diminish life's pleasures when there is no sound reason to do so (Graboys 1983).
4. **Care of the patient with a chronic rhythm problem requires patience, perseverance, and enthusiasm.**

REFERENCES

Graboys, T. B., B. Lown. 1983. Coffee, arrhythmias and common sense. *N Engl J Med* 308: 835–37.

Graboys, T. B. 1984. Stress and the aching heart. *N Eng J Me,* 311: 594–95.

Graboys, T. B. 1985. The treatment of supraventricular tachycardias. *N Eng J Med* 312: 62–64.

Harvey, W. 1628. *On the motion of the heart and blood in animals.* Translated by Robert Willis. New York: P.F. Collier & Son Company 1909.

15

Integrative Approach to Patients Undergoing Cardiac Surgery

GULSHAN K. SETHI

KEY CONCEPTS

- Despite significant improvements in drug therapy, technology, and reduction of risk factors for cardiovascular diseases, a select group of patients require cardiac surgery.
- Coronary artery bypass grafting (CABG) is one of the most common operations performed in the world.
- Surgery is always a stressful event, for patients and families alike.
- Various therapies drawn from complementary and alternative medicine (CAM) have been shown to reduce pain, anxiety, and stress associated with surgery.
- The American College of Cardiology (ACC) and the American Heart Association (AHA) have published guidelines for care of patients undergoing CABG.
- Combining ACC/AHA guidelines with various CAM therapies will provide more comprehensive care to patients undergoing cardiac surgery.

■

D espite significant improvements in drug therapy, in technology, and in reduction of risk factors for cardiovascular events, heart disease remains the leading cause of death for both men and women. For a select group of patients, heart surgery is and will remain a viable therapeutic option. Though the frequency of percutaneous coronary interventions have dramatically increased over the past few years, coronary artery bypass grafting (CABG) is still one of the most common operations performed in the world.

It accounts for more resource expenditure than any other single surgical procedure. For patients with valvular heart disease, heart valve repair and replacement are frequently performed.

For a select group of patients with end-stage heart disease, a heart transplant provides excellent long-term results. But for patients with end-stage heart disease who are not candidates for either a conventional surgical procedure or a heart transplant, implantation of a ventricular assist device as destination therapy may be necessary (Park, Tector, and Piccionis 2005). As the population ages, the demand for cardiac procedures will obviously continue to grow. The outcome after cardiac surgery is steadily improving, even though an increasing number of patients undergoing this surgery are much older, with a higher rate of coexisting morbid conditions. The improvement in cardiac anesthesia, operative techniques, cardiopulmonary bypass technology, myocardial preservation techniques, and postoperative care has resulted in very low operative mortality and morbidity rates after CABG. The widespread use of the left internal mammary artery for a graft, postoperative pharmacologic intervention with antiplatelet therapy and lipid-lowering drugs, aggressive measures to control diabetes, smoking cessation, behavioral modification, and cardiac rehabilitation programs has significantly improved long-term survival after CABG. Other improvements include the ability to perform CABG without using a heart-lung machine (beating heart, or off-pump coronary artery bypass), with minimally invasive techniques, and with robotics. Other technological advances include mechanical suture devices and graft to coronary and aortic connectors. Even though these newer modalities are still relatively controversial, well-designed studies will help determine their efficacy in the very near future.

Integrative medicine is healing-oriented medicine that takes into account the person as a whole: mind, body, and spirit. It combines mainstream medical therapies with complementary and alternative medicine (CAM), as long as scientific evidence supports the particular CAM therapy's safety and effectiveness. Patients take an active role in choosing various CAM practices that may aid their healing. Increasing evidence suggests that the integrative approach may lead to better short-term and long-term outcomes (Ai, Peterson, and Koenig 2002; Charlson and Isom 2003; Halpin et al. 2002; Kshettry et al. 2006; Tusek, Cwynar, and Cosgrove 1999).

Surgery is always a stressful time, for patients and families alike. Pain, anxiety, fear, helplessness, and uncertainty are common concerns before any operation. Like any other surgical procedure, cardiac procedures are associated with significant pain, which peaks within the first few days postoperatively and then gradually diminishes, and finally dissipates. If this pain is not adequately controlled, it causes stress and dissatisfaction and can compromise recovery. Pain also compromises patients' ability to breathe deep, thus exposing them to postoperative pulmonary complications, infections, and cardiac arrhythmias.

Various complementary therapies have been shown to reduce pain, anxiety, and stress by evoking the relaxation response through stimulation of the parasympathetic nervous system. They also complement patients' natural healing ability. Examples include guided imagery, music therapy, breathing exercises, massage therapy, meditation, yoga, and hypnotherapy. Nowadays, a few cardiac surgical centers offer some or all of these complementary therapies to patients undergoing cardiac surgery.

CABG is a palliative procedure that treats the manifestations of coronary artery disease. It does not cure the disease itself. Rather, it provides symptomatic relief of angina for most patients; for some, it has been proven to prolong life (Caracciolo et al. 1995; Takaro et al.1982; Yusuf et al.1994).

The American College of Cardiology (ACC), in association with the American Heart Association (AHA), has published guidelines for the care of patients undergoing CABG and for the management of various risk factors after revascularization (Eagle et al. 2004). The Agency for Healthcare Research and Quality (AHRQ) has also published recommendations for cardiac surgical patients, including that they undergo cardiac rehabilitation, exercise training, education, counseling, and behavioral modification (Wenger et al. 1995).

However, awareness is growing of the importance of providing a more patient-centered and holistic health care experience. The use of CAM therapies has steadily increased over the years. A recent survey by the National Center for Complementary and Alternative Medicine, of the National Institutes of Health, showed that four out of 10 Americans had used some form of CAM therapy in the past 12 months (Barnes, Bloom, and Nahin 2008). Ernst (2003) also reported that about half of the populations in the developed countries use CAM therapies.

According to Lui and colleagues (2000), patients undergoing cardiac surgery use CAM therapies as frequently as the general population, even if such patients do not discuss this use with their physicians. Patients who used CAM therapies believed that they were helpful. Patients also indicated that mental attitude was an integral part of the healing process.

Recently, Kshettry et al. (2006) reported that they were quite easily able to incorporate their CAM therapy protocol in treating their patients. This integration in no way compromised the safety of their patients. On the contrary, it helped alleviate their concerns and appeared to reduce pain and tension during early recovery.

This evidence suggests that following ACC/AHA guidelines and AHRQ recommendations and implementing various CAM therapies may provide

Table 15.1. Integrative Approaches for Patients Undergoing Cardiac Surgery

Preoperative Strategies	Postoperative Strategies
Prepare Patient and Family for Surgery	Use Pharmacologic and Behavioral Interventions
Develop Social Support	Take Aspirin and other Platelet Inhibiting Drugs
Manage Depression	Make Use of Beta-Blockers
Stop Smoking	Make Use of ACE Inhibitors
Use CAM Therapies to Reduce Stress and Anxiety, Including:	Make Use of Lipid-Lowering Drugs
Guided Imagery	Control Diabetes
Music Therapy	Control Hypertension
Breathing Exercises	Make Lifestyle Changes
Religious Belief and Prayer	Manage Depression
Massage Therapy	Undergo Cardiac Rehabilitation
Meditation	Make Use of Laughter Therapy
Yoga	
Hypnotherapy	
Laughter Therapy	

more comprehensive care to cardiac surgery patients, empowering them with various tools to improve their physical, mental, and spiritual health.

Table 15.1 summarizes the integrative approach to patients undergoing coronary artery bypass surgery.

Preoperative Preparation

Increasing evidence suggests that discussing decisions and treatment options with patients during preoperative visits influences early postoperative recovery as well as later outcome. Patients who perceive themselves as having strong social support have fewer depressive symptoms and less functional impairment postoperatively. For this reason, while waiting for surgery, patients should be encouraged to develop a healthy support system if they do not have one already. They should also be encouraged to bring family members and friends to pre- and postoperative visits (Oxman and Hull 1997). Depression affects almost half of all patients undergoing CABG and is a strong predictor of an adverse outcome; it increases operative mortality, decreases late survival, and may undermine quality of life even after technically successful surgery.

Blumenthal et al. (1997) reported that patients who adopt various approaches to manage stress have a significantly reduced incidence of cardiac events and an improved quality of life. In the preoperative care of patients undergoing cardiac surgery, it is well worth the effort to incorporate techniques to manage stress, depression, lack of social support, and anxiety. As a result, short- and long-term clinical outcome improves in terms of an increase in patient satisfaction, a better quality of life, and a decrease in later cardiac events.

SMOKING CESSATION

Smoking is, by far, the single most important risk factor for preventable premature cardiac mortality (Wasley et al. 1997). It is also associated with an increased incidence of postoperative pulmonary complications. All smokers should receive educational counseling. Patients who quit smoking not only are less likely to develop postoperative pulmonary complications, but also tend to have a lower incidence of recurrent angina or myocardial infarction and are less likely to require reoperations (Charlson et al. 1999; Wasley et al. 1997). CAM therapies such as acupuncture, guided imagery, and hypnotherapy have been very effective as smoking cessation tools.

In some patients, drug therapy may be necessary. For patients who are unable to quit smoking by behavioral modification or CAM therapies, transdermal nicotine patches and nicotine gum, which have been used widely with excellent results, should be considered (Kornitzer et al. 1995). For smokers who quit, bupropion, a sustained-release antidepressant, may help reduce the nicotine craving and anxiety. However, for patients with acute myocardial infarction, bupropion should be used with caution.

CAM Therapies

GUIDED IMAGERY

Guided imagery is a simple and non-pharmacologic but effective and powerful tool that can reduce stress and anxiety. It involves a deliberate daydream of positive sensory images encompassing sight, sound, smell, and taste. The goal is to teach patients to use their own imagination to influence their psychological and physiologic state. This form of relaxation can help overcome the anxiety, irritability, pain, and insomnia associated with stressful situations, such as open-heart surgery (Halpin et al. 2002; Tusek, Cwynar, and Cosgrove 1999). It may also reduce the requirement for postoperative narcotics, which are associated with hallucination, nausea, vomiting, and constipation. Use of guided imagery in this population may reduce the length of hospital stay as well (Tusek, Church, and Fazio 1997).

Guided imagery requires a minimal financial investment, yet its benefits are enormous. The equipment includes a headset, an audiocassette player, and cassettes. The cassettes are readily available; their contents vary, but usually include simple relaxation exercises, soothing music, and a general description of what will happen during the cardiac surgery procedure—reinforcing for patients that their physicians and caregivers are extremely competent, skilled, and experienced.

Guided imagery can be introduced to patients in various ways. The preoperative evaluation is an ideal time to ask patients if they would like to participate in the guided imagery program. Those who wish to do so are given a set of guided imagery cassettes specially designed for patients undergoing cardiac surgery. They are asked to listen to them preoperatively till the day of surgery, and then for a week or two postoperatively.

Patients with a very high level of anxiety may be helped by a session or two with a health care professional who is well trained in guided imagery and surgical preparation. The more relaxed and stress-free patients are, the better their outcome and the faster their recovery.

Many patients and even many health care providers are unaware of the value and benefits of guided imagery; they need to be educated about this very potent tool to prepare patients for cardiac surgery.

MUSIC THERAPY

Recommendations for pain management by the AHRQ include cognitive behavioral interventions such as relaxation, distraction, imagery, and music therapy (Wenger et al. 1995). Music can distract patients, diverting their attention away from anxiety and pain and toward something more pleasant and relaxing, thus producing a happier emotional state. For patients with angina and myocardial infarction, music therapy is associated with a decrease in heart rate, respiratory rate, blood pressure, and myocardial oxygen demand, resulting in a decrease in the frequency of cardiac complications (Sendelbach et al. 2006).

BREATHING EXERCISES

Because of postoperative pain, anxiety, and the prescription of narcotics, patients who have undergone cardiac surgery hesitate to take deep breaths. This shallow breathing may result in atelectasis and other pulmonary complications. Incentive spirometery is widely used to prevent atelectatsis. Various breathing exercises, with emphasis on the rhythmic control of breath (pranayama, in the yogic tradition), are relaxing and may help decrease postoperative pulmonary complications.

RELIGIOUS BELIEF AND PRAYER

Religion, prayer, and touch have been used as traditional healing therapy for centuries. Involvement in religious and communal activities has been positively related to all dimensions of social support and to a decreased likelihood of depression. The social network also reduces emotional distress and anxiety, aiding postoperative recovery and resulting in better physical health and longer survival time. Many studies have shown that stress, anger, hostility, and social isolation increase the risks for heart disease and impair recovery after myocardial infarction. Optimistic, relaxed, and confident patients seem to come through cardiac operations better than those who are anxious and depressed. Faith-based, positive coping styles may protect the psychological well-being of patients and have been associated with improved short-term postoperative overall functioning after heart surgery (Ai et al. 2002).

The role of spirituality and prayer for patients undergoing myocardial revascularization has not been fully evaluated. We do not know why some patients with a low surgical risk die while others with a high risk survive. Is it because of prayers, spirituality, willpower, supernatural power, luck, or a combination of all of these? The effect of prayers on patients with heart disease is controversial. A couple of notable studies reported a beneficial effect of prayer for patients in coronary care units (Byrd 1988; Harris et al. 1999).

Two excellent studies recently evaluated the efficacy of intercessory prayer for patients with coronary artery disease undergoing percutaneous intervention or surgery. Krucoff et al. (2004) did not find any benefit of intercessory prayer for patients undergoing percutaneous coronary intervention. Benson et al. (2006) studied the therapeutic effects of intercessory prayer for patients undergoing coronary artery bypass. The major postoperative events and the 30-day mortality were similar across the groups. However, complication rates were higher in patients who were certain (vs. noncertain) of receiving intercessory prayer than those who were uncertain of receiving it. Benson et al. had no explanation for their surprising findings. In any case, it seems reasonable to encourage patients who want to use their faith for coping to do so.

MASSAGE THERAPY

Massage therapy is a beneficial healing art that provides comfort to patients undergoing cardiac surgery. While helping to reduce postoperative pain, stress, anxiety, and tension, it also enhances patients' circulation, range of motion, and overall sense of well-being. Anderson and Cutshall (2007) reported that, for patients undergoing cardiac surgery, 20 minutes of massage therapy a day resulted in less discomfort, increased mobility, improved sleep, satisfaction with pain management, and a shorter hospital stay.

MEDITATION

Meditation is a form of conscious relaxation that makes the mind calm and peaceful. It teaches patients to reach a state of serenity, creating an inner mental space for clarity. In mindful meditation, the person sits comfortably and silently for 10 to 15 minutes, centering attention by focusing awareness on an object or process (such as on breathing or on a mantra). The practical purpose of focusing on breathing or on a mantra (which entails silent internal mental repetition of a word, phrase, or sound) is to deflect the mind from bothersome situations, leading to calmness and new insights. Meditation can lead to a decrease in blood pressure, heart rate, and stress.

YOGA

Yoga aims to create balance in the body through developing strength and flexibility. It involves meditation, spiritual discipline, stretching, diet, and the rhythmic control of breathing. It develops flexibility and muscular endurance by allowing muscles to be stretched and strengthened. It can decrease blood pressure, heart rate, and anxiety; it can increase agility and muscle relaxation.

HYPNOTHERAPY

Hypnotherapy produces an altered state of consciousness, inducing relaxation, guiding the imagination, and fostering the experience of being on a different plane of consciousness. It is a collection of methods that allows a person to access the mind–body connection and promotes self-healing. Hypnotherapy has been shown to be effective in smoking cessation, weight loss and pain management.

LAUGHTER THERAPY

Laughter therapy consists of three parts. These include a series of breathing exercises and stretching, a period of laughter exercises (unconditional laughter), followed by guided relaxation.

The laughter in laughter therapy is more than a vocal and muscular behavior. It is accompanied by a variety of physiological and neural manifestations. Various studies (in such areas as cardiac rehabilitation, pain perception, discomfort threshold, stress coping, and immune system enhancement) have shown measurable benefits of humor and laughter for patients. The mirthful laughter brings about reduced serum levels of cortisol, dopac, epinephrine, norepinephrin, and growth hormone (Berk et al.1989). It also increases natural killer cell activity and other immune markers (Berk et al. 2001; Takahashi et al. 2001).

One notable study found that people who fail to smile or laugh in stressful or uncomfortable situations may be more prone to heart problems. They interviewed 150 patients who had either suffered a myocardial infarction or had undergone aortocoronary bypass surgery. These patients' attitudes were compared with that of 150 age-matched controls. Each study participant was asked how he or she would react to a number of uncomfortable everyday situations. Miller et al. (2006) concluded that people with cardiac problems were more likely to get angry or hostile, rather than to laugh or use humor, in order to overcome the embarrassment or difficulty of the situation. In addition, people with cardiac problems were less likely to recognize humor or use it as an adaptive mechanism; they generally showed less ability to laugh, even in positive situations. Another finding was that brachial artery blood flow increased in study participants who watched movie clips that evoked humor and laughter, but decreased in those who watched movie clips that caused mental stress.

Tan, Tan, and Berk (1997) followed two groups of patients who had suffered a myocardial infarction in their cardiac rehabilitation program. Both groups were matched for pertinent patient characteristics, but the experimental group was allowed to view self-selected humorous movies for 30 minutes every day as an adjunct to standard therapy. The experimental group experienced fewer episodes of arrhythmias, lower blood pressure, lower urinary and plasma catecholamine levels, a lower incidence of beta-blocker and nitroglycerine use, and a lower incidence of recurrent myocardial infarction, as compared with the control group).

In a similar study, the same investigators assigned 20 adults with type II diabetes to either the control group or the laughter group. All 20 patients had hypertension and elevated cholesterol levels and were taking standard medication for diabetes, hypertension, and elevated cholesterol levels. At their one-year follow-up appointment, patients in the laughter group had a mean increase in their HDL cholesterol level of 26 percent (as compared with 3 percent in the control group), as well as a mean decrease in their C-reactive protein level of 66 percent (as compared with 22 percet in the control group); both differences were statistically significant (Tan, Tan, and Berk 2009).

Some investigators have raised the theoretical concern that, during laughter, the increase in heart rate and blood pressure could have a detrimental effect in patients with heart disease. However, given the lack of medical literature on myocardial infarction provoked by mirthful laughter, Fry (1994) suggested that a physiologic "sparing mechanism" in the body is associated with mirth and laughter.

Holistic and alternative approaches to patient care, which were first developed in the 1950s, stimulated interest in the use of humor in healing, though not specifically as a therapeutic modality per se. The humor therapy movement was not ignited until the late 1970s, with the publication of Norman Cousins now-classic book, *Anatomy of an Illness as Perceived by the Patient*, in which he detailed his personal experience of relieving pain due to ankylosing spondylitis with humor. In 1995, Kataria founded the Laughter Yoga Clubs in India; since then, they have mushroomed all over the world.

At the University of Arizona, we have modified Kataria's laughter yoga protocol and incorporated it into a program that consists of three parts:

- Part I: A series of breathing and stretching exercises to energize the body (5 minutes).
- Part II: Laughter exercises (unconditional laughter), along with chanting and clapping, followed by stretching and deep breathing (15 minutes).
- Part III: Breathing exercises and guided relaxation (10 minutes).

Laughter therapy can be used safely with all patients with heart disease. Postoperatively, before initiating the laughter therapy, the patients should have no incisional discomfort and they should also check with their physician and surgeon.

It is obvious that more research needs to be done in this field to make laughter therapy more acceptable to the public and caregivers alike.

Postoperative Care

PHARMACOLOGICAL INTERVENTIONS TO IMPROVE OUTCOMES

Aspirin and Other Platelet-inhibiting Drugs

Late postoperative results after CABG surgery depend on graft patency. Early postoperative administration of aspirin improves the graft patency rate for saphenous vein grafts and reduces the incidence of death, myocardial infarction, stroke, renal failure, and bowel necrosis (Goldman et al. 1990; Mangano et al. 2002). To achieve optimal results, aspirin should be administered within six hours postoperatively, either through the nasogastric (NG) tube or rectally; however, if the patient is bleeding, aspirin may be delayed for 24 hours. Aspirin therapy should be continued indefinitely. In case of aspirin allergy, Clopidogrel, a very effective platelet inhibitor that can be used.

Beta-Blockers

The perioperative use of beta-blockers is very effective in preventing postoperative arterial fibrillation. Their use has also been shown to improve survival in patients undergoing CABG after myocardial infarction (Chen et al. 2000).

Angiotensin-Cnverting Enzyme (ACE) Inhibitors

The use of ACE inhibitors is recommended for patients with left ventricular dysfunction (left ventricular ejection fraction, below 40 percent), hypertension, diabetes, or chronic renal disease. Their use has been shown to decrease the rates of myocardial infarction, stroke, and death in patients with coronary artery disease (Talbot 2000).

Lipid-Lowering Drugs

Elevated levels of serum triglyceride, low level of high-density lipoprotein (HDL), and elevated levels of low-density lipo-protein (LDL) are independent risk factors for coronary artery disease. Abundant evidence shows that all patients undergoing CABG should receive lipid-lowering therapy, unless otherwise contraindicated (Grundy et al. 2004). All individuals who have undergone CABG should aim for LDL levels at least below 100 mg/DL. Recently, the National Cholesterol Education Program recommended consideration of targeting LDL levels below 70mg/DL for people with a very high risk for coronary artery disease. These individuals are those with presence of established cardiovascular disease plus other risk factors, especially diabetes, \ poorly controlled risk factors, especially continued smoking or metabolic syndrome, or patients with acute coronary syndrome or elevated level of C-reactive protein (Post Coronary Artery Bypass Group Trial Investigators. 1997, Maron, Ridker, and Grundy 2008). The Post Coronary Artery Bypass Graft Trial also showed that patients aggressively treated with lipid-lowering agents (who achieved LDL levels below 100ml/DL) had lower atherosclerotic disease progression in their saphenous vein grafts and required fewer repeat revascularization procedures (Brown et al. 2006).

CONTROL OF DIABETES

Diabetic (vs. nondiabetic) patients tend to have higher rates of operative mortality, deep sternal wound infections, and strokes. They also have longer hospital stays and are at high risk for subsequent cardiovascular events (Estrada et al. 2003). Perioperative hyperglycemia, with or without diabetes, is associated with increased resource use for patients undergoing CABG (Furnary et al. 2003). Meticulous control of hyperglycemia with continuous intravenous infusion of insulin preoperatively has been shown to reduce the incidence of sternal wound infections, death, and morbidity (Hoogwerf et al. 1999). It is extremely important to aggressively control diabetes and have the patient take lipid-lowering drugs in order to achieve good long-term results (Domanski et al. 2000).

CONTROL OF HYPERTENSION

Hypertension is associated with cardiovascular diseases and stroke. It is well known that controlling blood pressure also reduces the extent of progression of atherosclerosis in patients who have undergone CABG with saphenous vein grafts (Goyal et al. 2005).

LIFESTYLE CHANGES

Lifestyle changes to reduce cardiovascular risks are extremely important after CABG. Patients should be encouraged to follow a heart-healthy diet. They should be advised to eat ample amounts of fruits, vegetables, and whole grains. Emphasis should be on reducing consumption of saturated fats and trans-fatty acids, cholesterol, and simple sugars. Fish consumption and supplementation with omega-3 fatty acids appear to promote cardiovascular health and especially to protect against sudden death. Being overweight and inactive tends to increase LDL levels and total cholesterol levels and to decrease HDL levels. Exercise and weight control are very important, especially for patients with metabolic syndrome.

MANAGEMENT OF DEPRESSION

Depression is associated with alterations in autonomic, neuroendocrine, immune, and platelet function. It is a risk factor for both the development of and the worsening of coronary artery disease. Major depressive disorders (as noted preoperatively) are related to subsequent mortality and morbidity as well as to less improvement in quality of life postoperatively (Musselman, Evans, and Nemeroff 1998). Depressed patients are also less physically active, less medically compliant, and more likely to engage in health-damaging behavior.

The incidence of preoperative major depression in cardiac patients ranges from 16 percent to 48 percent. Postoperatively, 18 percent of patients who were not depressed preoperatively develop significant depression. These newly depressed patients are at a higher risk for long-term cardiac events and death, as compared with patients who are not depressed (Peterson et al. 2002; Wellenius et al. 2008). Depressive symptoms are associated with atherosclerotic progression in patients' saphenous vein grafts; such patients have a significantly higher risk of cardiovascular events and of mortality related to heart disease (Miller 1998).

Preoperative education (aimed at helping patients better understand their illness, its treatment, and its effects) may reduce their psychological distress and improve their future well-being; depression may undermine their quality of life, despite successful cardiac surgery.

Potential Risks Associated with CAM Therapies

A large proportion of the American population uses CAM therapies, yet many patients do not disclose their use of CAM to physicians, even when they are prompted. Liu and colleagues (2000) surveyed 376 patients (mostly well-educated) undergoing cardiac surgery at Columbia-Presbyterian Medical Center in New York. Excluding prayer or the use of vitamins, 44 percent had tried some type of CAM therapy. Of those patients, only 17 percent said that they discussed their use of CAM therapy with their physicians, while 48 percent admitted that they did not want to discuss this topic with anyone

This lack of communication is potentially dangerous. Herbal medications, for example, possess significant pharmacologic activity; consequently, they may have potentially adverse effects and interact in harmful ways with other drugs. Some can speed up or slow down the heart rate, inhibit blood clotting, alter the immune system, or change the effect and duration of anesthesia. Several herbs directly affect platelet aggregation and bleeding time, while others interact with anticoagulation medications. Fish oil, garlic, onion, and vitamin E inhibit platelet aggregation. Feverfew, ginkgo biloba, coenzyme Q10, ginger, ginseng, and St. John's wort interact with warfarin. Hawthorn berry, kyusin, licorice, plantain, uzara root, ginseng, and St. John's wort interact with digoxin. St. John's wort also alters the metabolism of cyclosporine and increases the risk of rejection in heart transplant recipients.

Because of the extensive use of CAM therapies by the general population, physicians and patients must be open in their discussions, and bring up any use of such therapies. The surgeon should specifically ask patients about any herbal medications used, in order to prevent perioperative complications. The American Society of Anesthesiologists recommends that patients stop taking all herbal medication two weeks before undergoing cardiac surgery. Herbal medications may be resumed postoperatively, if they will not potentially interact with other prescribed drugs.

Conclusion

Despite improvements in drug therapy, percutaneous coronary interventions, and reduction of risk factors for cardiac diseases, many patients still need CABG either to resolve their symptomatic relief or to prolong their lives.

The ACC/AHA guidelines for care of patients undergoing CABG should be followed. Patients who prepare for surgery psychologically have less discomfort, fewer complications, and shorter hospital stays. Various CAM therapies have been shown to reduce pain, anxiety, stress, and depression, thereby further enhancing patients' natural healing abilities. Combining the ACC/AHA guidelines with various CAM therapies will provide more comprehensive care to patients, and empower them with an array of tools to improve their physical, mental, and spiritual health.

A large proportion of cardiac patients also take herbal medicine and dietary supplements. These may have adverse effects and may interact in harmful ways with other drugs. To avoid potential complications during surgery, all herbal medicines and dietary supplements should be discontinued before surgery and then closely monitored postoperatively.

REFERENCES

Ai, A. L., C. Peterson, S. F. Bolling, and H. Koenig 2002. Private prayer and optimism in middle-aged and older patients awaiting cardiac surgery. *Gerontologist* 42(1): 70–81.

Anderson, P. G., and S. M. Cutshall. 2007. Massage therapy a comfort intervention for cardiac surgery patients. *Clin Nurse Spec* 21(3): 161–65.

Barnes, P. M, B. Bloom, and R. Nahin. 2005. CDC National health statistics report No. 12. Complementary and alternative medicine use among adults and children: United States (2007). Dec. 10, (2008). *Lancet* 366(9481): 211–17.

Benson, H., J. A. Dusek, J. B. Sherwood, et al. 2006. Study of the therapeutic effects of intercessory prayer (step) in cardiac bypass patients: A multicenter randomized trial of uncertainty and certainty of receiving intercessory prayer. *Amer Heart J* 151(4): 934–42.

Berk, L. S., D. L. Felten, S. A. Tan, et al. 2001. Modulation of neuroimmune parameters during the eustress of humor-associated mirthful laughter. *Altern Ther Health Med* 7: 62–76.

Berk, L. S., S. A. Tan, W. F. Fry, et al. 1989. Neuroendocrine and stress hormone changes during mirthful laughter. *Am J Med Sci* 6: 298–390.

Blumenthal, J. A., W. Jiang, M. A. Babyak, D. S. Krantz, D. J. Frid, R. E. Coleman, R. Waugh, M. Hanson, M. Appelbaum, C. O'Connor, and J. J. Morris. 1997. Stress management and exercise training in cardiac patients with myocardial ischemia. Effects on prognosis and evaluation of mechanisms. *Arch Intern Med* 157(19): 2213–23.

Brown, J. R., F. H. Edwards, G. T. O'Connor, C. S. Ross, and A. P. Furnary. 2006. The diabetic disadvantage: historical outcomes measures in diabetic patients undergoing cardiac surgery—the pre-intravenous insulin era. *Semin Thorac Cardiovasc Surg* 18(4): 281–8.

Byrd, R. C. 1988. Positive therapeutic effects of intercessory prayer in a coronary care unit population. *South Med J* 81(7): 826–29.

Caracciolo, E. A., K. B. Davis, G. Sopko, et al. 1995. Comparison of surgical and medical group survival in patients with left main coronary-artery disease: Long-term CASS experience 91(9): 2325–34.

Charlson, M. E., and O. W. Isom. 2003. Clinical practice. Care after coronary-artery bypass surgery. *New Engl J Med* 348(15): 1456–63.

Charlson, M., K. H. Krieger, J. C. Peterson, et al. 1999. Predictors and outcomes of cardiac complications following elective coronary bypass grafting. *Proceedings of the Association of American Physicians* 111(6): 622–32.

Chen, J., M. J. Radford, Y. Wang, et al. 2000. Are beta-blockers effective in elderly patients who undergo coronary revascularization after acute myocardial infarction. *Arch Intern Med* 160(7): 947–52.

Clinical Practice Guideline Number 17: Cardiac Rehabilitation, Rockville, MD: Agency for Healthcare Policy and Research (AHCPR Publication No. 96-0672), October 1995.

Domanski, M. J., C. B. Borkowf, L. Campeau, G. L. Knatterud, C. White, B. Hoogwerf, Y. Rosenberg, and N. L. Geller. 2000. Prognostic factors for atherosclerosis progression in saphenous vein grafts: The postcoronary artery bypass graft (Post-CABG) trial. *J Am Coll Cardiol* 36(6): 1877–83.

Eagle, K. A., R. A. Guyton, R. Davidoff, et al. 2004. ACC/AHA (2004) guideline update for coronary artery bypass graft surgery: Summary article. *J Am Coll Cardiol* 44(5): 1146–54.

Ernst, E. 2003. Obstacles to research in complementary and alternative medicine. *Med J Aust* 179(6): 279–80.

Estrada, C. A., J. A. Young, L. W. Nifong, and W. R. Chitwood, Jr. 2003. Outcomes and perioperative hyperglycemia in patients with or without diabetes mellitus undergoing coronary artery bypass grafting. *Ann Thorac Surg* 75(5): 1392–99.

Fry, W. F. 1994. The biology of humor. *Humor* 7(2): 111–26.

Furnary, A. P., G. Q. Gao, G. L. Grunkemeier, et al. 2003. Continuous insulin infusion reduces mortality in patients with diabetes undergoing coronary artery bypass grafting. *J Thorac Cardiovascu Surg* 125(5): 1007–21.

Goldman, S., J. Copeland, T. Moritz, et al. 1990. Internal mammary artery and saphenous-vein graft patency effects of aspirin. *Circulation* 82(5): 237–42.

Goyal, T. M., E. L. Idler, T. J. Krause, et al. 2005. Quality of life following cardiac surgery: Impact of the severity and course of depressive symptoms. *Psychosom Med* 67(5): 759–65.

Grundy, S. M., J. I. Cleeman, C.N. Merz, et al. 2004. Coordinating Committee of the National Cholesterol Education Program. Implications of recent clinical trials for the National Cholesterol Education Program Adult Treatment Panel III Guidelines. *J Amer Coll Cardiol* 44(3): 720–32.

Halpin, L. S., A. M. Speir, P. CapoBianco, and S. D. Barnett. 2002. Guided imagery in cardiac surgery. *Outcomes Management* 6(3): 132–37.

Harris, W. S., M. Gowda, J. W. Kolb, et al. 1999. A randomized, controlled trial of the effects of remote, intercessory prayer on outcomes in patients admitted to the coronary care unit. *Arch Intern Med* 159(19): 2273–78.

Hoogwerf, B. J., A. Waness, M. Cressman, J. Canner, L. Campeau, M. Domanski, N. Geller, A. Herd, A. Hickey, D. B. Hunninghake, G. L. Knatterud, and C. White. 1999. Effects of aggressive cholesterol lowering and low-dose anticoagulation on clinical and angiographic outcomes in patients with diabetes: The Post Coronary Artery Bypass Graft Trial. *Diabetes* 48(6): 1289–94.

Kornitzer, M., M. Boutsen, M. Dramaix, et al. 1995. Combined use of nicotine patch and gum in smoking cessation—a placebo-controlled clinical-trial. *Prev Med* 24(1): 41–47.

Krucoff, M. W., S. W. Crater, D. Gallup, J. C. Blankenship, M. Cuffe, M. Guarneri, R. A. Krieger, V. R. Kshettry, K. Morris, M. Oz, A. Pichard, M. H. Sketch, Jr., H. G. Koenig, D. Mark, and K. L. Lee. 2004. Music, imagery, touch, and prayer as adjuncts to interventional cardiac care: The Monitoring and Actualisation of Noetic Trainings (MANTRA) II randomised study. *N Engl J Med* 350: 21–28.

Kshettry, V. R., L. F. Carole, S. J. Henly, S. Sendelbach, and B. Kummer. 2006. Complementary alternative medical therapies for heart surgery patients: Feasibility, safety, and impact. *Ann Thorac Surg* 81(1): 201–05.

Liu, E. H., L. M. Turner, S. X. Lin, L. Klaus, L. Y. Choi, J. Whitworth, W. Ting, and M. C. Oz. 2000. Use of alternative medicine by patients undergoing cardiac surgery. *J Thorac Cardiovasc Surg* 120(2): 335–41.

Mangano, D. T., L. Saidman, J. Levin, et al. 2002. Aspirin and mortality from coronary bypass surgery. *N Engl J Med* 347(17): 1309–17.

Maron, D. J., P. M. Ridker, and S. M. Grundy. 2008. *Prevention strategies for coronary heart disease. Hurst's The Heart,* ed. V. Fuster, R. A. O'Rourke, R. A. Walsh, et al., 1203–34. New York: McGraw-Hill Professional.

Miller, L. G. 1998. Herbal medicinals—Selected clinical considerations focusing on known or potential drug–herb interactions. *Arch Int. Med* 150(20): 2200–11.

Miller, M., C. Mangano, Y. Park, et al. 2006. Impact of cinematic viewing on endothelial function. *Heart* 92: 261–62.

Musselman, D. L., D. L. Evans, C. B. Nemeroff. 1998. The relationship of depression to cardiovascular disease: Epidemiology, biology, and treatment. *Arch Gen Psychiatry* 55(7): 580–92.

Oxman, T. E., and J. G. Hull. 1997. Social support, depression, and activities of daily living in older heart surgery patients. *J Gerontol Series B-Psychological Sciences & Social Sciences* 52(1): P1–14.

Park, S. J., A. Tector, and W. Piccionis. 2005. Left ventricular assist devices as destination therapy—a new look at survival. *J Thorac. Cv. Surg* 128: 9–17.

Peterson, J. C., M. E. Charlson, P. Williams-Russo, K. H. Krieger, P. A. Pirraglia, B. S. Meyers, and G. S. Alexopoulos. 2002. New postoperative depressive symptoms and long-term cardiac outcomes after coronary artery bypass surgery. *Am J Geriatr Psychiatry* 10(2): 192–98.

Post Coronary Artery Bypass Group Trial Investigators. 1997. The effect of aggressive lowering of low-density lipoprotein cholesterol levels and low-dose anticoagulation on obstructive changes in saphenous-vein coronary-artery bypass grafts. The Post Coronary Artery Bypass Graft Trial Investigators. *N Engl J Med* 336(3): 153–62.

Sendelbach, S. E., M. A. Halm, K. A. Doran, E. H. Miller, and P. Gaillard. 2006. Effects of music therapy on physiological and psychological outcomes for patients undergoing cardiac surgery. *J Cardiovasc Nurs* 21(3): 194–200.

Takahashi, K., M. Iwase, K. Yamashita, et al. 2001. The elevation of natural killer cell activity induced by laughter in a crossover designed study. *Int J Molecular Med* 8: 645–50.

Takaro, T., P. Peduzzi, K. M. Detre, et al. 1982. Survival in subgroups of patients with left main coronary-artery disease Veterans Administration cooperative study of surgery for coronary arterial occlusive disease. *Circulation* 66(1): 14–22.

Talbot, P. 2000. Effects of an angiotensin-converting-enzyme inhibitor, ramipril, on cardiovascular events in high-risk patients. *N Engl J Med* 342(10): 748.

Tan, S. A., L. G. Tan, and L. S. Berk. 1997. Mirthful laughter an effective adjunct in cardiac rehabilitation. *Canadian J Cardiol* 13: 190.

Tusek, D., J. M. Church, and V. W. Fazio. 1997. Guided imagery as a coping strategy for perioperative patients. *AORN J* 66(4): 644–49.

Tusek, D. L., R. Cwynar, and D. M. Cosgrove. 1999. Effect of guided imagery on length of stay, pain and anxiety in cardiac surgery patients. *J Cardiovasc Manag* 10(2): 22–28.

Wasley, M. A., S. E. McNagny, V. L. Phillips, et al. 1997. The cost-effectiveness of the nicotine transdermal patch for smoking cessation. *Prev Med* 26(2): 264–70.

Wellenius, G. A, K. J. Mukamal, A. Kulshreshtha, S. Asonganyi, and M. A. Mittleman. 2008. Depressive symptoms and the risk of atherosclerotic progression among patients with coronary artery bypass grafts. *Circulation* 117(18): 2313–19.

Wenger, N. K., E. S. Froelicher, L. K. Smith LK, et al. 1995. Cardiac rehabilitation as secondary prevention. *Am Fam Physician* 52(8): 2257–64.

Yusuf, S., D. Zucker, and P. Peduzzi, et al. 1994. Effect of coronary-artery bypass graft-surgery on survival—overview of 10-year results from randomized trials by the coronary-artery bypass graft-surgery trialists collaboration. *Lancet* 344(8922): 563–70.

ADDITIONAL RESOURCES

O n behalf of all the chapter authors, we hope that this volume has been helpful to those seeking to incorporate aspects of integrative cardiology into clinical care and research. Adopting this new approach can be challenging, however, as it involves a data set not typically part of current medical training. Furthermore, since the field is relatively new, reliable reference material may be difficult to identify.

For these reasons, we have compiled a focused list of resources that the authors have found to be most useful.

Continuing Education

AMERICAN COLLEGE OF CARDIOLOGY

The report of the American College of Cardiology Foundation task force, titled "Integrating Complementary Medicine Into Cardiovascular Medicine" is an excellent overview of research involving integrative approaches to cardiovascular disease. This document can be found at: http://content.onlinejacc.org/cgi/reprint/46/1/184.pdf.

FELLOWSHIP PROGRAM IN INTEGRATIVE MEDICINE AT THE UNIVERSITY OF ARIZONA

The two-year fellowship program in Integrative Medicine offered by the University of Arizona Center for Integrative Medicine combines distance learning with three weeks of activities in Tucson. The program is designed for physicians, nurse practitioners, and physician assistants in all stages of their careers. More information is available at http://integrativemedicine.arizona.edu/education/fellowship/.

NATIONAL INSTITUTES OF HEALTH: THE NATIONAL CENTER FOR COMPLEMENTARY AND ALTERNATIVE MEDICINE

The Web site of the National Center for Complementary and Alternative Medicine, sponsored by the National Institute of Health, contains reference material as well as information about government-funded research opportunities: www.nccam.nih.gov.

Journals

The authors have found the following journals to be especially helpful and informative:

- *Alternative Therapies in Health and Medicine*
- *Explore: The Journal of Science & Healing*
- *Journal of Alternative and Complementary Medicine*

Nutritional Supplements

CONSUMERLAB

This group provides an independent laboratory analysis of the content and purity of various supplements. Many practitioners find this information to be helpful in the selection of the brand of supplement to recommend. This service is available for a fee. More information is available at: http://www.consumerlab.com.

NATURAL MEDICINES DATABASE

This resource, available online and in hard copy, is a highly useful reference for learning about the science and practical use of supplements including mechanism of action, dose, and interactions with drugs and supplements. This service is available for a fee. More information is available at: www. naturaldatabase.com.

NATURAL STANDARD

This searchable database of supplements (which requires a fee for access) includes a ranking of the quality of supporting evidence: www.naturalstandard.com.

OFFICE OF DIETARY SUPPLEMENTS

This Web site provides dietary supplement fact sheets and a link to the International Bibliographic Information on Dietary Supplements (IBIDS). It can be accessed for free at: http://ods.od.nih.gov/.

HERBAL GRAM

The Web site is sponsored by the American Botanical Council, a nonprofit organization that provides reference material on herbal medicine. It contains an Herb Clip section which summarizes current research on herbal preparations. Some content is free content, but a fee is required for full access: www. herbalgram.org.

INDEX

Note: Page numbers followed by "*f*" and "*t*" denote figures and tables, respectively.